D0891033

Performance Nutrition for Winter Sports

Monique Ryan MS, RD, LDN

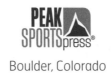

PEAK
SPORTSpress®

Boulder, Colorado

Performance Nutrition for Winter Sports
© 2005 Monique Ryan

The information and ideas in this book are intended to be for instructional and educational purposes, and are not intended as prescriptive advice.

Printed in the United States of America.

Interior and cover design by Anita Koury
Cover photo by Chris Milliman, www.chrismilliman.com
Interior photos by Tom Moran, Tim Hancock, gettyimages.com, and istockphoto.com

10 9 8 7 6 5 4 3 2 1

Distributed in the United States and Canada by Publishers Group West.

Library of Congress Cataloging-in-Publication Data

Ryan, Monique, 1962–
    Performance nutrition for winter sports / Monique Ryan.
       p. cm.
    ISBN 0-9746254-5-0 (pbk. : alk. paper)
  1. Athletes—Nutrition. 2. Winter sports. I. Title.

TX361.A8 R94 2005
613.2'024'796—dc22

                      2005011349

Peak Sports Press, an imprint of VeloPress®
1830 North 55ᵗʰ Street
Boulder, Colorado 80301–2700 USA
303/440-0601 • Fax 303/444-6788 • E-mail velopress@insideinc.com

To purchase additional copies of this book or other VeloPress® books, call 800/234-8356 or visit us on the Web at velopress.com.

Contents

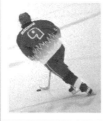

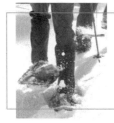

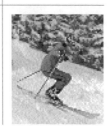

Introduction: A Guide to Using this Book

Never has participation in winter sports been so popular. Males and females alike at the junior high school, college, and adult levels now regularly participate in alpine skiing, snowboarding, cross-country skiing, snowshoeing, and hockey—the sports detailed in this book. Chances are that you are reading this book because you or a family member derives great satisfaction from participating, training, and competing in a winter sport and appreciates that the proper fuel can greatly enhance your athletic accomplishments. Focused athletes realize that the daily food choices they make are highly interconnected with how they train, recover, and compete. Ultimately, consuming a quality training diet allows you to make the most of each training session and subsequently leaves you best prepared for extended days on the slopes, snow, and ice, and for competition.

Performance Nutrition for Winter Sports is designed for the athlete interested in the everyday application of respected, cutting-edge sports nutrition science. Whether you are training on the slopes, snow, or ice, providing your body with the proper food choices, consumed in the right amounts at the right times, lays a solid nutrition foundation for your chosen playing level, sport and competition goals, and optimum health. The high-quality training diet outlined in this book is designed to optimize your recovery, assist you in building muscle and strength, and sustain your energy during exercise, training, and competition.

Performance Nutrition for Winter Sports has several unique features. First, it is designed to be a practical book and provides a bridge between sports nutrition science and real-life application of practical sports nutrition and health-related guidelines. In addition to the chapters that outline nutrition choices for good health and optimal fueling, specific advice for popular winter sports are included. To provide this information, this book has been divided into two parts.

Part I, "High-Performance Nutrition," emphasizes that good training and performance begins with a solid nutrition foundation of quality food choices. A quality diet consisting of the highest nutrient and food choices on a daily basis provides fuel and hydration for both training and competition, as well as nutrients for optimal health. Also addressed are the unique considerations of the many age groups of athletes that may participate in winter sports, from high school to the masters athlete.

This section takes sound nutrition choices and outlines how food and fluid intake can address the diverse nutrition training concerns of athletes participating in winter sports, such as fueling before and during practice, optimal food and fluid choices for recovery, and nutritional strategies to optimize muscle building. A full chapter on meal planning is provided to assist the high school, collegiate, and adult athlete in putting together the sport diet suited to their sport, training and body composition goals, and lifestyle. Supplement use and the research behind many products marketed to athletes are also covered in this section.

Part II, "Sport-Specific Nutrition," outlines specific nutritional considerations for the endurance sports of cross-country skiing and snowshoeing, the power sports of alpine skiing and snowboarding, and the power/middle-distance endurance team sport of hockey. This section addresses nutritional strategies unique to training programs and competition for these sports.

I hope that the information provided in this book will enhance your health, enjoyment of your sport, and athletic accomplishments.

Part I

High-Performance Nutrition

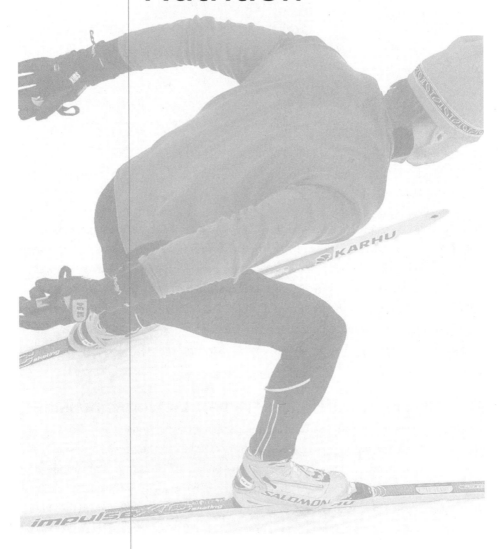

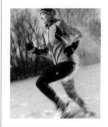

1 The Daily Performance Diet

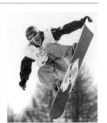

Winter athletes often participate in a variety of activities and sports year-round and are aware that the foods and fluids they crave and consume change with the seasons. Winter nutrition conjures up images of warm, comforting foods that fuel your fit body and provide nutrients that keep you healthy through the cold season. Whether you train and focus on your chosen winter sport year-round or switch into winter training mode with the onset of cold weather, your daily food intake directly impacts your energy levels, recovery from training, and overall good health.

DAILY FOOD AND FLUID CHOICES FOR OPTIMAL WINTER TRAINING

Whether you are an enthusiastic recreational participant or serious competitor preparing both indoors and outdoors, choosing the proper foods in the portions designed for your training program replaces the body fuel you burn during training and supplies the ingredients required to build strength and muscle. When you focus on optimal nutritional recovery from day to day, your efforts are rewarded when you arrive for a day on the slopes, snow, or ice in the best nutritional shape possible. When you are focused on winter training, you must meet the nutritional demands placed on your body in order to derive the maximum benefit from your exercise program.

Bodies trained and primed for winter sports also require premium fuel for staying healthy throughout the season. If you suffer from lackluster training days, injuries, and more than a fair share of colds, flu, and the various viral and respiratory infections that can plague winter, you may not be making the highest-quality fuel choices possible. When it comes to your daily diet, as a winter sport athlete you should focus on quality, variety, and balance in order to obtain the more than forty-five different nutrients required for optimal functioning in your body.

Quality, Variety, and Balance

Daily eating that places an emphasis on quality foods, variety, and balance of all food groups creates the panorama that is the big-picture focus of your winter training diet. Many categories of foods are complex and provide several nutrients that work in tandem with other food categories to keep your body well nourished and healthy. Eating a variety of food choices at meals and snacks throughout the day, and incorporating variety into your weekly grocery shopping, sets the stage for a quality training diet. Within each category of foods are nutrient-packed choices that are minimally processed, fresh, and wholesome (Table 1.1). It is best for your lasting good health that you avoid the highly processed foods so prevalent in the North American diet and eating environment.

Quality eating for training and good health takes knowledge and planning. Food groups provide a bird's-eye view of how you can balance your diet. Often foods are grouped under the three major categories of carbohydrate, protein, and fat content, as the proper balance of these nutrients is required for a winter sport athlete's optimal training and recovery.

TABLE 1.1 » BASIC TRAINING FOOD GROUPS

Carbohydrates	Proteins	Fats
Fruits and fruit juices	Fish	Nuts and seeds
Green vegetables	Poultry	Liquid oils
Starchy vegetables	Lean red meat	Avocado
Whole grains	Beans and lentils	
Cereals	Soy proteins	
Breads	Eggs	
	Skim milk and	
	low-fat yogurt	
	Low-fat cheeses	

Every winter sport athlete has his or her own optimal combination of food groups that come together to produce a cutting-edge diet. Some individuals may choose to place a strong emphasis on their fruit and vegetable intake, especially for the excellent immune system boost provided by these foods. Other athletes may highlight plant protein sources and obtain most of their fat intake from nuts and seeds rather than oils, or they may or may not prefer to have a significant amount of dairy products in their diet.

While grouping and categorizing foods can be useful in planning a healthy winter sport diet, it can also be an oversimplification of what nutrients foods provide. For example, some oils are highly processed and make a very poor nutritional choice. Animal proteins can contain varying levels of fat, some much too high in fat to be a regular part of your diet, while skim milk and yogurt also contribute carbohydrate in addition to high-quality protein. Grains can be wholesome, high in fiber, and even provide small amounts of protein, or they can be highly processed and nutritionally very poor.

The next step in planning a healthy training diet is to look at some of the food choices available within each of these designated food groups, so that you can appreciate which choices are the most nutritious. How you portion and time these healthy foods is what distinguishes your winter sport nutrition diet from an everyday diet geared toward good health. Table 1.2 outlines functions and food sources of nutrients. More information on food portioning and timing in conjunction with your training program is provided in the subsequent chapters.

Drinking in the Fluid
Water: The First Nutrient

With the arrival of cold weather, many athletes are often not as focused on daily hydration as they prepare for their training sessions. Much research and emphasis is placed on fluid intake directly before, during, and after training, but you shouldn't ignore your daily fluid intake at work, school, or rest either.

Fluid is the most essential nutrient for any athlete, including those participating in the cold outdoors and gym setting for winter sport training. Dehydration quickly results in adverse performance effects that are readily apparent and easily measured. While sweat losses of athletes competing in the cold outdoors are not always obvious to the eye, fluid losses during training, excursions, and competition taking place in colder temperatures can be significant enough to drag down your performance. Studies demonstrate that athletes competing even in thirst-inspiring hot weather routinely replace less fluid than is lost in sweat during training and especially during competition.

To obtain positive performance effects, adequate daily hydration is crucial for both general well-being and athletic performance, and every winter athlete should arrive for

TABLE 1.2 » NUTRIENTS AND THEIR FUNCTIONS

Nutrient	Functions	Food Sources
Water	Carries oxygen and nutrients to cells Plays a role in digestion Cools the body through sweat production Important role in many cellular processes Important part of muscle tissue	Tap water Bottled water Fruit juices, dairy, and soy milk Solid foods that contain water: fruits, vegetables, yogurt
Carbohydrate	Primary high-energy fuel source during exercise Replenishes body stores of carbohydrate Provides dietary fiber	Grains, breads, cereals, rice, pasta Fruit and fruit juices Vegetables Dairy and soy milk, yogurt
Protein	Provides essential amino acids Required for maintaining and developing muscle and other body tissue Essential component of enzymes, hormones, antibodies Needed for the formation of hemoglobin	Meat, poultry, fish, cheese, eggs Soy, dried beans, lentils Dairy and soy milk, yogurt
Fat	Provides essential fatty acids Provides fat-soluble vitamins Adds flavor to foods Used as a fuel source Protects and insulates body organs Component of cell structures	Liquid oils Margarine and butter Nuts and seeds Avocado Fish
Vitamins	Enhance energy production Involved in tissue repair and protein synthesis Role in red blood cell formation Act as antioxidants	Fruits and vegetables Lean protein foods Whole grains Nuts and seeds
Minerals	Involved in energy production Role in building body tissue Play role in muscle contraction Involved in oxygen transport Maintain acid-base balance of blood	Fruits and vegetables Lean proteins Whole grains Nuts and seeds

training sessions optimally hydrated. In fact, even though it deserves top priority, daily water intake is often a secondary nutrition consideration, and many athletes frequently fall short on the everyday consumption of the most important nutrient in their diet. Don't ignore daily hydration essentials. (Strategies regarding optimal fluid intake around exercise are covered in Chapter 3, "Body Fuel: Eating for Training and Recovery.")

Much marketing fuss has been made about the optimal fluids that athletes require. But before the plethora of sports drinks flooded the market, there was simply water. Water is basic and unpretentious and flows naturally into your active sport life with no packaging or gimmicks attached. Don't take water for granted. Just as you don't want to arrive to training and competition with a low fuel tank, your fluid stores should be topped off as well.

Water is both a significant part of your body and plays an integral role in its optimal functioning, whether you are training or not. Anywhere from 60 to 70 percent of your total body weight is water. Well-hydrated muscle tissue is also high in fluid content, with about 70 to 75 percent of your muscle composed of water. In comparison, fat tissue is low in water content at about 10 percent. Consequently, muscular athletes will have high body water content when adequately hydrated.

Water is stored in many body compartments, and it moves freely between these various spaces. About two-thirds of your body's water is stored inside your body's cells, giving them their shape and form. The rest of the water in your body surrounds these cells and flows within your blood vessels. Even your relatively solid bones are about 32 percent water. Water plays a role in cooling the body and also provides structure to body parts, consequently protecting important tissues such as your brain and spinal cord, and lubricating your joints. When fluid becomes depleted through sweating, both your cells and blood decrease in water content and volume.

Athletes should appreciate that water is also the main component of their blood. Blood performs the important functions of carrying oxygen, hormones, and nutrients such as glucose to your cells and is linked to important body fuel and nutrient stores such as protein, carbohydrates, and electrolytes. The protein content of blood, muscle, and other tissues also holds water in those tissues. Muscle glycogen also holds a considerable amount of water, and water removes lactic acid from exercising muscles, which can be an advantage to athletes. Water is involved in digestion through saliva and stomach secretions, and it eliminates waste products through urine and sweat. Water is essential for all your senses, such as hearing, sight, and sound, to function properly.

Clearly the role water plays in maintaining your overall health is extremely important. That's why you can't live without water for more than a few days. But the role that water plays in your performance is also essential. Being even slightly underhydrated is unacceptable for top athletic performance. As the primary component of sweat, water plays a major role in body temperature regulation. You are able to maintain a constant body temperature under various environmental conditions by continually making adjustments to either gain or lose heat. Your fluid balance is simply the result of your intake of fluids versus output of fluids. Intake is the net result of the water and hydrating fluids we consume, water in some of the foods we eat, and the metabolic water produced by your body. When you are not training, urine output represents your greatest fluid loss, while sweating during exercise can result in significant fluid losses, even in cold weather and during intense workouts in the gym. Fluid is also lost in feces and the air you exhale.

Warm or humid weather, living in a dry climate, or living and training at altitude all increase fluid losses. Traveling, especially by plane, can boost water loss. In general, your body loses about 64 to 80 ounces or 8 to 10 cups (2 to 2.4 liters) of fluid daily through the urine, feces, skin, and lungs.

Your daily water requirements are based on the amount of calories you consume. Winter sport athletes can have very high nutritional requirements, especially during periods of growth, during intense practices, and when participating in all-day or two-a-day training sessions. At rest, your body water levels can be slowly replenished, requiring a conscious effort to drink every 1 to 2 hours to replace these fluid losses.

What About Sweat?

Chapter 4 covers the science of sweat as it relates to winter sport athletes in more detail, but you may be wondering how your daily fluid intake fits into your fluid needs during exercise. This all depends on how much you sweat when training.

One of water's functions in the body is to maintain adequate blood supply to the skin. This blood transfers heat to the environment outside your body through sweating. When sweat evaporates, it cools the skin, blood, and your body's inner core. Athletes who are in top shape actually sweat more than their sedentary counterparts, often resulting in fluid needs that are quite high. So while it may appear that your tolerance to heat buildup improves with increased training and improved fitness, your fluid losses are actually higher for the same type of workout in the same weather conditions. Though sweating does the important job of keeping your body core cool and safe, the resulting minor to large fluid losses can impair your athletic performance during training, excursions, and important competitions.

Unfortunately, thirst is not a very good indicator of the amount of fluid that your body requires, during exercise or at rest. Some early signs and symptoms of dehydration are light-headedness, headaches, decreased appetite, darkly colored urine, and fatigue (see sidebar on next page). Pay attention to how you feel during the day. An annoying headache may indicate the need to up your fluid intake.

» SIGNS AND SYMPTOMS OF DEHYDRATION

Physiological Effects	Symptoms
Decreased levels of:	**Mild dehydration**
Blood volume	Dark urine
Cardiac output	Decreased appetite
Skin blood flow	Headache
Sweat rate	Fatigue
Urine output	Heat intolerance
	Light-headedness
Increased:	Small amount dark urine
Body temperature	Nausea
Heart rate	
	Severe dehydration
	High temperature
	Delirium, disorientation, dizziness
	Difficulty swallowing
	Dry, shriveled skin
	Muscle spasms
	Sunken eyes

Daily Hydration Essentials

It is essential that you stay on top of your fluid needs by drinking a minimum of 60 to 80 ounces (1.8 to 2.4 liters) of fluid daily for basic hydration requirements when away from the slopes, snow, and ice. Try to drink on a schedule of 8 ounces (240 milliliters) every hour. Water should comprise about half of your daily fluid intake, but you can also receive hydration benefits from other fluids. Hydrating choices include juice, dairy milk, soy milk, soup, and various sports nutrition supplements. Some foods also contribute fluid to your daily diet, such as fruits and vegetables.

Winter sport athletes with very high energy requirements can consume high-calorie drinks such as juices and smoothies to assist them in meeting their fluid, carbohydrate, and energy needs. Caffeinated beverages can be incorporated into your diet in reasonable amounts, but they should not be your first choice for training hydration purposes and for several hours following training. Overdoing your caffeine intake can also interfere with your sleep patterns and make you nervous and jittery. Excess caffeine may also act as a mild diuretic in your daily diet shortly after you drink a caffeine-containing beverage. However, overall, caffeine-containing beverages are not as dehydrating as they were once thought to be and can be included in moderate amounts with other fluids in the diet. You can monitor your hydration status by checking the color and quantity of your urine. Clear or lemonade-colored urine reflects adequate fluid intake, while darker or apple-juice-colored urine in smaller volume indicates that you need to step up your fluid intake. Urine tends to be more concentrated when you first wake up but should be clearer throughout the day. You should urinate at least four full bladders every day. Certain vitamin supplements can darken urine, so volume rather than color may be a better indicator of hydration status if you take these urine-coloring products. You can also consider regular monitoring of your weight during heavy training periods. If you notice significant weight losses at a morning weigh-in, this may also be an indicator of chronic dehydration.

Focusing and practicing to improve your daily fluid intake is definitely worthwhile. Athletes who have developed techniques for increasing their fluid intake have consistently found that improved hydration resulted in enhanced recovery and higher energy levels. Improving your hydration levels is really very simple. Just plan ahead and make sure that water and other hydrating fluids are available for consumption throughout the day. This will ensure that you begin your training sessions with a well-hydrated body.

» DAILY WINTER HYDRATION STRATEGIES

Start your day with hydration in mind. Consume liquids such as juice, dairy or soy milk, or hot chocolate at breakfast. Drink 8 to 16 ounces (240 to 480 milliliters) of water or hydrating fluid when you start your day. Don't overdue caffeinated beverages in the morning.

Don't rely mainly or solely on caffeinated beverages for daily hydration needs. Younger athletes should avoid or limit caffeine. Have plenty of decaffeinated hot drinks such as decaffeinated coffee, decaffeinated tea, and herbal tea.

Carry water with you at all times—when you drive or commute, at work or school, and wherever the opportunity to drink presents itself.

Incorporate fruit juices, milk, soy milk, hot decaffeinated drinks, or water into meals or snacks.

Spruce up your water with lemon, lime, or a small amount of juice for flavor.

Adults should consume any serving of alcohol with a full 8 to 12 ounces (240 to 360 milliliters) of hydrating fluid.

Consider consuming foods high in fluid such as fruits and vegetables, cooked cereals, and yogurt.

Consume 24 ounces (720 milliliters) of fluid 2 hours before exercise and 8 to 16 ounces (240 to 480 milliliters) of fluid 30 minutes before exercise to ensure adequate hydration prior to exercise.

» FILTERED, BOTTLED, OR TAP?

With the advent of the extensive bottled water market, you may have wondered whether it is in the best interest of your health to consume water other than tap water. For healthy adults, tap water in the United States is very safe, but that doesn't mean that you shouldn't make water safer, and many American consumers are considering new water options. Over the past several years, purchases of home filtration systems has increased, and Americans consumed more than 5 billion gallons of bottled water in the year 2000 alone. Currently, the Environmental Protection Agency (EPA) estimates that 90 percent of the country's drinking water is safe.

Tap water does contain substances other than water. Depending on where you live it can provide varying levels of minerals such as calcium, sodium, magnesium, iron, zinc, lead, and mercury. While calcium may be a beneficial mineral obtained from water, lead and mercury are not. As a health-minded athlete and consumer, you may also be concerned about microbial contamination and pesticide residues in water.

Tap water is regulated under the strict standards of the EPA, but there are some contaminants that the EPA does not regulate. Your local water municipality is required to supply you with an annual "Right to Know Report" every July, which lists contaminants detected in your drinking water and notes any violations that have occurred in the past year. Your water provider is also required to test for microbes several times daily. In addition, you can contact your local water municipality to obtain the names and numbers of certified testing labs to have the water from your own tap checked. Levels of lead and copper in your water may be higher than official reports due to leaching from household plumbing and faucets.

Filtered water may be a viable option. Many filters attach right to the tap and filter lead and other contaminants. Another convenient filter method is a pour-through filter that can be placed in a special pitcher and kept in your refrigerator. More expensive filters include an under-sink model that requires a permanent connection to your water pipe. Reverse osmosis is the best type and filters out lead, mercury, minerals, some pesticides, and microorganisms. Whole-house filters are the most expensive and are installed where the water meets the main water pipe, and they cover all the water used in the house.

Carbohydrates: The Athlete's Fuel
Classifying Carbohydrates: From Simple to Complex to Indexing

Winter athletes should appreciate that carbohydrates are a major source of fuel. Carbohydrate recommendations for athletes can be hard to reconcile with the numerous diet books and programs that extol the pitfalls of consuming a high-carbohydrate diet. While nutrition plans should always be personalized to an athlete's training program, medical history, and genetics, if your carbohydrate intake does not provide a sufficient amount of fuel for your training and recovery, you will not perform at your best. Of course, your carbohydrate choices should be of the highest quality possible.

You may also determine that bottled water is a convenient option for reaching your recommended daily water intake, though there is no guarantee that it is microbe-free or safer than tap water. About one-quarter of all bottled water comes from municipal water supplies. Bottled water can also be spring water, mineral water, well water, or distilled water. Unlike tap water, which is regulated by the EPA, bottled water is regulated by the Food and Drug Administration (FDA), is not tested for the parasites cryptosporidium and giardia, and is tested only once weekly for microbes. The advantages of bottled water may simply be its taste and convenience.

Both water filter systems and bottled water can be certified by an independent organization called the National Sanitation Foundation (NSF). The NSF sets standards for and certifies water filtration systems. Its Web site at www.nsf.org lists filters and the contaminants that the filter is certified to reduce in your water. Look for a filter with a pore size less than 1 micron in diameter. Be sure to follow the manufacturer's directions for replacement of the filter cartridge. The best and most expensive systems are reverse osmosis.

It is also a good idea to look for brands of bottled water that maintain the NSF certification.

In order to maintain this certification, water bottlers must send daily samples for microbial testing to an independent lab and maintain records of filter changes and other quality checks. You can also determine whether your brand of water is NSF certified by visiting the NSF's Web site.

New varieties of bottled water include fortified waters, fitness water, waters supplemented with vitamins and herbs, and oxygen-enriched water. Some of these waters simply provide flavor for individuals who do not want to drink plain water and encourage good fluid intake. Some contain only a small number of calories, while others may provide more calories per bottle than consumers realize. Check labels to determine the number of calories per serving and the number of servings per bottle. Some of the new designer waters may contain artificial sweeteners. Herbal and vitamin-enhanced waters may not provide significant amounts of these nutrients per serving; however, you could potentially consume enough servings in a day and take in too much of some of these substances. Currently there is no apparent value or scientific backing to consuming oxygen-enriched water, which claims to boost energy by increasing the oxygen content of red blood cells.

Many athletes are familiar with the traditional classification of carbohydrates. *Simple carbohydrates*, which are often called "sugars," consist of one or two molecules; *complex carbohydrates* or *starches* are composed of up to thousands of carbohydrate molecules joined together. What was long advised regarding these foods was that simple carbohydrates such as fructose and other sugars cause a rapid rise and subsequent fall in blood sugar that results in fatigue and that these sugars are less nutritious. Conversely, it was maintained that complex carbohydrates resulted in a more gentle blood glucose rise and are more nutritious foods. In summary, simple carbohydrates were considered "bad" and complex carbohydrates "good."

Although this classification might seem logical, scientific data from the past decade indicate that this carbohydrate advice is an outdated concept. What winter sport athletes should truly be concerned about is the quality of the carbohydrate they consume, emphasizing nutritious and wholesome sources while decreasing nutrient-poor refined sources in their diet. Wholesome carbohydrates provide vitamins, minerals, and fiber, while refined carbohydrates are processed foods that provide little other than calories.

What you should also appreciate is that wholesome carbohydrates are not always of the complex variety, and refined carbohydrates are not always simple sugars and are often overly processed grain sources that were much more nutritious in their natural state. Fruit is a simple carbohydrate and is packed with nutrients, while products made from complex white flour such as white bread often have a much lower vitamin and mineral content. For optimal training and good health, wholesome carbohydrates are a very important component of your diet, because they are higher in nutritional value.

In addition to being wholesome or refined, carbohydrates can also be categorized according to how they affect your blood sugar or blood glucose levels. The belief that simple carbohydrates cause a rapid rise in blood glucose and that complex carbohydrates cause a slower rise in blood glucose is outdated. Research has demonstrated that each carbohydrate food produces its own unique blood glucose profile that does not correlate with the simple-versus-complex classification.

The ranking system that describes the blood glucose profile of a food is referred to as the glycemic index. In this system, the blood glucose profile of 50 grams of pure glucose has been designated a glycemic index of 100. Other carbohydrates are tested in 50-gram doses and compared to glucose. High-glycemic foods are generally considered to have a glycemic index of greater than 70. Moderate-glycemic index foods are in the 55 to 70 range, and low-glycemic index foods have a score of less than 55.

Table 1.3 provides a glycemic index ranking of high-carbohydrate foods. Interestingly, fruits generally have a low glycemic index, despite being simple carbohydrates, whereas white potatoes, a complex carbohydrate, have a high glycemic index. Many factors influence the glycemic index of a food, including the type of fiber in the food, how the glucose molecules in the food are connected, and the form in which the food is prepared.

Individuals with specific health concerns such as diabetes who need to control blood glucose and elevated blood lipids can manipulate their carbohydrate intake according to their benefit based on the glycemic index of the foods. The glycemic index can also play a role in treating individuals diagnosed with a condition referred to as *metabolic syndrome* that is characterized by a resistance to using the body's insulin appropriately. Ongoing research for individuals with these health concerns will fine-tune appropriate dietary recommendations that consider the glycemic index.

TABLE 1.3 » GLYCEMIC INDEX OF FOODS

Food	Serving Size	Grams of Carbohydrate (CHO)	Glycemic Load	Glycemic Index (50 g)
High-Glycemic Foods (GI >70)				
Potato, baked	6.5 oz. (200 g)	29	27.3	94
Rice, instant	50 oz. (200 g)	42	36.5	87
Cornflakes	1 oz. (30 g)	25	215	86
Rice Krispies	1 oz. (30 g)	29	24	82
Total cereal	1 oz. (30 g)	25	19	76
Waffle	2 oz. (60 g)	25	19.3	76
Cheerios	1 oz. (30 g)	25	18.5	74
Watermelon	8 oz. (240 g)	12	8.6	72
Bagel, white	2.25 oz. (70 g)	35.5	25.5	72
Millet	5 oz. (150 g)	34.8	24.7	71
Bread, white	2 oz. (60 g)	26.8	18.8	70
Moderate-Glycemic Foods (GI 55–70)				
Shredded Wheat	1 oz. (30 g)	21.7	14.6	67
Pineapple	4 oz. (120 g)	9.6	6.3	66
Oat kernel bread	2 oz. (60 g)	25.6	16.6	65
Raisins	2 oz. (60 g)	42.7	27.3	64
Couscous	5 oz. (150 g)	14.3	8.7	61
Muffin	1.9 oz. (57 g)	27.7	17.2	62
Spaghetti, white, durum wheat	6 oz. (180 g)	44.3	25.6	58
Muesli	2 oz. (60 g)	32	17.9	56
Oat Bran, raw	2 oz. (60 g)	30	16.5	55
Low-Glycemic Foods (GI <55)				
Buckwheat	5 oz. (150 g)	28.8	14.6	51
Bread, whole-grain	2 oz. (30 g)	23	12	51
Banana, ripe	4 oz. (120 g)	23.9	12.1	50
All-Bran	2 oz. (60 g)	36.8	18.4	50
Rice, brown	5 oz. (150 g)	47.7	23.9	49
Porridge oatmeal	8 oz. (250 g)	20.3	9.94	48
Sweet potato	5 oz. (150 g)	26	12.5	48
Grapefruit juice	8 oz. (260 g)	15.7	7.5	41
Pear, Bartlett	4 oz. (120 g)	11.3	4.6	40
Apple	4 oz. (120 g)	14.6	5.9	33
Yogurt, fruited	6.5 oz. (200 g)	33	10.9	32

CONTINUED

TABLE 1.3 continued

Food	Serving Size	Grams of Carbohydrate (CHO)	Glycemic Load	Glycemic Index (50 g)
Low-Glycemic Foods (GI <55)				
Milk, skim	8 oz. (259 g)	13	4.1	32
Spaghetti, whole-meal	4 oz. (120 g)	30	9.6	28
Peach	8 oz. (240 g)	15	4.2	28
Lentils	5 oz. (150 g)	14.9	4.1	28
Kidney beans	5 oz. (150 g)	24	5.5	23

» CONSIDER THE GLYCEMIC LOAD

While the glycemic index (GI) is a ranking of carbohydrates based on their immediate blood glucose effect, the glycemic load (GL) builds on the GI of a food and provides a more meaningful measure of how your body truly responds to the carbohydrates you consume. That's because the glycemic load takes into consideration the portion of the food. Not all your carbohydrate food portions will supply the 50-gram dose used in glycemic index testing; often you may consume a much smaller amount.

Glycemic load is the glycemic index of a food multiplied by the total grams of carbohydrate in the portion of the food, which is then divided by 100. One GL unit is approximately equal to the glycemic effect of 1 gram of glucose. The GL of all carbohydrate foods can be added up for the day. The total GL range for the day is typically 60 to 180. A low GL day is less than 80, while a high GL day is greater than 120.

GL = GI x grams of carbohydrate per serving divided by 100

Let's compare the GL of carrots to corn. Carrots have a glycemic index of 92, a high GI, while corn has a more moderate glycemic index of 60. Let's assume that ½ cup (120 ml) cooked of each is consumed, which is a reasonable and commonly eaten portion.

1. Carrots have a GI of 92, and you eat ½ cup cooked, which has 6 grams of carbohydrate.
   92 x 6 = 552 divided by 100 = a glycemic load of 5.52

2. Corn has a GI of 60, and you eat ½ cup cooked, which has 20 grams of carbohydrate.
   60 x 20 = 1,200 divided by 100 = a glycemic load of 12

Although carrots have a higher glycemic index than that of corn, because of the portion consumed, the glycemic load of carrots is lower than a similar portion of corn. This example illustrates that many moderate- to high-GI carbohydrate foods may not be consumed in the 50-gram portion test dose and could potentially have a low GL. A low GL for a carbohydrate serving is 10 or less, moderate GL is 11 to 19, and high GL is 20 or more.

Athletes may also be able to utilize the glycemic index to their performance advantage in regard to specific recommendations before, during, and after training. These sports nutrition applications of glycemic index will be reviewed in Chapter 3 and 4. For their daily diet, winter athletes should experiment with various nutrient-dense carbohydrate foods to determine what works best with their food preferences and schedules.

Go for the Grains—The Wholesome Ones!

With the advent of carbohydrate-restricted diets, the group of carbohydrates most often eliminated and heavily restricted are grains. This is unfortunate because wholesome grains are good sources of carbohydrate, fiber, and B vitamins. Because they are so concentrated in carbohydrate, they are excellent choices for replenishing your body's carbohydrate stores—namely, muscle and liver glycogen, which become depleted from intense and demanding training sessions. Grains are easily obtained in the North American diet, but unfortunately many of these choices are refined grains rather than whole grains. Just as many of us have chosen diets based on the good fat, bad fat concept (which we explore later), it is obvious that in the North American diet there are good carbohydrates and bad carbohydrates.

For both optimal health and a top winter sport diet, choose whole grains whenever possible. Whole grains literally come from the entire grain that includes the endosperm, germ, and bran portion of the grain, thereby retaining all the desirable nutrients. In contrast, when refined grains are produced, the bran and germ are separated from the starchy endosperm. The endosperm is then ground into flour.

Whole grains are packed with vitamins, minerals, and phytochemicals, which have powerful antioxidant and disease-fighting properties that you won't obtain from white bread, processed cereals, white rice, and even many "enriched" multigrain breads. Some of the phytochemicals found in whole grains include oligosaccharides, flavinoids, lignans, phytates, and saponins, many of which have powerful antioxidant properties. Whole grains also provide vitamin E and selenium. Studies have shown that regular consumption of whole grains is linked to prevention of heart disease, diabetes, and certain cancers, yet surveys indicate that most Americans consume less than one serving of whole grains daily. Consuming grains such as whole oats, barley, and bran can also reduce the glycemic load of your diet. High-fiber whole-grain breads that contain whole seeds will also have a lower glycemic index.

A variety of whole grains can be included in your diet. Even just making simple changes such as having brown rice instead of white rice and whole-wheat pasta rather than semolina pasta is beneficial. Buy 100-percent whole-grain breads, and look for "whole grain" on the health claim packages, which indicates that more than half of the weight of the product comes from whole grains.

» GETTING IN THE GRAINS

Aim for three servings of whole grains each day. One slice or 1 ounce (30 g) of bread equals a serving, and 1 ounce (30 g) of cereal equals a serving.

Find a whole-grain cereal that you enjoy. Good choices include oatmeal or bran flakes.

Buy breads that list 100-percent whole-grain flour as the first ingredient and for all other listed flours as well.

Use brown rice instead of white and whole-wheat pasta instead of semolina.

Add All-Bran or wheat germ to your yogurt, in smoothies, or in other cereals.

Look for the "whole-grain" health claim on the package, which indicates that more than half the weight of the products comes from whole grains.

Athletes who are tired of the same wheat- and rice-based grain choices also have a few more adventuresome options. There are many whole-grain alternatives, including amaranth, kasha (buckwheat), quinoa, spelt, teff, and triticale (see Table 1.4). They may take a bit more cooking time than pasta, rice, and potatoes, but they are nutritious and add variety to the diet. You can experiment with various seasonings to further flavor these wholesome grains.

Whole grains should be an important part of your diet for the nutrients and carbohydrates that they provide. But you should also place a strong emphasis on fruits and vegetables, not only for their carbohydrate content but also the great health benefits that they offer. In fact, some health organizations and health researchers believe that fruits and vegetables should comprise the *majority* of our carbohydrate intake. Studies have shown that eating more fruits and vegetables can reduce your risk of heart disease, stroke, and some types of cancer. How you put together your sport diets will ultimately depend on your food preferences, convenience, your personal health considerations, and your carbohydrate training requirements. But chances are that boosting fruit and vegetable intake would be a step in the right direction for any athlete interested in optimal performance on the slopes, snow, and ice and dedicated to lifelong good health.

Fruits and Vegetables: The Harvest of Champions

Fruits and vegetables are especially distinguished by the thousands of substances that they provide that protect our bodies from disease. These phytonutrients act as antioxidants and counteract the cellular damage that we encounter every day. Fruits and vegetables are

TABLE 1.4 » WHOLE-GRAIN ALTERNATIVES

Grain	Description	Tips
Amaranth	High in protein and fiber; good source of vitamin E	Boil and eat as a cereal. Cook 1 cup grain in 3 cups water for ½ hour.
Barley	High in soluble fiber	Cook 1 cup of grain per 3 cups water, for 45 minutes.
Spelt	A distant cousin to wheat; high in fiber and B vitamins	Used to make breads and pastas. Can be used in pilafs. Cook 1 cup with 4 cups water 30–40 minutes.
Millet	A staple in Africa; high in minerals	Cook 1 cup grain with 2.25 cups water 25–30 minutes. Serve with meat or cook as a cereal.
Bulgur	High in fiber, folate, magnesium, and iron	Cooks in 10–12 minutes. Use 1 cup grain to 2 cups liquid.
Kasha (buckwheat groats)	Excellent source of magnesium; high in fiber	Serve as a cereal, pilaf, or pancakes. Simmer 1 part groats to 2 parts water for 15 minutes.
Oats	Source of a cholesterol-lowering fiber; high in protein.	Steel-cut oats cook for 20 minutes, using 1 cup oats for 4 cups liquid. Avoid instant varieties.
Quinoa	Excellent source of B vitamins, copper, iron, and magnesium	Can make an oatmeal-like cereal. Rinse before cooking to remove bitter coating. Cook 1 cup quinoa in 2 cups water for 20 minutes.
Brown rice	High in fiber, B vitamins, iron, and magnesium	Cooks in 24–45 minutes. Use 1 cup rice to 2.5 cups water.
Teff	The world's smallest grain; rich in protein and calcium	Serve as a hot breakfast cereal or part of a stew. Cook 1 cup of teff in 3 cups water for 15–20 minutes.

also great sources of the immune-boosting vitamin A and antioxidant beta-carotene, as well as other health-enhancing carotenoids. They also supply ample amounts of vitamin C, another important antioxidant and vitamin that performs many essential functions in your body, and the mineral potassium. In this chapter we will review not only some nutrient-packed fruit and vegetable choices for winter but also excellent sources of specific vitamins, minerals, and antioxidants.

Filling Up on Fruit

Because fruits are so packed with disease-fighting nutrients, a high number of daily fruit servings is strongly recommended by the American Heart Association and the American Cancer Society. Fresh fruits, dried fruit, and fruit juice can also provide the winter sport athlete with a significant and concentrated source of carbohydrates that provide energy for training and fuel for recovery.

All fruits are nutritious, but some choices are extremely nutritious. Tropical fruits such as papaya, mango, kiwifruit, and guava have wonderfully high levels of vitamin C and carotenoids, which are potent antioxidants. Carotenoids are also found in significant amounts in deep-colored fruits such as apricots, cantaloupe, and nectarines. Citrus fruits such as oranges and grapefruits are known for being great sources of vitamin C. Phytonutrients, which appear increasingly important to maintaining good health, such as catechins, flavonols, stilbenes, allicin, quercetin, ellagic acid, anthocyanins, limonin, zeaxanthin, and lutein are also found in fruits.

The best way to obtain a variety of phytonutrients is to consume a variety of fruits. Dried fruits and real fruit juices will provide the most concentrated sources of carbohydrate for athletes with higher energy needs. Dried fruit, however, will not be as great a source of vitamin C, though it may provide more minerals and fiber than fresh because they are so concentrated. Try to avoid dried fruits prepared with sulfites if you are sulfite-sensitive. (Sulfites are preservatives that trigger allergic reactions in some individuals.) Fresh fruits are also great sources of fiber and the highest in nutrients.

While the warm summer months are associated with a wide variety of fresh fruits, fresh produce is often not as abundant or reasonable in cost during the winter months. While you should choose fresh and eat fresh whenever possible, don't disregard frozen and canned choices to keep a healthy supply of fruit in your diet. The nutritional value of fresh fruits is too high to ignore, but any source of fruit is better than none. Flash freezing and other new technologies trap vitamins, minerals, and phytochemicals in fruit immediately after they are harvested when produce is at its peak. When you peruse the supermarket aisles, purchase enough fresh fruits and vegetables to last three to four days, the amount of time it takes fresh fruit to lose its nutritive value when sitting in your refrigerator. If you shop twice weekly, pick up another fresh fruit stash later in the week.

» TOP WINTER FRUIT CHOICES

Individuals who consume more colorful fruits have lower rates of cancer and heart disease due to the vitamins, minerals, and hundreds of phytochemicals that they contain. While fresh fruit is still readily available in the winter, it is not in as abundant supply during the warmer months. Frozen and canned varieties are also sources of important nutrients. Consider these choices:

Bananas—available year-round and a good source of vitamin B6, potassium, and vitamin C

Red grapefruit—an excellent source of vitamin C and carotenoids

Tangerines—a source of vitamin C, vitamin A, beta-carotene, and other carotenoids

Red grapes—a good source of potassium, beta-carotene, and lutein

Apples—a good source of fiber and flavonoids

Cranberries—a good source of vitamins A, C, and K, and carotenoids

Pomegranate—high in antioxidants, potassium, fiber, and vitamin C

Berries (frozen)—provide vitamins A and C, potassium, folate, and a wide variety of phytonutrients

During the winter season, try to incorporate a variety of fruits into your diet. Aim for at least three servings daily. A serving is one medium to large piece of fruit, 1 cup of fruit, or 8 ounces of fruit juice.

If you shop once a week (and it can be challenging to keep up a healthy sport diet if you shop any less frequently), buy a variety of frozen or canned fruit. Fresh oranges, apples, and grapefruits are available year-round and tend to retain their nutritive value a bit longer than other fruits. Other great fresh fruit choices during the winter include red grapes, bananas, red grapefruits, and pears.

Choose your frozen and canned fruits carefully. Avoid frozen brands that add extra sugar or syrup and canned varieties that are packed in heavy syrup, as this preparation adds non-nutritive calories. Opt for fruit canned and packed in light juice and frozen fruit where the fruit is the sole ingredient on the package.

If you miss those delicious summer raspberries and blueberries, don't forget the frozen version; organic fruit is available frozen also. Frozen fruits should also move about freely in the package; when they have fused into a solid block of ice, some nutrient loss has already occurred. Also avoid packages that are sweating or stained with the fruit inside; this appearance indicates that it has been partially thawed and refrozen before reaching the supermarket. Once-thawed frozen fruit can be a bit more waterlogged than its fresh counterparts. Frozen fruits can work great on top of hot cereals, pancakes, and waffles, and they are perfect for smoothies, which are so appreciated and useful to athletes.

Finding Veggie Heaven

Like fruits, vegetables provide a wide variety of vitamins, minerals, and phytonutrients, and fiber that enhance your health. Great winter vegetable choices include broccoli, bok choy, Brussels sprouts, potatoes, sweet potatoes, and of course winter squash.

All vegetables are good healthy choices, but some stand out nutritionally speaking, and are even more concentrated in nutrients than fruit. Color is often a good indicator of a higher nutrient content in vegetables. Some stellar options include carrots, sweet potatoes, and red peppers, which are high in carotenoids. Spinach and Romaine lettuce are good leafy choices for their vitamin C, folate, and phytonutrient content. Another group of vegetables that contain not only beta-carotene and vitamin C but also the cancer-fighting phytonutrients indoles are broccoli, cauliflower, bok choy, collards, Brussels sprouts, and kale.

Each day try to consume a variety of colorful vegetables that are yellow, orange, red, and deep green. Choose large servings of vegetables when you eat at home, as it can be challenging to obtain quality vegetable choices when eating out. Buy fresh vegetables when you know you will consume them in a few days and store them in the refrigerator crisper drawer. When buying fresh, carrots tend to retain their nutritive value a bit longer, whereas kale, broccoli, and green beans lose nutrients a bit more quickly.

Frozen vegetables are a good second choice. Frozen produce may even provide more beta-carotene, as it is protected from light by packaging. Fresh tomatoes contain lycopene, a powerful antioxidant, canned and jarred tomatoes and tomato sauces contain even higher levels of available lycopene. Frozen and canned vegetables are preferable to fresh choices that have been sitting in your crisper too long, and they are a good winter alternative to your delicious summer farmer's market produce. Frozen vegetables, like frozen fruits, should also move freely about the package, indicating they have retained the full force of their nutritional value.

Avoid overcooking your vegetables in order to preserve all the wonderful nutrients they contain. Steaming above water level is the best choice for preserving nutrients in cooked vegetables, while boiling or any contact with water results in the highest nutrient losses. When microwaving vegetables, use as little water as possible to preserve nutrient content and check frequently to avoid overcooking them.

Fitting in the Fiber—Every Day!

Wholesome and unprocessed foods also provide the highly important nutrient fiber. Despite the wide selection of high-fiber food choices at the supermarket, Americans obtain only about half of the recommended intake of 20 to 35 grams daily, which is not enough to obtain all the known health benefits of fiber. Diets high in fiber can help prevent heart disease, diabetes, stroke, high blood pressure, cancer, diverticulitis, and constipation. Fiber

» TOP WINTER VEGETABLE CHOICES

Individuals who consume a wide variety of nutrient-dense vegetables have a lower incidence of heart disease and cancer and other diseases. Many highly nutritious vegetables are available during the winter season. Try to incorporate a variety of choices into your diet. Many areas have a winter farmer's market that sells fresh choices. When fresh is not available, purchase frozen vegetables. Here are some top choices:

Tomato—high in the antioxidant lycopene and beta-carotene

Winter squash—excellent source of vitamins A and C, and a good source of folate

Bok choy—excellent source of vitamins A and C, and folic acid

Broccoli—high in phytonutrients; good source of vitamin C and calcium

Brussels sprouts—source of iron, lutein, and zeaxanthin, and beta-carotene

Sweet potato—high in beta-carotene and vitamin A

from food is your best choice, rather than supplements, so that fiber can work its wonder with the other nutrients in foods.

Fiber is a group of indigestible carbohydrates found in plant foods divided into two main categories, water-soluble and water-insoluble fiber. Both types of fiber are found in every fiber-rich food, though one usually predominates. Insoluble fiber is the most familiar form and is found in wheat bran, whole-grain cereals, dried beans and peas, vegetables, and nuts. This type of fiber aids digestion, moves potentially cancerous substance through the colon, and keeps colon function regular. Water-soluble fiber acts more like a sponge and can help control blood glucose and blood cholesterol levels. Good sources of water-soluble fiber include whole oats, oat bran, some fruits, and dried beans. Fiber can also increase your feeling of fullness after consuming a meal, a useful tool for individuals trying to reduce their caloric intake and lose weight.

If you need more fiber in your diet, increase your intake slowly and drink plenty of water. Most fruits and vegetables average 2 to 3 grams of fiber per serving. Dried peas and beans are loaded with fiber, providing 6 to 8 grams per ½ cup. Whole grains can provide 2 to 3 grams of fiber per serving. Check labels to make the best choices. Nuts and seeds are also great sources of fiber.

High-fiber foods should be part of your daily diet but may not be the best choices immediately before training and close to competition as they may cause intestinal discomfort with exercise. For the athlete who benefits from a comfortable stomach and intestinal system during exercise, fiber intake is not only about health but also about consuming the correct amounts at the safest times.

Protein Power

While wholesome carbohydrates are a staple in an athlete's diet, winter sport athletes interested in maximizing power and strength and building endurance also need adequate

» SIFTING THROUGH THE SUGARS

For many of us, sugar is contained in foods that we view as treats or even comfort foods. Perhaps as an active athlete, you feel that there is a little bit of room for sugar in your diet. There is no denying that sugar is a significant part of our diet, with Americans estimated to consume over 60 pounds (27 kilograms) yearly.

The term sugar commonly refers to simple carbohydrates composed of single and double carbohydrate molecules. Glucose, fructose, and galactose are monosaccharides, or single carbohydrate molecules that are the building blocks for carbohydrates found in our diet. Disaccharides are composed of two sugar molecules and include sucrose (table sugar) and lactose (milk sugar).

Depending on the food choices you make, sugar in your diet is either added sugar, which is simply sugar added to food, and naturally occurring sugar, which is a natural component of foods and therefore not added in processing, preparation, or at the table. The key to smart sugar consumption is choosing the healthy natural sugars and downplaying the nonnutritive added sugars.

Naturally occurring sugars are the fructose found in fruits and the lactose found in milk and yogurt. The health benefits of these foods are reviewed in other sections of this chapter. Food sources of these sugars are highly nutritious and contain a wide range of vitamins and minerals.

Added sugars are quite the opposite and are often found in foods quite low in nutritional value. Sucrose, commonly referred to as table sugar, is found mainly in dessert and snack foods with very limited nutritional value. Particularly prevalent is the added sugar high-fructose corn syrup (HFCS), which is produced by chemically altering cornstarch and is cheaper and sweeter than sucrose. HFCS is made up of about 55 percent fructose and 45 percent glucose. Some HFCS has higher fructose levels, at 90 percent, for an even sweeter flavor. HFCS is added to a variety of food products, including baked goods, breads, cereals, ketchup, and soft drinks, and many other items, so read labels carefully. One-third of all the sugar consumed in the United States is the HFCS in soft drinks.

Recently health concerns have been raised regarding HFCS. Some experts contend that increased intake of HFCS is directly linked to the growing rate of obesity and type 2 diabetes in the United States. Other experts counter that it is simply the empty calories consumed from HFCS-containing products that contribute to obesity, and weight gain is not inherent and unique to the sweetener itself. Of course, all experts agree that this sugar is found in foods with very little nutritional value protein for top performance. Protein plays an important role in the growth, repair, and maintenance of muscles and other tissues in your body is also required to form hormones, enzymes, and neurotransmitters. It is the key component of your immune system, is needed for hemoglobin formation (the substance that carries oxygen to the exercising muscles), and can even serve as a fuel source during endurance exercise if your body's carbohydrate stores run low.

and is high in refined carbohydrates.

In many cases, fruit juice is an excellent example of a natural sugar product gone bad. Any fruit juice you consume should be 100-percent juice and not a juice drink or blend that provides some HFCS. But real fruit juice is still higher in simple sugar than whole-fruit counterparts. Fruit juice also provides no fiber. Look for 100-percent fruit juice on labels, and try to avoid the cheap fillers of apple juice and white grape juice. Read the ingredient list carefully. Juices listed at the beginning are present in the greatest quantity. Juices with color tend to have more antioxidants and phytonutrients, so purple grape juice is better than white grape juice.

Sugars can make foods more palatable and need not be completely eliminated from your diet. But how much added sugar is too much? Nutritional surveys and logic indicate that as added sugar intake increases, intake of several vitamins and minerals decreases. Processed sugar calories should not replace appropriate servings of fruits, vegetables, whole grains, and low-fat dairy products, or the quality of your diet will suffer. The World Health Organization recommends limiting free sugars, which includes added sugars and the sugar present naturally in fruit juice, to no more than 10 percent of daily calories, a recommendation significantly lower than the National Academy of Science guideline of 25 percent. One recent study estimates that 20 percent of our carbohydrate intake and 10 percent of our total calorie intake comes from corn syrup alone.

Try to minimize sugar in your diet, not eliminate it completely. The occasional dessert or candy after a meal is fine, as part of a well-balanced diet. If your active lifestyle demands an intake of 2,400 calories daily, your sugar intake should not exceed 240 calories, leaving room for some treats in a daily diet filled with wholesome choices. You can also aim for an intake of no more than 10 teaspoons of sugar daily. One teaspoon of sugar equals 4 grams.

The Nutrition Facts label does not distinguish between added sugar and natural sugars in a food, as only the "total sugars" are listed, and can include natural sugar choices in the food as well. But you can determine whether added sugars are a major ingredient by referring to the ingredient list. The closer the terms are to the beginning of the ingredient list, the greater the amount of added sugar in the product. Some added sugars to look for on the label include beet juice, brown rice syrup, cane syrup, corn syrup, corn sweetener, crystalline fructose, dextrose, evaporated cane juice, fructose, high-fructose corn syrup, invert sugar, malt syrup, maltodextrin, and sucrose.

Proteins are composed of amino acids, which are the building units that create protein-based tissues. We obtain amino acids from the protein-containing foods we consume and from the breakdown of our muscle tissue. Amino acids that can be manufactured by our body are considered nonessential, as it is not required that we consume them from food. Conversely, amino acids that we cannot manufacture in our body are considered essential and must be obtained in our diet for good health and optimal performance. Proteins that we consume are digested into amino acids and go to the amino acid pool in our bodies. These amino acids can then be drawn upon to synthesize protein-based tissues or to use as energy if carbohydrate stores run low.

Your sport diet protein intake can easily comprise 15 to 20 percent of your daily energy consumption with a well-balanced and even typical North American diet. Generally, many athletes exceed their protein intake, most likely due to large protein portions encouraged in our food culture. An exception would be weight- or body fat-conscious athletes who restrict certain foods in attempts to limit or avoid fat intake, possibly placing themselves at risk for consuming inadequate protein.

Animal protein in the form of lean meats, poultry, fish, and eggs are the foods most concentrated in protein. Many of these animal proteins are also good sources of iron and zinc. High-quality plant sources of protein include soy products such as tofu and tempeh, dried peas and beans, and lentils. Low-fat dairy foods are also an excellent source of protein and the mineral calcium.

What is important for optimal health is to choose lean protein sources, as this will reduce your intake of saturated fat. Too high an intake of saturated fat is a risk factor for developing heart disease. (See Table 1.5, which lists the protein content of certain foods per specified portion.) Try to emphasize leaner choices of beef, lamb, pork, and other red meats to limit your intake of saturated fat. Cheese can also add significant amounts of saturated fat to the diet. More discussion on choosing protein and protein requirement for specific types of training will be provided in Chapter 3.

Fat: Facts and Figures

Fat is an important part of an athlete's diet. Although fat is somewhat renowned for being a concentrated source of calories, it does play several key roles in keeping you healthy. Most important, fat is a source of nutrients known as essential fatty acids. Just as you need to obtain vitamins and minerals in your daily diet, the two essential fatty acids, linoleic acid and alpha-linolenic acid, must also come from the food you eat. Another important function of fat is its role in the transport and absorption of fat-soluble vitamins and carotenoids. Of course, fat can also add a wonderful flavor to our meals and make meals more filling and satisfying.

TABLE 1.5 » PROTEIN CONTENT OF SELECTED FOODS

Food	Serving Size	Protein (g)
White fish, cooked	3 oz. (100 g)	20
Chicken, white, cooked	3 oz. (100 g)	25
Pork, lean, cooked	3 oz. (100 g)	23
Beef, lean, cooked	3 oz. (100 g)	21
Tofu, firm	4 oz. (120 g)	20
Lentils, cooked	1 c. (240 ml)	18
Soy milk	1 c. (240 ml)	10
Milk	8 oz. (240 ml)	8
Peanut butter	2 tbsp. (40 ml)	8
Cheese	1 oz. (30 g)	7

» BEING A VEGETARIAN ATHLETE

In recent years, many nutritionally aware athletes have decreased their intake of specific proteins, such as meats high in saturated fat. Some have gone a step further and replaced animal proteins with plant proteins. Vegetarians are individuals who have consciously made the choice to completely exclude or include only specific animal foods in their diet, such as dairy products, eggs, or fish, and obtain a significant portion of the protein from plant foods. Whether these dietary modifications are for health, environmental, animal rights, or taste-related issues, you need to pay attention to your vegetarian nutrition program to ensure that your diet is adequate in protein, provides specific vitamin and minerals, and is well balanced for your training program.

Vegetarianism is a term that actually incorporates a range of dietary exclusions. A plant-based vegetarian diet may refer to one of the following descriptions:

Semi- or near vegetarians eat small amounts of fish, poultry, eggs, and dairy, and avoid red meat.

Pesco-vegetarians eat fish, dairy, and eggs.

Lacto-ovo-vegetarians eat dairy foods and eggs.

Ovo-vegetarians eat eggs.

Vegans eat no animal foods whatsoever.

Depending on what type of vegetarian diet you follow, you need to carefully choose foods that provide specific nutrients in your diet. These nutrients include protein, of course, but also iron and zinc, and, particularly if you exclude dairy products, vitamin B12, calcium, and vitamin D.

CONTINUED

Throughout this book, the unique considerations of vegetarian athletes will be addressed in regard to specific nutrients. Of course, all athletes, vegetarian or not, can choose to include more plant sources of specific nutrients in their diet, including high-quality plant proteins. Plant foods are filled with health-promoting minerals and other nutrients. Vegetarians appear to have a lower risk of hypertension, certain cancers, and a decreased risk for developing heart disease and diabetes. A plant-based diet also supplies plenty of carbohydrates for replenishing body fuel stores after training. Filling up on whole grains, fruits, and vegetables benefits any winter sport athlete. Milk and yogurt, though sources of high-quality protein, add nice amounts of carbohydrate to your diet as well.

However, athletes training seriously for winter sport should pay close attention to their vegetarian diet. Like a diet containing meat and other animal protein, a vegetarian diet can be well planned and support your training efforts, or it can be overly restrictive and ill conceived and hamper your training efforts.

Much has been made of the quantity of fat consumed in the North American diet. A high-fat content is often characterized by consuming many convenience foods, frequent restaurant meals, and especially fast foods. Fats are a concentrated source of calories, and excess fat beyond your requirement does not provide optimum fuel for your body and can even crowd out valuable carbohydrates and proteins. While consumption of less fat may take planning and knowledge of hidden fats, many North Americans consume too much of the wrong types of fats.

Fat comes in several chemical forms, some of which are healthier than others. Depending on their composition, fats are categorized as saturated or unsaturated. Unsaturated fats include both polyunsaturated and monounsaturated fats. Currently the American Heart Association sets the recommended range of fat intake from 15 to 30 percent of total calories. Exceeding this range may increase the risk of heart disease, while going below this range could result in essential fatty acid insufficiency in some individuals. For winter sport athletes, a diet in which 20 to 30 percent of the calories are supplied from fat should be appropriate. This amount provides adequate fat to replenish fuel stores after training and leaves room for adequate carbohydrate and protein in the diet.

Most important, limit the amount of saturated fat and hydrogenated fat that you consume to 10 percent or less of your total calorie intake in order to prevent heart disease. Saturated fats and the "trans" fat produced from hydrogenation of liquid oils raise the harmful low-density lipoprotein (LDL) cholesterol, and trans fat can also lower the beneficial high-density lipoprotein (HDL) cholesterol. Undesirable saturated fat is found mainly in fatty animal foods such as cheese and whole milk products, fatty cuts of meat, highly processed lunch meats, butter, lard, and shortening. Palm, palm kernel, and coconut oil are three highly saturated plant oils, which can sometimes be found in processed foods and commercially baked goods.

Trans-fatty acids are created from liquid oils that are "partially hydrogenated." Hydrogenation turns liquid corn oil into margarine sticks and increases the shelf life of commercial products that contain these altered oils. Some common sources of trans fat include cookies, crackers, and snack chips. Check labels to limit hydrogenated oils as much as possible, particularly if they are listed as one of the first several ingredients. If you do consume margarine, choose products that list "liquid oil" as the first ingredient.

Unsaturated fat can help lower LDL cholesterol when they replace saturated fat in your diet. Sources of polyunsaturated oil include corn, safflower, sunflower oil, and walnuts and sunflower seeds. These oils should make up no more than one-third of your total fat intake and should be consumed in liquid form. Most health care professionals advocate that monounsaturated fats comprise the majority of your fat intake. Many cultures that consume ample amounts of olive oil seem to have a decreased risk of heart disease, and monounsaturated fat seems to be the fat of choice for other health concerns. Good sources of monounsaturated oils include olive oil, canola oil, avocados, almonds, and hazelnuts. Table 1.6 outlines the types of fats contained in various oils.

Unfortunately what has gotten lost in some of this heart-healthy advice is recommendations regarding the types of polyunsaturated fats that you should emphasize in your diet. Linoleic and alpha-linolenic essential fatty acids are both polyunsaturated fats, but they differ greatly in how they affect our health. Linoleic acid is from a family of fats known as "omega-6" fats; alpha-linolenic is from the "omega-3" family of fats. Two other omega-3 fats, docosahexanoic (DHA) and eicosapentaenoic (EPA) are abundant in fish oils such as salmon and tuna. The body can convert alpha-linolenic acid to DHA and EPA, though the conversion is not the most efficient.

DHA and EPA are of great interest to health experts. Consuming these fats, as well as alpha-linolenic acid, is necessary to produce hormone-like compounds that can reduce unnecessary blood clotting, boost immune function, and reduce inflammation. Conversely, excess linoleic acid can produce hormones that lead to inflammation, promote blood clotting, and constrict arteries. Because linoleic and alpha-linolenic acid compete in the body for use by the body, it is best not to consume an excess of linoleic acid.

Keep in mind that both of these essential fats are good for you. What is desirable is to obtain the proper balance of the two essential fatty acids in your diet. However, most North Americans consume an excess of linoleic fat (omega-6) and need to increase their

TABLE 1.6 » PERCENTAGES OF FAT OF VARIOUS OILS

Oil	Saturated	Polyunsaturated	Monounsaturated
Canola	6	32	62
Hazelnut	7	11	82
Flaxseed	7	75	18
Safflower	7	79	14
Almond	8	19	73
Walnut	9	67	24
Grapeseed	10	73	17
Sunflower	11	69	20
Corn	13	62	25
Olive	14	9	77
Pumpkin seed	15	53	15
Soybean	15	61	24
Sesame	15	44	41
Margarine (tub)*	17	34	24
Wheat germ	17	61	22
Peanut	18	34	48
Rice bran	26	28	46
Cottonseed	27	54	19
Lard	41	12	47
Palm kernel	85	2	11
Coconut	92	2	6

*Also contains some trans-fatty acids. Different brands of margarine contain varying levels of hydrogenated oils. Choose those labeled as trans fat-free.

intake of alpha-linolenic acid (omega-3). Table 1.7 will guide you in choosing food sources of these fats. Try to emphasize fatty fish and use soy and canola oils. Olive oil supplies very little of these essential fats, but it is an excellent source of the healthy monounsaturated fat. Other good sources of alpha-linolenic acid include leafy green vegetables, walnuts, and flaxseed. Several foods are listed under both of these fat sources, as they are rich in both essential fatty acids. While scientists are still formulating specific recommendations, aim for a minimum of 2.0 grams of the alpha-linolenic acid daily.

To emphasize the best fat choices, you can balance your intake in the following way:

• Consume fish such as salmon, light tuna, sole, and tilapia two times weekly or more.

• Emphasize soy and canola oils and related products, and use olive oil as well.

- Have green leafy vegetables, walnuts, and ground flaxseed in your diet.
- Choose the leanest cuts of red meat possible.
- Limit fatty cheeses.
- Emphasize poultry, beans, lentils, and soy protein in your diet.
- Control margarine intake and choose products with liquid oil as the first ingredient.
- Avoid processed foods that contain partially hydrogenated oil and trans fat.

TABLE 1.7 » FOOD SOURCES OF ESSENTIAL FATTY ACIDS

Foods Rich in Alpha-Linolenic Acid

Food	Serving Size	Alpha-Linolenic Acid (g)
Flax oil	1 tbsp. (20 ml)	6.6
Canola oil	1 tbsp. (20 ml)	1.6
Soybean oil	1 tbsp. (20 ml)	1
Walnut oil	1 tbsp. (20 ml)	1.4
Flaxseed, ground	1 tbsp. (20 ml)	1.8
Soy nuts, roasted	½ c. (120 ml)	1.8
Tofu, firm	½ c. (120 ml)	0.7
Soy milk	1 c. (240 ml)	0.4
Legumes	½ c. (120 ml)	0.05
Oat germ	2 tbsp. (40 ml)	0.2
Wheat germ	2 tbsp. (40 ml)	0.1
Sardines	2 oz. (60 g)	0.28
Spinach, cooked	1 c. (240 ml)	0.15
Kale, cooked	1 c. (240 ml)	0.13
Almond butter	2 tbsp. (40 ml)	0.12

Foods Rich in Linoleic Acid

Food	Serving Size	Linoleic Acid (g)
Safflower oil	1 tbsp. (20 ml)	10.1
Sunflower oil	1 tbsp. (20 ml)	9.2
Corn oil	1 tbsp. (20 ml)	7.8
Soybean oil	1 tbsp. (20 ml)	6.9
Walnuts	1 oz. (30 g)	11

CONTINUED

TABLE 1.7 continued

Foods Rich in Linoleic Acid

Food	Serving Size	Linoleic Acid (g)
Soy nuts, roasted	½ c. (120 ml)	9
Brazil nuts	1 oz. (30 g)	7
Pecans	1 oz. (30 g)	6
Tofu, firm	4 oz. (120 g)	5.4
Peanuts	1 oz. (30 g)	4.5
Peanut butter	2 tbsp. (40 ml)	4.4
Almonds	1 oz. (30 g)	3
Almond butter	2 tbsp. (40 ml)	3.8
Wheat germ	2 tbsp. (40 ml)	0.8
Flaxseed, ground	1 tbsp. (20 ml)	0.5

Alcohol: The Nonnutritive Nutrient

Alcohol may very well play a moderate role in your current lifestyle if you are of legal age to drink. But it is important for an athlete to use alcohol sensibly, because it does not play any important role in your recovery and could have detrimental effects on your performance. Obviously alcohol abuse can affect your health and that of others by contributing to liver cirrhosis and irresponsible and drunk driving. Alcohol is also a widely abused drug in North America, with a significant number of problem drinkers or abusers. Of course, alcohol should never be consumed during pregnancy. Let's take a look at the implications of alcohol in regard specifically to your training diet and athletic performance.

While alcohol is a drug, it provides calories just as foods do and makes for fairly caloric beverages. As far as your body is concerned, alcohol is merely a bunch of empty calories as these calories are not used for energy in the same way as carbohydrates, proteins, and fats. Beer and wine contain only small amounts of carbohydrates and only trace amounts of protein, vitamins, and minerals. In fact, alcohol can interfere with how your body uses vitamins and minerals. One-half ounce of pure ethanol is the equivalent of one drink that equals 12 ounces (240 milliliters) of beer (150 calories), 4 ounces (120 milliliters) of wine (100 calories), and 1.25 ounces (38 milliliters) of liquor (100 calories).

Despite originating from fermented carbohydrates, alcohol is metabolized in your body as fat. Alcohol by-products are converted into fatty acids, which are stored in your liver

» CONSUMING FISH OILS SAFELY

Fish is good for you because it is a great source of omega-3 fatty acids, which can reduce disease risk and enhance health. But when you consume fish, it would be appropriate to take into consideration choices that will reduce your mercury intake. Mercury is present in our air and water, and when converted to methyl-mercury, it can accumulate in fish and humans. Methyl-mercury is a known toxin to developing fetuses, babies, and children, and it is now considered a potential threat to adults as well. Mercury can damage the brain and nervous system, and cause symptoms such as fatigue and hair loss.

The health benefits of eating fish do outweigh these risks, if you make good choices regarding the type and amount of fish consumed. Currently the American Heart Association recommends eating fish twice weekly. Generally you can keep your total fish portions to about 12 ounces weekly, though mercury's effects are somewhat dose related based on body weight.

Next, try to choose fish lower in mercury. Fish highest in mercury include shark, swordfish, king mackerel, and tilefish. Other high-mercury fish are fresh tuna, red snapper, orange roughy, and marlin. Some of the fish lower in mercury include shrimp, salmon, pollack, catfish, tilapia, sardines, and sole. Canned white albacore tuna contains more mercury than canned light tuna and should be limited. Tuna lovers can switch to the light tuna. Other fish fairly low in mercury include haddock, herring, and whitefish.

Many salmon lovers are also concerned about the cancer-causing polychlorinated biphenyl (PCBs) in fish. Testing indicates that both farmed and wild salmon are contaminated with PCBs, with the farmed varieties containing much higher amounts. Farmed varieties from both the United States and Canada contain lower amounts of PCBs than those from European countries, but all levels were much higher than wild varieties. When in season, wild Alaska salmon, which is lowest in PCBs, is the best choice. You can also choose canned salmon, which comes almost exclusively from the wild Alaskan variety. Since September 2004, all seafood has been labeled as farmed or wild, and with the country of origin, which should assist you in making decisions around fish choices.

and sent to your bloodstream. Obviously alcohol is not the best nutrient choice if your goal is to be a lean athlete. Much has been made of alcohol's protective effects against heart disease. But while moderate amounts may raise the desirable and protective HDL cholesterol, too much alcohol may actually increase your risk of heart disease. Too much alcohol can raise your blood pressure and raise the harmful blood fats called triglycerides, which, when combined with a low amount of HDL cholesterol, makes for a health profile associated with an increased risk of heart disease. Consumed in excess over a long period, alcohol may not only elevate blood pressure but also increase the risk of stroke and certain cancers, and of course result in liver damage.

Too much alcohol too soon after training and competition can impede recovery. Though you may rehydrate well after training, alcohol is a diuretic that causes your body to lose more fluid than it takes in. That's why you need to replace losses even after drinking moderate amounts of alcohol. Alcohol may also interfere with glycogen synthesis. Athletes with soft-tissue damage or bruising may also want to consider that alcohol is a blood vessel dilator. Consuming alcohol after exercise may aggravate swelling or bleeding and impair healing. These types of injuries are usually treated with ice, which is designed to constrict blood flow to the injured parts.

Excessive alcohol consumed the night before or alcohol consumed shortly before training can impair fine-motor ability and coordination, increase risk of dehydration, and impair fuel stores. Reaction times are delayed, as your brain's ability to process information is impaired. Know your limits and how they change with your training and fitness level.

Keep in mind, too, that how fast you metabolize alcohol varies with body size. Average-sized men metabolize slightly less than one drink per hour, while smaller men and women take longer to metabolize this amount.

Underage drinking is also a problem for today's teenager and may adversely affect the high school and college athlete participating in winter sports. Besides the obvious short-term risks involved, parents should emphasize that there are long-term health risks involved with alcohol consumption, such as liver damage and certain types of cancers. But they should also understand that there are clear adverse performance effects with alcohol consumption and a subsequent hangover. Alcohol will disrupt fluid balance and temperature regulation, affect fine-motor skills, and can cause athletes to have a subpar practice or competition. Alcohol should never be consumed in the middle of a winter sport day, such as a return to the slopes and snow in the afternoon, as this behavior could place you and others at risk.

Alcohol can be a small part of a healthy sport diet for adults, but drink in sensible amounts. Have a large glass of water with each drink. Consider that your top priority as an athlete is recovery. Too much alcohol can compromise how effectively you do recover.

NUTRIENTS FOR OPTIMAL WINTER TRAINING

As an athlete, you are understandably interested in consuming an optimal amount of vitamins and minerals in your diet for both maximum performance and good health. You may find yourself questioning just how your training program may alter or increase your requirements of these important nutrients. And, as an athlete, you have a highly vested interest in keeping your immune system healthy so that illness does not put a halt to training, especially during the winter. While athletes have long been advised by sports nutritionists to consume high-quality foods for an optimal nutrient intake, advertising that targets active individuals would suggest they require a daily vitamin and mineral supplement.

Why Vitamins and Minerals Matter

Of course, choosing foods that provide you with adequate amounts of vitamins and minerals is necessary for optimal performance. Correcting any dietary inadequacies could even improve your performance. Depending on your health status, typical dietary intake, and specific nutrient needs, you may need to supplement your diet in an educated fashion. Certain groups of athletes might benefit from nutrient supplementation beyond the basic assurance of a daily multivitamin mineral supplement. However, research has not conclusively proven that taking "extra" amounts of vitamins and minerals when no deficiency is present will enable you to train harder and longer.

Balanced Eating

While all vitamins and minerals are important, winter sport athletes should be aware of nutrients that are especially important to an athlete. As Table 1.8 indicates, balanced eating clearly provides variety and ample amounts of vitamins, minerals, phytochemicals, and quality carbohydrates, particularly in view of an athlete's higher energy needs for training. You should also keep in mind that nutrients exist together in foods in the proper balance.

Vitamin Basics

Vitamins consist of thirteen organic compounds found in small amounts in most foods. They play important roles in many physiological processes, many of which are greatly enhanced during exercise. Therefore, it is wise to ensure that you have high levels of body reserves of these nutrients in order for these body processes to function optimally. Although it is true that inadequate intake of vitamins may result in deficiencies, whether or not it will adversely impact your performance depends on the extent of that deficiency. Extreme deficiencies are not very commonplace in North America, and many dietary inadequacies can be corrected by making the proper food choices.

Athletes most likely to have problems with an inadequate vitamin intake are those following a restricted calorie diet for weight loss, athletes who have adopted an extreme or fad diet, and perhaps those on a very restrictive vegetarian diet. Overall, however, athletes training and competing in team sports can greatly minimize their risk of vitamin deficiency by consuming a wide variety of nutrient-dense foods and adequate calories to match their training needs.

TABLE 1.8 » BALANCE OF FOODS FOR ATHLETES

Food Group	Serving Size	Number of Servings	Nutrients
Fruits	1 c. fruit (240 ml) 1 medium piece	3 daily	Carotenoids, Vitamin A, Vitamin C, Phytonutrients
Vegetables	1 c. cooked (240 ml) 2 c. raw (480 ml)	2-3 daily	Carotenoids, Vitamin A, Vitamin C, Phytonutrients, Calcium
Dairy milk, yogurt, fortified soy milk	8 oz. milk (240 ml) 6-8 oz. yogurt (200-240 ml)	2-3 daily	Calcium, Riboflavin, Vitamin A, Vitamin D
Poultry, fish, lean red meat	3-4 oz. (100-120 g)	2-4 daily	Thiamin, Niacin, Iron, Zinc
Whole grains and starch	2 oz. bread (60 g) 1½ c. cereal (360 ml) 1 c. cooked (240 ml)	6-12 daily	Thiamin, Niacin, Iron, Riboflavin
Fats and oils	1 t. to 1 tbsp. (7-20 ml)	4-6 daily	Vitamin A, Vitamin D, Vitamin E

Vitamins play a major role in catalyzing energy production reactions from body fuel stores. For instance, a number of B vitamins are essential to converting carbohydrate into energy for muscular contraction. Vitamins themselves do not directly provide energy, which must be obtained from consuming carbohydrates, protein, and fat. The vitamins B12, B6, and folic acid play an important role in the development of red blood cells that deliver oxygen to the exercising muscles. Vitamins are also involved in tissue repair and protein synthesis. Several vitamins such as E and C are antioxidants that protect cells from potentially toxic free radicals. *Free radicals* are unstable molecules produced by oxygen-related reactions in the body and have been implicated in contributing to a number of diseases. Each vitamin is unique in the functions it performs in the body and in how it interacts with other dietary nutrients.

Vitamins are separated into two classifications: fat-soluble and water-soluble. Your body may contain large stores of the fat-soluble variety—A, D, E, and K. Deficiencies of these nutrients are rare, though excessive intakes may have toxic effects. The water-soluble variety—which include vitamin C and the eight B vitamins, thiamin (B1), riboflavin (B2), pyridoxine (B6), niacin, B12, folacin, biotin, and pantothenic acid—are not stored in

» OPTIMAL HEALTH AND DIETARY REFERENCE INTAKES

The Dietary Reference Intakes (DRIs), developed by the Food and Nutrition Board of the National Academy of Sciences in the 1990s, are designed to reflect the health goals of the twenty-first century. Rather than merely preventing nutrient deficiencies, these latest guidelines for nutrient intakes were set with the goal of optimizing health by reducing risk of chronic diseases such as heart disease, cancer, and osteoporosis.

Each nutrient is assigned a number of terms under the umbrella heading of DRI. The DRI include the four following classifications:

Recommended Daily Allowance (RDA).

The RDA is the amount of a nutrient that should decrease the risk of chronic disease for most healthy individuals in a specified age group and gender. It is based on estimating the average requirement plus an increase to account for individual variation. It is to serve as a goal for individuals only.

The RDA is a good starting point for athletes to determine the nutritional adequacy of their diet. Athletes of all ages are likely to have energy requirements higher than the average person, and some vitamins and minerals are required to process this energy. Athletes may also have a higher nutrient intake than the average person, simply because of their high energy needs and quality food choices.

Adequate Intake (AI).

The AI is used when there is not enough scientific evidence to set an RDA. It is a recommended daily intake based on observed or experimentally determined approximations of nutrient intake by a group of healthy people. The AI can be used as a goal for individual intake when an RDA does not exist.

Estimated Average Requirement (EAR).

The EAR is the nutrient value estimated to meet the requirements of half the healthy individuals in a group. The EAR represents the average nutrient intake required to maintain a specific body function. For example, the EAR for vitamin C is set at a level that prevents scurvy, a deficiency disease. The EAR is used to develop the RDA, assess adequacy of intakes, and plan diets for population groups.

Tolerable Upper Intake Level (UL).

The UL is the highest level of a daily nutrient intake recommended, from both food and supplements, which should not be exceeded, or individuals may experience adverse or toxic health effects. This is not a recommended amount but rather an upper limit. For most nutrients, the UL refers to the total amount obtained from your food intake, fortified foods, and supplements. This number may be of interest to athletes who consume a number of such fortified foods, take various vitamin and mineral supplements, and frequently use sports nutrition products that are supplemented with nutrients as well.

your body in significant amounts. Harmful effects of excessive intakes of these water-soluble vitamins are not as likely, though there are exceptions. Appendix B provides a list of vitamins, their functions, DRIs, and food sources.

Important Vitamins
B Vitamins

Because of their role in processing energy from the metabolism of carbohydrate, B vitamins have received much attention from athletes. However, several of these vitamins are easily obtained from a variety of carbohydrate-rich foods such as breads and whole grains, and other foods that are found in relatively high amounts in the high-energy athlete's diet. Often intake of nutrients easily exceeds the RDAs when an athlete consumes the calories required for training and competing.

Thiamin and Riboflavin

Thiamin, or vitamin B1, is present in a wide variety of food sources besides whole grains, including nuts, dried peas and beans, and pork. It plays an important role in deriving energy from carbohydrates. A thiamin deficiency is unlikely to occur in athletes. Many athletes with high energy needs likely consume thiamin above the current RDA of 1.2 milligrams daily.

Riboflavin is also involved in energy production from carbohydrates, proteins, and fat. Vegetarians should pay attention to their riboflavin intake, as milk, meat, and eggs are good sources. Some plant sources include brewer's yeast, wheat germ, soybeans, avocados, green leafy vegetables, and enriched bread and cereals. Training for your sport may slightly increase your riboflavin requirements, but the higher amounts are easily met in a well-balanced diet.

Pyridoxine and Niacin

Pyridoxine, or vitamin B6, is found mainly in whole-grain cereals, brown rice, wheat germ, bananas, legumes, fish, and poultry. This vitamin is closely linked to protein metabolism, the manufacture of muscle and hemoglobin, and in the breakdown of muscle glycogen. Athletes who consume adequate calories should get plenty of vitamin B6 in their diets. Though most water-soluble vitamins are easily excreted, excess supplementation of B6 can present a problem. Doses of more than 1 gram daily over several months may cause numbness and even paralysis. Symptoms have also been experienced with chronic doses as low as 200 milligrams.

Niacin is involved not only in carbohydrate, protein, and fat metabolism but also in glycogen synthesis and cellular metabolism. Good food sources of niacin are meat, whole or enriched grains, nuts, seeds, and dried beans. Because it is in such a wide variety of foods, it is relatively easy to obtain enough niacin in your diet. In fact, excess niacin from over-supplementation can block the release of free fatty acids, resulting in greater use of muscle glycogen and thereby depleting a limited energy source for exercise. Large doses may actually reduce performance.

Vitamin B12

Vitamin B12 plays a major role in red blood cell development among other important functions. Vegetarian athletes who are strict vegans should pay close attention to their B12 intake.

Your vitamin B12 needs are easily met by consuming animal foods. So if you consume eggs and dairy foods, your intake should be fine. But the only plant foods that can be counted on for their B12 content are those that have been fortified with this vitamin, such as soy milk, soy burgers, and some breakfast cereals. Plant proteins such as tempeh and miso may not contain the active form of vitamin B12. The human intestinal tract does make some vitamin B12, but this form is generally not well absorbed.

While requirements of this vitamin are relatively low, deficiencies can have serious implications and even lead to irreversible nerve damage. Vegans who do not regularly consume fortified foods should take a vitamin B12 supplement.

Folacin

Folacin is a B vitamin that has deservedly received much increased attention from health professionals over the past several years. *Folacin* is the collective term for folate, folic acid, and other forms of the vitamin. Folate is the form found naturally in foods, and folic acid is the form of the vitamin found most often in your body and added to foods and supplements. Folic acid is actually absorbed twice as well as the folate that occurs naturally in foods.

Since January 1998, manufacturers were required to add folic acid to all enriched products including flour, bread, rolls, grits, cornmeal, rice, pasta, and noodles. There is good reason for this fortification. Obtaining enough folic acid in the early weeks of pregnancy can significantly reduce the risk of neural tube defects such as spina bifida in newborns. Prior to fortification, most Americans consumed only about 200 micrograms of folic acid daily, falling short of the recommended 400 micrograms. Fortification will prevent a significant number of all neural tube defects.

But this fortification may not only benefit pregnant women and newborns. Evidence is building that folic acid may reduce the risk of heart disease, stroke, and certain cancers. Folic acid helps reduce blood levels of the amino acid homocysteine. High levels of homocysteine appear to be a strong predictor for heart disease and stroke. Keeping homocysteine low also requires adequate intake of the vitamins B6 and B12. Thirty percent of all older Americans don't produce enough stomach acid to absorb the B12 found in foods. Synthetic B12, however, doesn't have this stomach acid dependency. Connections between folic acid and the prevention of cervical cancer and colorectal cancer, through prevention of damage to DNA, have also been suggested.

Many researchers suggest that individuals over the age of 50 take a supplement providing the RDA (high doses are not advised) of folic acid, B12, and B6. Older individuals are also more likely to take medications that interfere with folic acid absorption.

Of course, every active individual should increase the intake of folate-rich foods because of folate's relationship to maintaining red blood cells (see Table 1.9). Folate is easily destroyed by long storage times and common cooking techniques. Try to obtain folate from fresh foods.

Vitamin C

Another water-soluble vitamin of interest to and heavily marketed to athletes is vitamin C. Several important functions of this vitamin impact athletes. It is necessary for the formation of connective tissue and scar tissue, and certain hormones and neurotransmitters that are secreted during exercise. Vitamin C plays a role in iron absorption and in the formation of red blood cells. This vitamin is also strongly promoted because of its role as a powerful antioxidant. Symptoms of vitamin C deficiency could impair athletic performance.

Despite being a water-soluble vitamin that is easily excreted, the human body actually has a pool of vitamin C ranging from 1.5 to 3.0 grams. Serious vitamin C deficiencies are rare because fresh or frozen fruits and vegetables are so abundant in our food supply. Though vitamin C is readily available from food, athletes often consume vitamin C supplements. Correcting a deficiency clearly improves performance, but research does not demonstrate that vitamin C supplements enhance performance when a vitamin C deficiency is not present.

On the other hand, because exercise places stress on the body, moderate amounts of vitamin C, above the RDA of 75 to 90 milligrams, may be appropriate for athletes. Some scientists have recommended 200 to 300 milligrams daily, which can be obtained from a diet abundant in fruits and vegetables. Research indicates that 200 milligrams daily of vitamin C leads to full saturation of plasma and white blood cells, which supports optimal immune function. Vitamin C supplements may also reduce the symptoms and duration of upper respiratory tract infections often seen after strenuous physical efforts. Vitamin C also plays an important part in the healing process when there is injury or muscle soreness. However, most studies have not found vitamin C supplementation to prevent the common cold.

TABLE 1.9 » FOLATE CONTENT OF FOODS

Food	Serving size	Folate (micrograms)
Lentils, cooked	1 c. (240 ml)	358
Yeast, brewer's	1 tbsp. (20 ml)	312
Liver, beef	3 oz. (100 g)	285
Garbanzo beans, cooked	1 c. (240 ml)	282
Kidney beans, cooked	1 c. (240 ml)	229
Turnip greens, cooked	1 c. (240 ml)	171
Asparagus, boiled	6 spears	131
Beans, white, baked	1 c. (240 ml)	122
Orange juice	1 c. (240 ml)	110
Spinach, raw, chopped	1 c. (240 ml)	108
Mustard greens, cooked	1 c. (240 ml)	103
Broccoli, cooked	1 c. (240 ml)	78
Romaine lettuce	1 c. (240 ml)	76
Endive	1 c. (240 ml)	72
Wheat germ, raw	¼ c. (60 ml)	70

A diet rich in fruits and vegetables provides ample amounts of vitamin C (see Table 1.10) and other healthful substances found in those foods. Avoid excessive intakes of vitamin C supplements reaching 1,000 to 3,000 milligrams daily, which can cause side effects such as diarrhea and kidney stones.

Vitamin E

Vitamin E receives much attention from athletes because of its major role as an antioxidant. It prevents the oxidation of unsaturated fatty acids in cell membranes and protects the cell from damage. Vitamin E is widely distributed in foods and stored in the body, so vitamin E deficiencies are rare. The current RDI is 22 International Units (IU). Polyunsaturated oils such as soybean, corn, and safflower are the most common sources of vitamin E. Other good sources are fortified grain products and wheat germ (see Table 1.11).

Experiments on vitamin E supplementation at altitude have produced some interesting results, but more research is required, especially to determine whether any real performance benefits are possible. Vitamin E may also be beneficial to athletes training in high-pollution areas due to its antioxidant effects. Though no performance benefits have been established, vitamin E supplements may be recommended for possible prevention of chronic diseases, especially heart disease. Some researchers currently feel that a daily supplement dose of 100 to 200 IU is safe and appropriate, though more research on the highest safety dose is required. People with a bleeding disorder or on anticoagulant medication or statin medications designed to lower elevated blood lipids should be cautious and first check with their physician before taking vitamin E. If you do take a vitamin E supplement, choose one that provides the natural source of the vitamin.

TABLE 1.10 » VITAMIN C CONTENT OF FOOD

Food	Serving Size	Vitamin C (mg)
Pepper, green	1 large	130
Orange juice	1 c. (240 ml)	124
Cranberry juice	1 c. (240 ml)	108
Grapefruit juice	1 c. (240 ml)	94
Broccoli, cooked	⅔ c. (200 ml)	90
Brussels sprouts, cooked	7	85
Strawberries, raw	1 c. (240 ml)	85
Orange, navel	1	80
Kiwi	1 medium	75
Cantaloupe, pieces	1 c. (240 ml)	70
Cauliflower, cooked	1 c. (240 ml)	65

TABLE 1.11 » VITAMIN E CONTENT OF FOODS

Food	Serving Size	Vitamin E (IU)
Wheat germ oil	1 tbsp. (20 ml)	25
Sunflower seeds	1 oz. (30 g)	21
Almonds	1 oz. (30 g)	11
Sunflower oil	1 tbsp. (20 ml)	10
Wheat germ	1 oz. (30 g)	5
Margarine, soft	1 tbsp. (20 ml)	3
Mayonnaise	1 tbsp. (20 ml)	3
Brown rice	1 c. (240 ml)	3
Mango	1 medium	3
Asparagus	4 spears	2

Other Important Food Components
Carotenoids

Beta-carotene is one of six hundred carotenoid pigments that give fruits and vegetables their yellow, orange, and red colors. Carotenoids are also abundant in green vegetables. While carotenoids are not vitamins, many act as antioxidants and also protect cells from free radicals.

Carotenoids most commonly found in blood and tissues are alpha-carotene, beta-carotene, beta-cryptoxanthin, lycopene, lutein, and zeaxanthin. Only alpha-carotene, beta-carotene, and beta-cryptoxanthin can be converted to vitamin A in the body. Research is just beginning to determine how specific carotenoids can boost immunity and protect the heart and eyes from chronic disease.

To obtain a variety of carotenoids in your diet, aim for at least five servings combined of fruits and vegetables daily, focusing mainly on yellow-orange, red, or dark green choices. You can easily obtain ample amounts in your diet.

Taking a supplement with carotenoids requires some caution, particularly in the case of beta-carotene supplements, which were found to increase cancer in smokers. If you do supplement, stay under 3 milligrams daily. You should also keep in mind that carotenoids interact with one another. Supplementing with one carotenoid may impair the absorption of others. Carotenoids are converted to vitamin A as the body requires. But vitamin A supplements can be highly toxic at greater than the daily RDA of 5,000 IU. Besides, foods high in carotenoids may provide health-promoting substances not found in supplements. It's quite possible that these protective nutrients work best when they are packaged together, as in food.

Phytochemicals

While vitamin A can be formed from some carotenoids, this group of nutrients is actually one of many that fall under the broader classification of phytochemicals. Many important disease-fighting properties have been attributed to these plant chemicals. Unlike vitamins and minerals, phytochemicals are not nutrients. Most phytochemicals are found in carbohydrate-containing foods such as fruits, vegetables, and grains. Some phytochemicals you may have heard about include allylic sulfides found in garlic, flavonoids found in citrus fruits, genistein found in soybeans, indoles in broccoli and cauliflower, and phytoestrogens in soy products, to name a few.

To take advantage of these phytochemicals, eat plenty of fruits and vegetables, dried peas and beans, and soy products. In the future, probably even more phytochemicals will be discovered.

» SUPER SOURCES OF CAROTENOIDS

Apricot halves, 6 dried

Broccoli, ½ cup cooked
(120 milliliters)

Cantaloupe, 1 cup chunks
(240 milliliters)

Carrot, 1 medium raw

Collard greens, ½ cup cooked
(120 milliliters)

Grapefruit, ½ medium

Kale, ½ cup cooked
(120 milliliters)

Mango, 1 medium

Mustard greens, ½ cup cooked
(120 milliliters)

Orange, 1 medium

Papaya, ½ medium

Pepper, red, ½ raw

Pumpkin, ½ cup cooked or canned
(120 milliliters)

Spinach, ½ cup raw
(120 milliliters)

Sweet potato, ½ cup mashed
(120 milliliters)

Tangerine, 1 medium

Tomato sauce, ½ cup (120 milliliters)

Mineral Basics

Like vitamins, minerals are involved in energy metabolism and also play important roles in building body tissue, forming the base of the strength and structure of the skeleton, contracting muscles, transporting oxygen, maintaining acid-base balance of the blood, and regulating normal heart rhythm—all important for top athletic performance. Weak bones can contribute to development of stress fractures, and acid-base imbalance affects endurance and energy metabolism, so that fuel is not utilized as efficiently during training. Minerals are involved in the metabolism of carbohydrates, proteins, and fats and in obtaining energy from an important fuel source, phosphocreatine.

There are two classes of minerals, both important to optimal body functioning. The macrominerals are present in relatively large amounts in the body and include calcium, phosphorus, and magnesium. Trace or microminerals include iron, zinc, chromium, copper, and selenium. Altogether there are twenty-five essential minerals, all with their own unique functions.

Minerals are obtained in our diet from the water we drink and from both plant and animal foods. Training-induced mineral losses can occur through urine, sweat, and gastrointestinal losses.

Important Minerals

Two very important minerals to the athlete are calcium, because of its essential role in maintaining healthy bone structure, and iron, which plays a crucial role in oxygen transport. Sodium is also an important mineral because of potential sweat losses.

Calcium. This is the most abundant mineral in the body. Ninety-eight percent of calcium is found in bone, a dynamic tissue that is constantly being broken down and rebuilt. The remaining 2 percent of calcium in your body is in your teeth and circulates in your bloodstream.

This circulating calcium has a significant effect on metabolism and physiological functions. It is involved in all types of muscle contraction, including the heart muscle, skeletal muscle, and smooth muscle found in blood vessels. By activating a number of enzymes, calcium also plays a role in both the synthesis and breakdown of muscle and liver glycogen. It is also involved in nerve impulse transmission, blood clotting, and secretion of hormones. These physiological functions of calcium take precedence over formation of bone tissue. If the diet is low in calcium, it can be pulled from the bone for these functions.

Calcium deficiency can develop from inadequate intake or increased calcium excretion. Strenuous exercise increases sweat loss of calcium. One of the major health concerns associated with inadequate intake of calcium is osteoporosis, a disorder in which bone mass decreases and susceptibility to fracture increases. Optimal bone building takes place until age 25, but you can continue to build some bone until 35 years of age. After this age, your efforts should focus on maintaining your current level of bone mass.

Hormonal status, more specifically estrogen loss, also contributes significantly to the development of osteoporosis, making women more susceptible to this disease after menopause occurs, though men can also develop osteoporosis. Hormonal status in younger female athletes also plays an important role in bone health. Extra calcium is recommended for female athletes with absent or irregular menstruation and for post-menopausal athletes. Weight-bearing exercise such as running and weight training enhances calcium skeletal absorption, increases bone mass, and can help prevent bone loss at any age. Calcium recommendations for various ages are provided in Table 1.12.

Dairy products are very concentrated sources of calcium and for most individuals provide about three-fourths of their total calcium intake. Athletes who do not have a high intake of dairy products and vegan athletes need to focus on alternative plant sources of calcium intake and increase their intake of calcium fortified foods. Try to choose low-fat options as much as possible. Some good plant sources of calcium include dark leafy greens, broccoli, bok choy, dried beans, and dried figs (see Table 1.13). Some good fortified sources (check labels) are soy and rice milk, orange juice, cereals, tofu processed with calcium

TABLE 1.12 » CALCIUM AND VITAMIN D NEEDS		
Age	**Calcium (mg)**	**Vitamin D (IU)**
19–50 years	1,000	200
51–70 years	1,200 (on hormone replacement therapy) 1,500 (not on HRT)	400
> 70 years	1,200 (on HRT) 1,500 (not on HRT)	600

sulfate, and various energy bars. Look for products marked as "high" or "rich in" or an "excellent" source of calcium. They contain more than 200 milligrams per serving.

Individuals who are lactose-intolerant can buy specially formulated lactose-free milk, or take lactase supplement enzymes before consuming milk products. Yogurt and cheese have lower lactose levels than milk and may be well tolerated. You may also be able to tolerate small amounts of lactose-containing foods.

A well-balanced training diet should provide many of the essential nutrients needed to build and maintain healthy bones; however, a calcium supplement may also be indicated if your food intake is not adequate. If you do take a calcium supplement, find one that provides more than 500 milligrams per pill, and take one pill at a time. Amounts greater than 500 to 600 milligrams will not be fully absorbed. Calcium carbonate should be taken with meals to increase absorption, while the calcium citrate form can be taken at any time. Avoid calcium made from oyster shells, bonemeal, or dolomite as it may contain lead.

Vitamin D recommendations are also provided in Table 1.12, because this vitamin is essential for adequate calcium absorption. When there is inadequate vitamin D, we absorb only 10 to 15 percent of the calcium that we consume, compared to the typical 30 percent. Calcium and vitamin D also work together to prevent colon cancer in some high-risk individuals, and vitamin D may also help prevent prostate cancer. Vitamin D seems to play a role in the prevention of autoimmune diseases such as type I diabetes, rheumatoid arthritis, and multiple sclerosis. As we age, our bodies become less efficient at converting sunlight to vitamin D.

Good food sources of vitamin D are relatively limited. They include fatty fish, such as cod, mackerel, salmon, and sardines, and egg yolks. Fortified sources include milk, soy milk, butter, margarine, and many cereals. Some athletes may spend a considerable

TABLE 1.13 » FOOD SOURCES OF CALCIUM

Great Sources (300-mg serving)	Good Sources (200-mg serving)	Fair Sources (100-mg serving)
1% milk, 8 oz. (240 ml)	Cheddar cheese, 1 oz. (30 g)	Skim milk, dry, 1 tbsp. (20 ml)
Skim milk, 8 oz. (240 ml)	Brick cheese, 1 oz. (30 g)	Cottage cheese, 1%, 1 c. (240 ml)
Yogurt, 6 to 8 oz. (200-240 ml)	Colby cheese, 1 oz. (30 g)	Parmesan, grated, 1½ tbsp. (30 ml)
Swiss cheese, 1 oz. (30 g)	Edam cheese, 1 oz. (30 g)	Frozen yogurt, ½ c. (120 ml)
Mackerel, canned, 3 oz. (100 g)	Mozzarella cheese, 1 oz. (30 g)	Pudding, ½ c. (120 ml)
Sardines, canned, w/bones, 3 oz. (100 g)	Instant breakfast, 1 packet	Shrimp, cooked, 6 oz. (200 g)
Salmon, canned, w/bones, 3 oz. (100 g)	Broccoli, cooked, 1 c. (240 ml)	Lobster, cooked, 6 oz. (200 g)
Rhubarb, cooked, 1 c. (240 ml)	Kale, cooked, 1 c. (240 ml)	Tofu, ½ c. (120 ml)
Collard greens, cooked, 1 c. (240 ml)	Turnip greens, cooked, 1 c. (240 ml)	Navy beans, cooked, 1 c. (240 ml)
Blackstrap molasses, 2 tbsp. (40 ml)	Mustard greens, cooked, 1 c. (240 ml)	Pinto beans, 1 c. (240 ml)
Orange juice, calcium fortified, 1 c. (240 ml)	Bok choy, fresh, 1 c. (240 ml)	Orange, 1 large
	Sesame seeds, 2 tbsp. (40 ml)	Tempeh, cooked, 1 c. (240 ml)
	Soybeans, cooked, 1 c. (240 ml)	Swiss chard, cooked, 1 c. (240 ml)
		Figs, dried or fresh, 5 medium

amount of time outdoors during certain times of the year, and your bodies can make enough vitamin D when your skin is exposed to sunlight. However, sun exposure may not be adequate from October to April in the northern parts of the United States and in Canada. If you spend a considerable amount of time in direct sunlight when participating in your winter training, you could make adequate vitamin D from sunlight. Sunscreen may block some vitamin D production, however. If you tan when outdoors, you should be making sufficient amounts of vitamin D in your skin. But because our ability to make vitamin D from sunlight also decreases as we age, older athletes and individuals with limited sun exposure living in northern climates, as well as vegetarians, may want to consider taking a vitamin D supplement. Vitamin D is often conveniently combined with calcium in supplement form and can also be obtained from a multivitamin.

Other nutrients besides vitamin D that are also an important part of building healthy bones:

- Vitamin C—Plays a role in collagen production that helps hold bone together. A diet with plenty of fresh fruits and vegetables provides ample amounts.
- Vitamin K—Activates osteocalcin, which is needed for optimal bone strength. Good sources are dark, leafy green vegetables.
- Magnesium—Another important mineral for bone formation. Good sources are almonds, bananas, avocados, dried beans, lentils, nuts, tofu, wheat germ, and whole grains.

In contrast, some dietary factors are actually harmful to calcium absorption. Excess sodium, protein, and caffeine, for example, increase calcium excretion. Alcohol can also be damaging to bone cells. Try not to consume excessive sources of caffeine. Excessive intakes of phosphorus—namely, from carbonated beverages—should also be limited, because too much of this mineral can upset calcium balance in the body. Keep your protein intake at an appropriate level for training, but do not consume excessive and unneeded amounts from supplements.

Obtaining adequate calcium in your diet takes planning. Here are some tips for maximizing your calcium intake:

- Have a breakfast every day that includes high-calcium milk, yogurt, or calcium-fortified soy product.
- Plan a high-calcium food into three meals or snacks daily.
- Prepare or order low-fat milk and soy milk smoothies whenever possible.
- Make some great stir-fried vegetables for dinners that include one of the following: bok choy, kale, broccoli, and leafy greens.
- Add reduced-fat cheeses to sandwiches.
- Drink a glass of calcium-fortified orange juice on a regular basis.
- Buy tofu high in calcium for stir-fries and other recipes.

Iron. Many athletes are aware of the important role that iron plays in exercise metabolism. Hemoglobin transports oxygen in the blood, and myoglobin transports oxygen in the muscle. Both of these oxygen-carrying molecules require iron for optimal formation. Many muscle enzymes involved in metabolism require iron. Other iron compounds facilitate oxygen use at the cellular level. It makes sense, then, that poor iron status could impair these functions and exercise performance.

The body storage form of iron, ferritin, is used as an indicator of iron stores, as are transferrin and hemoglobin. About 70 percent of the iron in your body is involved in oxygen transport, while the other 30 percent is stored in the body. This has been demonstrated when an athlete has iron deficiency that has progressed to anemia. Anemia causes fatigue and intolerance to exercise.

Iron deficiency is the most common nutrient deficiency in the United States. It is estimated that 22 to 25 percent of female athletes are iron-deficient, with 6 percent having full-blown anemia. When iron stores are low, total hemoglobin drops, and the muscles do not receive as much oxygen. Normal hemoglobin levels for males are 14 to 16 grams per deciliter, with anemia classified as less than 13. The normal range for women is 12 to 14 grams deciliter, with anemia diagnosed at less than 12 grams per deciliter. Blood work can be interpreted to determine whether you have early iron deficiency or full iron deficiency anemia. However, remember that endurance training can affect your blood measurements of iron. Training produces an increased blood volume, which dilutes hemoglobin, making it appear low in some athletes when iron stores are adequate. This increased blood volume often occurs at the start of a training program and has no harmful effect on performance. In fact, this increased blood volume means that your heart can pump more blood to your working muscles, enhancing oxygen delivery.

Data clearly indicate that true iron deficiency anemia will impair exercise performance. Although we have less information regarding the performance effects of a low ferritin level, athletes may experience symptoms of fatigue and poor recovery with this condition. Of course, it makes sense to treat low ferritin levels so that full-blown iron deficiency anemia does not develop and to improve any reoccurring symptoms. Your blood work should be monitored by a physician and treated as appropriate.

Inadequate dietary intake of iron is the most common cause of iron deficiency or anemia. Women with heavy menstrual blood loss may also experience iron deficiency. Strenuous exercise can also increase iron sweat loss, precipitate gastrointestinal bleeding, and decrease iron absorption. Heavy training may also accelerate red blood cell destruction from mechanical trauma, such as during running. Training at altitude can also place you at risk for developing iron deficiency. Development of iron deficiency is also associated with low-calorie diets, vegetarian diets, very high-carbohydrate diets containing only small amounts of animal protein, and various fad and unbalanced diets.

Iron is obtained from food in two forms. Heme iron is found in animal foods—good sources are lean meat and dark poultry (see Table 1.14). About 10 to 30 percent of heme iron is absorbed from the intestines. Nonheme iron is found in plant foods—dried peas and beans, whole grain products, apricots, and raisins are good sources. About 2 to 10 percent of nonheme iron is absorbed. Nonheme iron absorption is compromised by the phytates that are found in many vegetables and whole grains.

Consuming meats and plant iron sources together can enhance iron absorption from plant foods. Small amounts of red meat in bean chili, spinach with chicken, and turkey with lentil soup combine heme and nonheme iron. Vitamin C—containing foods also enhance plant iron absorption. Try having orange juice or strawberries with fortified cereal.

To boost iron intake, try these recommendations:

- Incorporate lean meat regularly into your diet. Have small amounts several times weekly.
- Try adding small amounts of red meats to your favorite recipes like stir-fry, soups, pasta sauces, and casseroles.
- Mix heme-iron foods with nonheme choices, such as bean chili with dark turkey meat.
- Incorporate iron-fortified cereals into your diet.
- Consider increasing fish and shellfish in your diet for their iron content.
- Increase your intake of plant irons such as whole grain cereals, legumes, and green leafy vegetables. Have them with a vitamin C—containing food to improve iron absorption.
- Athletes training at altitude, female athletes, and vegetarians may want to consider a supplement that provides 100 percent of the Daily Values (DV) for iron and other trace minerals such as zinc and copper to ensure that they obtain adequate amounts of these nutrients.

Many multivitamins contain this amount of iron, so check labels. You should also have your hemoglobin, hematocrit, and ferritin stores monitored regularly. Taking excess iron from supplements, however, does carry some risk.

It is important that you do not self-diagnose low iron stores, but rather have your blood work evaluated by a physician. If you take a supplement providing greater than 100 percent of the RDA for iron and zinc, your hemoglobin, hematocrit, and ferritin should be monitored regularly. Higher doses of iron, even as little as 25 milligrams, can inhibit absorption of zinc and another mineral, copper.

Excess iron supplementation may also adversely affect individuals who have a genetic predisposition to iron overload. Iron overload, a condition known as *hemochromatosis*, is a genetic disorder that affects one in every two hundred people. This condition can result in excess iron deposits in the heart, liver, joints, and various body tissues, with the potential for damaging these tissues. High levels of iron supplements can also lead to gastrointestinal intolerance and constipation.

TABLE 1.14 » IRON CONTENT OF SELECTED FOODS

Food	Serving Size	Iron (mg)
Sources of Heme Iron		
Liver, beef, cooked	3 oz. (100 g)	6.0
Beef, cooked	3 oz. (100 g)	3.5
Pork, cooked	3 oz. (100 g)	3.4
Shrimp, cooked	3 oz. (100 g)	2.6
Turkey, dark, cooked	3 oz. (100 g)	2.0
Chicken, breast, cooked	3 oz. (100g)	1.0
Tuna, light	3 oz. (100 g)	1.0
Flounder, sole, salmon	3 oz. (100 g)	1.0
Sources of Plant Iron		
Cereal, iron-fortified	1 oz. (30 g)	2-18
Cream of wheat	¾ c. (200 ml)	9
Lentils	1 c. (240 ml)	6
Instant breakfast	1 envelope	4.5
Kidney beans, canned	1 c. (240 ml)	3.2
Baked potato, with skin	1 medium	3.0
Prune juice	8 oz. (240 ml)	3.0
Wheat germ	¼ c. (60 ml)	2.6
Apricots, dried	10 halves	1.7
Spaghetti, enriched, cooked	½ c. (120 ml)	1.4
Bread, enriched	1 slice	1.0

Zinc. This is another important mineral for athletes who train hard. An adequate amount of zinc keeps your immune system strong and promotes healing of wounds and injuries. Zinc is also a component of several enzymes involved in energy metabolism and is involved in protein synthesis. Like iron, though, excess zinc can be too much of a good thing: oversupplementing with zinc can interfere with absorption of other minerals.

Good sources of zinc include red meat, turkey, milk, yogurt, and seafood—especially oysters. The zinc from animal foods is better absorbed than that found in plant foods. Plant sources of zinc include garbanzo beans, lentils, lima beans, brown rice, and wheat germ.

Multivitamin Mineral Supplements

Athletes training in winter sports have the distinct advantage of being able to eat more than their sedentary counterparts. With a focus on quality food choices, this generally means a diet filled with variety and nutrients. While a multivitamin mineral supplement does guarantee that you will obtain all the Daily Values for vitamins and minerals, it is not the same as eating food. Nutrients from foods tend to be optimally absorbed and will provide you with all the phytochemicals, undiscovered or otherwise, that are not in your supplement.

However, a broad-range, reasonable-dose supplement may just be that little extra insurance that athletes who care about their health often seek. Active individuals who may want to seriously consider taking a vitamin and mineral supplement might include athletes who consume fewer than 1,500 calories daily; have food allergies that restrict a significant number of choices from one food group; travel frequently; have disordered eating and erratic diets; are vegans or vegetarians who may need additional vitamin D, zinc, iron, B12, and riboflavin; are picky eaters who may restrict many foods; are at risk for osteoporosis; or are pregnant or planning a pregnancy.

If you decide to take a multivitamin mineral supplement, try to stick to the following guidelines:

- Choose a broad-range, balanced supplement of vitamins and minerals that provides 100 percent of the Daily Values. These doses are known to be safe.
- Avoid supplements that contain an excess of minerals or any one mineral, as these nutrients compete with one another for absorption.
- Choose a supplement with the USP stamp of approval on the label to guarantee that it dissolves properly in your body.
- Choose a supplement in which the majority of vitamin A is actually beta-carotene, the precursor to vitamin A.
- A blend of natural and synthetic supplements is fine. Don't pay more for "timed-release" or "chelated" products.
- Calcium and magnesium may need to be purchased separately as they are too bulky for a regular multivitamin pill.
- If you take antioxidant supplements, keep doses to 100 to 200 IU vitamin E and 250 milligrams vitamin C.
- Take your multivitamin with a meal or snack and plenty of water.
- Don't double up on one-a-day vitamins. You may get too much of certain nutrients.
- Avoid megadoses, and be sure to account for any vitamins and minerals you may be taking from sports nutrition supplements.
- Individuals over 50 years of age can opt for iron-free formulas, and look for B6 and B12 content in the higher range.

Antioxidant supplements are strongly marketed to athletes, but it is actually diets abundant in foods that contain antioxidant nutrients that have been shown to prevent cancer and other diseases. So don't discount the importance of increasing food sources of these nutrients. You may also wonder whether training increases the effects of free radicals or whether athletes learn to cope with these negative by-products. Probably both situations occur. It is impossible to directly measure free radical production in humans. Free radical by-products do increase with exercise, but trained athletes may dispose of them more effectively.

Moderate doses of vitamin C, beta-carotene, and other carotenoids are easily obtained with educated food choices. However, one nutrient that may be difficult to obtain at antioxidant levels on a diet under 30 percent fat is vitamin E. Good sources are high in fat, and you would need to consume large amounts of them to reach even the low antioxidant dose of 100 IU. Researchers still need to determine the optimal doses of antioxidant supplements needed for preventing heart disease and cancer.

If you do supplement, do so wisely. A multivitamin mineral supplement providing 100 percent of the DV should be safe, though not always necessary. But keep in mind that the hazards of vitamin and mineral overdosing are real and can be subtle. If you take a supplement, understand the good reasons for taking it, consume appropriate doses, and discontinue its use when it is no longer needed.

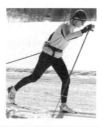

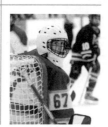

| 2 | # Perfomance Nutrition for All Ages |

Athletes of all ages participate in winter sports, from grade school, to high school, through college, and later as a masters athlete who wants to stay fit and healthy, and perhaps compete at some level. Many professional athletes in certain winter sports continue to compete at a high level in their sport into their 30s. It is important to appreciate some of the differences in nutritional requirements not only between the various winter sports as covered in Part II but also between athletes of all ages, and between men and women, so that winter sport athletes can experience optimal growth, increased strength, and nutritional recovery, and meet specific nutrient requirements. Age- and gender-specific nutrition considerations also provide a sound framework to support and enhance enjoyment of an athlete's sport and competitive endeavors. Table 2.1 summarizes the nutritional concerns of specific athletic population groups.

FUEL FOR THE PREADOLESCENT ATHLETE

Many children develop an appreciation and enjoyment of their winter sport at an early age. They may hit the slopes with their parents and develop a lifelong love for skiing or participate in hockey in junior leagues. It is important that these active children be well

TABLE 2.1 » NUTRITIONAL CONSIDERATIONS FOR SPECIFIC POPULATION GROUPS

Athlete Group	Nutritional Considerations
Children	Must monitor growth curve to assess nutritional adequacy Need quality protein sources to meet high requirements At higher risk of overheating and becoming dehydrated Require good calcium and iron intake Must learn sound eating habits
Adolescents	Body image affected by significant growth spurt and varying rates of growth Protein needs met in well-balanced diet Calcium and iron intake very important May want to try various sports supplements for muscle building and decreasing body fat Often eat on the run and are involved in own meal preparation Sound nutrition education very beneficial
Collegiate	May bring fast-food eating habits to college Benefit from nutritional assessment and monitoring Supported by healthy training table programs Benefit from nutrition team seminars and individual counseling Require healthy guidelines for eating on campus and eating out Benefit from education on proper food and fluid intake before, during, and after practice/games
Masters	Changes in physiology that affect performance Often include strength training in their program May have decreased energy needs Have higher protein needs than sedentary counterparts Require higher amounts of calcium and iron Require higher amounts of vitamins B6 and B12 Should pay close attention to adequate daily and training hydration
Females	At higher risk for developing disordered eating At higher risk of anemia Need to pay careful attention to adequate calcium intake May require special nutrition considerations during pregnancy and lactation

nourished and properly fueled for their activity and competition. Athletes aged 5 to 12 years must consume a diet designed to support both growth and development, and training and performance.

When feeding these athletes, it is important that we appreciate that they are not miniversions of adolescent or adult athletes. The preadolescent athlete's nutritional needs cannot be easily quantified as one-diet-fits-all because of the wide variation in growth rates among children, variety in exercise and training programs, and the lack of scientific data on child athletes. Parents and coaches need to be sensitive to these children's nutritional needs and provide the food choices and direction required by their young bodies. Young athletes require more nutrients per body weight, have smaller stomachs, and need to consume the additional calories and nutrients required for training in their sport. Consequently, they require energy- and nutrient-dense foods to fuel their bodies and growth.

Young athletes between the ages of 5 and 10 attain 20 percent of their adult height, and physical activity is just as important as calcium for developing optimal bone density. Young girls and boys store extra fat before the start of puberty as it provides energy for growth. Young female athletes should appreciate that changes in body weight are related to bone, body tissue, and muscle, not just increases in body fat.

Calories

Children involved in winter sports and year-round exercise should be observed in regard to their growth and energy levels to effectively determine whether they are consuming adequate calories or energy. Chronic poor calorie intake can result in many health concerns such as short stature, delayed puberty, poor bone health, menstrual irregularities, increased susceptibility to injury, fatigue and poor performance, and higher risk of developing an eating disorder. Energy requirements in children are not only affected by growth and training. Their energy needs are also increased because children are not as metabolically efficient and also waste calories by being more mechanically inefficient due to a relative lack of coordination.

Children often do the best job of determining their caloric intake simply by choosing foods and eating in accordance with their hunger and fullness levels. Calorie intake is affected by the training program, as well as other lifestyle issues, and may vary throughout the season as sport involvement changes from family to club involvement and participation in other seasonally related sports. The parents' role is to provide three regular, structured meals, healthy between-meal snacks, and foods and fluid around practice times.

Children involved in sports may be unaware of the important role nutrition plays in the enhancement of their athletic performance, but they can also be encouraged to take some responsibility for their own food and fluid choices. Education in this area may benefit both the parent and child, as it is easier to adopt healthy eating practices earlier in life.

The child athlete's growth should be monitored at regular intervals and can include height, weight, skinfold, and circumference measurements. If children are growing appropriately for their own specific growth curve, their energy needs are likely being met. Any substantial deviation from this growth curve should be investigated. Growth may be affected by an increase or decrease in training intensity, and various medical or psychological problems can affect food intake.

Children sometimes develop eating patterns that are counterproductive to meeting their energy and nutritional requirements. Many school-age children skip breakfast, an important meal that helps them perform better in school and during exercise. Breakfast fills up carbohydrate stores in the liver, an important fuel source that becomes depleted overnight when sleeping. Maintaining this fuel source with a steady supply of fuel from breakfast, lunch, and an afternoon snack ensures adequate stores for afternoon training.

A balanced school lunch is also important. Parents should consider the choices offered at school or pack a lunch as appropriate. The child's friends can often influence food choices. Parents should ask children what they eat at school, whether they eat the entire lunch packed, and find out what snacks are consumed away from home. Many child athletes exercise after school, making an afternoon snack appropriate and well timed. This snack provides fuel for training and can prevent extreme hunger during practice. This is also a convenient time for the athlete to hydrate prior to practice.

Protein

Child athletes have higher protein requirements than adults because of the extra amounts required for growth. The younger the child, the more protein required per pound (or kilogram) of body weight. However, these higher protein amounts are easily met with good food choices and a well-balanced diet. The child athlete who consumes enough calories will also use the protein provided in the diet more efficiently and for important unique protein functions.

Children may often gravitate toward lower-quality protein sources such as hot dogs, fatty luncheon meats, and fast foods. Adding choices such as nonhydrogenated peanut butter, lean poultry meat, and yogurt or milk to meals and snacks can contribute to their total protein intake, laying the foundation for good eating habits early in life.

Fluids

Younger children are more likely than older children to become dehydrated, and consequently active children need to consume plenty of fluids. Because children don't sweat as easily as adults, their bodies do not cool as efficiently. Even in the colder winter months, children should arrive for exercise fully hydrated and drink at regular pauses during the training session. Cooled beverages can be more appealing when exercising in hotter weather, and they are well accepted by children, as well as being absorbed more quickly. Children are less likely to drink than adults, even when pushed to do so during exercise. Checking weight before and after exercise can also provide information on how well children are meeting their fluid needs. Any weight loss during exercise can completely be attributed to fluid loss. Though not directly applicable to winter sports, parents and coaches should appreciate that young children also need more time than adults to acclimatize to hot weather. When children start practice in hotter weather, they should be given time to adjust. Adequate fluid intake is imperative.

While water is adequate for rehydration, children are more likely to drink adequate amounts when provided flavored drinks. Real fruit juice, dairy and soy milk, and foods that are high in water such as oranges, watermelon, and apples can also be used to rehydrate the body. Some of the fluid and high-water food choices cannot only replace lost fluid but provide carbohydrates for replenishment as well. Fluids consumed during exercise that provide carbohydrate and sodium, such as sports drinks, are also appealing to children.

Minerals

Calcium is a very important mineral for the child athlete because of its role in developing strong, hard bones and teeth properly. Adequate calcium also reduces the risk of fractures and is essential to the healing of broken bones. Calcium requirements are very high during childhood, and many young athletes have an inadequate calcium intake, perhaps as consumption of milk has decreased in favor of less nutritious fluids. Children need at least three servings of calcium-rich foods daily. (Good sources of calcium have been presented earlier, in Table 1.13.)

Iron is also an essential mineral for the child athlete, as iron requirements are extremely high at this stage of life, mainly because of its role in the formation of hemoglobin. (A list of iron-rich foods was provided in Table 1.14.) Children should be encouraged to consume low-sugar, iron-fortified cereals and other high-iron foods such as raisins, iron-enriched grains, and protein sources such as lean beef and poultry.

Vitamin and mineral needs of young athletes are easily met through a well-balanced diet. Achieving nutrient balance over the week is what is important. If a child athlete is provided with a basic multivitamin mineral supplement, it should not provide children with a false sense of security, and nutritious foods should still be encouraged and consumed. Ergogenic aids such as creatine are not suitable for child athletes for a number of reasons, but particularly for their potential short-term and long-term harmful effects.

Weight Control

Prepubescent athletes can be sensitive to the normal body changes that occur with growth and development. Young athletes may be skilled at their sport before going through puberty. As the body starts changing, some athletes may attempt to control food intake and maintain their current "competitive" weight. Even young children can experiment with fad diets and disordered eating behavior. Coaches and parents can help by appreciating the normal growth stages of the prepubescent athlete and by being prepared to help children cope with normal body changes.

Unhealthy weight management strategies should not be practiced when trying to achieve top athletic performance. A diet that is restricted in calories and nutrients and that may compromise the health of a child should not be promoted. Parents should not inappropriately eliminate food groups or overly restrict foods in an attempt to control weight or prevent disease later in life. Instead, parents can encourage long-term healthy eating habits that support growth, provide fuel for sport, and reduce unnecessary amounts of saturated fat, hydrogenated fat, and sugars in the diet.

Children with very high energy needs may find it difficult to consume adequate calories and may require concentrated food sources. Smoothies, low-fat milkshakes, concentrated starches, and dried fruits may help them consume adequate calories. These children should consume three meals and at least two snacks daily to stay in calorie balance.

Conversely, child athletes should not be encouraged to eat excessively in the belief that they will build strength and endurance more quickly. Genetics mainly determines the course of a child's growth spurt and cannot be pushed ahead with nutrition strategies. Inappropriate calorie consumption can lead to the start of a lifelong struggle of being overweight. Parents who require some nutritional guidance for their child athlete can consult a qualified sports nutritionist.

» ASSESSING BODY COMPOSITION IN YOUNG ATHLETES

Body composition in young athletes can differ greatly from that of adults in several important areas. While changes in body composition are related to body fat changes, significant changes also occur in lean body tissue and bone mass. Often in adults, various body composition techniques are used, including skinfold calipers (see Chapter 5). Skinfold measurements in young athletes are greatly influenced by their stage of development and changes in lean body tissue. If skinfold assessments are taken on these young athletes, they should be done by a skilled professional and interpreted appropriately based on age and growth.

Body composition assessment in young athletes should never be used to determine strict weight loss or body fat loss guidelines, which could adversely affect growth and development of young athletes. Children should be assessed according to their own growth curve, and further evaluation can occur if they deviate greatly below or above their own growth curve or from the norms for their age.

FUEL FOR THE HIGH SCHOOL ATHLETE

The adolescent or high school athlete will experience a significant growth spurt and body changes that may concern or even frustrate them. Every high school athlete will develop and grow at the individual's own pace. In any one high school grade, you will see a wide variety of normal body shapes and sizes.

Teenagers can be very sensitive about their changing bodies. Girls may desire to be both lean and fast, while boys may focus on being stronger and bigger for increased strength. This may conflict with the fact that acquiring increased body fat is normal for a developing female athlete, and that some boys may develop later than their classmates. It is important that high school athletes appreciate good nutrition practices, the physical demands of their sport, and how nutritional decisions affect both their short- and long-term health.

Calories

The energy requirements of the high school athlete depend on the basic (basal) energy expenditure for adolescence, growth requirements, daily activities, and of course the energy burned when training and competing for their sport. Many teenage athletes have high calorie needs, and eating enough to support all their activities is important.

Table 2.2 reviews daily calorie intake for preadolescents and teenagers. These caloric intakes do not include calories that need to be consumed for exercise and training. The longer and harder these young athletes train, the more food they should consume. (Estimation of energy needs is described in Chapter 3, with the energy expenditures for various sports listed in Table 3.5.)

An ideal calorie level for growing teen athletes will reflect all of their energy expenditure, but it should be interpreted with caution as these numbers are only an estimate. Calorie needs vary greatly from teenage athlete to athlete depending on growth, age, and type of training. The athlete's energy level, recovery, body weight, growth, and general health should

TABLE 2.2 » AVERAGE DAILY CALORIE INTAKES FOR TEENAGERS

	Age	Calories
Male	11-14	2,500
	15-18	3,000
Female	11-14	2,200
	15-18	2,200

all determine whether adequate calories are being consumed. When an athlete does not eat enough food, her metabolism slows down, resulting in fewer calories being burned. This in turn means that an athlete requires less food for the same amount of activity, which could lead to future eating and weight control problems. Athletes with a slowed metabolism may also feel tired, underperform in their sport, and not grow to their full potential.

Estimates of energy requirements for adolescent athletes range from 2,200 to 4,000 calories per day for females and 3,000 to 6,000 daily for males in high school, depending on their total energy expenditure. Let's say we have a 16-year-old male cross-country skier who trains for 90 minutes at a pace of 2.5 miles per hour (4 kilometers/hour). His weight is 140 pounds (64 kilograms). He burns 7.0 calories per minute for 90 minutes of practice for a total of 630 calories. Add this to the basic energy expenditure of 3,000 calories, and his energy needs for a heavy practice day are over 4,000 calories. Now consider a 14-year-old female downhill skier who skis a total of 60 minutes one day. At a weight of 130 pounds (59 kilograms), she burns 510 calories on the slopes at 8.5 calories per minute. Added to 2,200 calories daily, her total calorie needs are approximately 2,710 daily.

Protein

Healthy teenagers require about 0.4 to 0.45 grams of protein per pound of body weight (0.8 to 1.0 gram/kilogram body weight) daily. No scientific data are available to indicate whether teenage athletes require additional protein. Winter sport athletes who may require additional protein include athletes who are just starting a training program and athletes who are actively weight training as part of their overall program. As for most North Americans, the protein intake of teenagers usually exceeds the recommended amounts. While exceeding their protein requirements does not build more muscle in teenagers, consuming adequate calories ensures that protein is used for unique protein functions and will not be wasted as a fuel source during exercise. High-quality protein sources should be emphasized, such as lean meats, fish, poultry, eggs, and dairy products. Vegetarian teenage athletes need to emphasize soy and dairy protein sources, and consume plenty of dried peas and beans.

Iron and Calcium

Even teenagers not involved in sports have a high risk of developing low iron stores, but athletes are at risk due to increased demands of growth, sports-related blood loss, poor iron absorption, menstruation in female athletes, and possibly poor nutritional intake and unbalanced eating. Good sources of iron should be emphasized.

Calcium is also a very important mineral for the teenage athlete, as this is one of the most critical times for building bone. It is not usual for teenagers to consume inadequate

» IRON TIPS FOR THE HIGH SCHOOL ATHLETE

Teenagers who do not have a variety of foods in their diet such as meat, fish, and poultry may be at greater risk for developing poor iron status.

Restrictive eating, fad diets, and poorly balanced vegetarian diets can significantly decrease iron intake.

Full-blown iron deficiency in adolescents will impair athletic performance. While iron deficiency without anemia may not have the same effect, it should be treated with appropriate food intake and supplementation to prevent the more serious condition of anemia from developing.

Nutritional intake of iron must be adequate to meet needs for training, support growth and development, and produce adequate hemoglobin and ferritin to maintain iron status.

Teenage athletes should appreciate that poor iron status can result in symptoms such as fatigue when training, breathlessness, paleness, slightly elevated heart rate, and inability to keep warm.

Iron deficiency is more common in female athletes because of menstrual losses, rapid growth in the early high school years, and inadequate dietary iron intake.

Iron loss can also be associated with weight-bearing exercise as seen in team sports, gastrointestinal losses, and excessive sweating.

amounts of calcium. Female athletes who restrict calories often restrict more concentrated food sources of calcium such as dairy products. Dairy products are usually the main source of calcium in the adolescent's diet.

Poor calcium intake may not be apparent until the athlete experiences a stress fracture, and it is often not apparent until identified with laboratory or bone density tests. Female athletes with irregular periods and amenorrhea, or cessation of menstruation, are at great risk for poor bone status. Amenorrhea is often related to inadequate calorie intake for growth and training needs, and it may also reflect disordered eating. The recommended daily calcium intake for adolescents is 1,300 milligrams, but high school–age females may consume just 400 to 700 milligrams daily, and males may consume only half their calcium requirements. High school athletes should be educated on good sources of calcium, ways to increase calcium absorption, and the number of food servings required for meeting their calcium needs. Teenagers may respond better than younger children to the more immediate concerns of poor calcium intake such as stress fractures, as well as the long-term concern of osteoporosis.

Other Supplement Use

High school athletes may take a daily multivitamin mineral supplement for a variety of reasons, including the desire to improve athletic performance. Supplements can offset any uneven eating habits; still, good food choices should be encouraged whenever possible. Supplements themselves will not improve athletic performance, though they can correct marginal deficiencies that may impact exercise performance. Adolescent athletes who may benefit from a vitamin and mineral supplement include vegetarians, girls who are iron-deficient, and those who are amenorrheic. Misuse and overuse of supplements is possible and could have adverse effects on health. These supplements should be taken only as directed.

Young athletes participating in winter sports should also be advised that athletic performance is dependent on a number of important factors, such as years of good training, sound nutrition practices, skill acquisition, and growth stages, and they should be advised to not place unrealistic and high expectations on the use of nutritional supplements. Supplements designed to specifically enhance performance such as ergogenic aids, described in Chapter 7, are often supported by flashy advertising and anecdotal success stories. Many of these ergogenic aids are frequently used by male adolescent athletes interested in building muscle or female athletes interested in losing body fat. These products may include protein powder, creatine, and hydroxyl-methyl butyrate or HMB, with the short- and long-term effects of these on adolescents not known. They may often contain banned ingredients due to poor product purity and quality control and could have harmful side effects, as well as result in a positive drug test. Many of these products are often not backed by scientific testing and appropriate safety data and have not been tested on young athletes. It has been suggested that athletes under 18 years of age do not consume ergogenic aids.

Fluid and Hydration

During the off-season from winter sports when adolescents often participate in other, warmer-weather sports, they should be monitored closely for signs of heat stress and dehydration. Younger bodies and smaller bodies are at greater risk for developing dehydration due to greater heat production. Athletes with higher levels of body fat and heavier builds are more susceptible to heat stress because they are less efficient in dissipating heat when exercising. Adequate fluid consumption during exercise is essential to preventing heat-related problems.

Athletes should start training in a well-hydrated state at any time of the year, particularly for training situations where ideal fluid consumption practices during exercise may not allow them to keep up with their fluid losses. Starting the training session well hydrated can lessen the degree of dehydration that can develop during training. Dehydration in adolescents will result in a greater increase in core body temperature than in adults. (Guidelines for fluid intake during training will be covered in Chapter 4.)

Developing Good Eating Habits

Adolescents often have distinct eating habits from both younger children and adults. Older adolescents, particularly girls, may become regular breakfast skippers and not rely as much on snacking to meet their daily nutrient intake. Older adolescents are also more likely to obtain and consume food away from home.

A number of factors influence the food choices of adolescent athletes, including convenience and time considerations around busy school and training schedules, hunger and cravings, food appeal and appearance, peer and parental influences, beliefs about health often influenced by the media, moods and feelings, body image, and cost. Girls are more likely to obtain their nutrition and weight loss information from magazines that may not be accurate and factual. Other, more positive sources of nutrition information include physicians, the school environment, and coaches. Adolescent athletes may also have exposure to accurate information from sports nutritionists, usually as a result of parental initiation, though some schools may include this as a free service in their programming for athletes.

Body Image Concerns

Body image is an important issue for many adolescents because this is a period of fast and often unpredictable growth, as well as significant emotional changes. Becoming self-conscious about the body starts at an early age as many males strive for a muscular physique, whereas many females attempt to be small, lean, and thin.

These body image concerns can sometimes translate into poor nutrition practices. Males may consume large and unnecessary amounts of protein in the belief that this will build more muscle, while females may develop restrictive eating patterns in hopes of losing weight and body fat. Disordered eating patterns can also occur in hopes of enhancing performance, attempting to change body type to reach an ideal for their chosen sports, and attaining the physique idealized in society. Athletes who are at a healthy weight and attempt to lose or drastically decrease body fat can resort to weight loss techniques that have negative effects on nutrient intake and balance in the diet, as well as harmful effects on physical and psychological health. Some ill-advised and unhealthy techniques can be skipping meals, decreasing meals, eliminating food groups, use of laxatives, purging after meals, and using over-the-counter weight loss supplements.

Nutrition Education

Adolescent athletes can benefit from repeated and regular sound nutrition advice. Support in preparing or purchasing healthy school lunches, consuming healthy snacks, and taking responsibility for meal preparation should be encouraged. Adolescents can become quite independent in meeting their nutritional needs, and this practice is often essential due to demanding school and training schedules, and conflicting schedules for various family members. Education of other family members, particularly the person responsible for food shopping and meal preparation, is also indicated.

Specific strategies may be required for athletes with high energy requirements, such as nutrient-dense food choices in the form of smoothies, low-fat shakes, and concentrated carbohydrate choices. These athletes may need to base most meals and snacks on carbohydrate-rich foods, pack foods for school, and make good use of high-carbohydrate liquids. Filling foods that are low in nutrients and calories should be kept to appropriate levels.

Athletes identified as having weight management concerns should be referred to a sports dietitian who can provide healthy nutrition guidelines so that restrictive eating and disordered eating behaviors are prevented. Rapid weight loss is not recommended; when indicated, gradual weight loss is recommended. Regular monitoring is also essential. Vegetarian adolescent athletes and their families could also benefit from qualified nutritional guidance.

FUEL FOR THE COLLEGIATE ATHLETE

In the United States, hundreds of thousands of male and female collegiate athletes participate in a variety of sports and activities year-round, including winter sports. College athletes often appreciate the importance of nutrition in athletic performance but may have had limited exposure to sound sports nutrition advice. Many of these athletes may have gone through high school sports thriving on convenience items and fast food and have not developed the sports nutrition practices required for optimal performance.

Eating in the school's dining hall, which provides a variety of food choices, may or may not support a positive change in nutrition habits. These athletes may not always like college dorm food choices or may have trouble adapting a vegetarian diet to college life. Moreover, class schedules often require that some meals be eaten on campus, where a variety of food choices may be offered, including fast food. Athletes may opt to consume some meals in their room or on their dorm floors, with options limited to microwaving and other simple food preparation techniques. Most college athletes are not proficient cooks and may lack some of the equipment and facilities previously utilized at home.

Even for collegiate athletes motivated to shop for healthy foods and comfortable with meal planning and cooking, time may be a great limitation in achieving these tasks.

Frequently, these athletes have very busy schedules with little free time for off-campus activities such as food shopping. Between training (sometimes more than once a day), class time and studying requirements, and participation in other hobbies and interests, they have heavy demands on their time.

Nutrition Assessment Education

Nutrition education and support programs can vary widely among locations, with some of the larger universities more likely to offer comprehensive programming. Ideally a sports nutritionist is available to offer a variety of services and is part of a comprehensive program, working closely with the athletic department and the food service staff. Collegiate athletes are also exposed to a variety of nutrition information sources, both accurate and healthy, and inaccurate and perhaps risky. For example, these athletes have exposure to the Internet and advertising for supplement use, as well as weight loss products.

In addition to the risk of nutrition misinformation, research indicates that collegiate athletes may experience other health risks. These athletes may be focused on an ideal weight that may conflict with good health and appropriate nutrition habits. Males in team sports may be preoccupied with building muscle and may be exposed to and use anabolic steroids. They are also more likely to consume alcohol, engage in binge drinking, and be a passenger in a vehicle driven by a driver under the influence of alcohol. Female athletes can also be at risk. Preoccupation with weight and disordered eating habits can result in a higher rate of irregular and absent menstruation and a higher incidence of stress fractures which obviously does not enhance athletic ability.

Sports nutrition evaluation and services that the collegiate athlete can be offered include the following:

- Assessment of body composition and evaluation to determine weight and body fat goals. This can include body fat loss and ongoing monitoring of a strength and conditioning program designed to build muscle mass.
- Evaluation of blood chemistry and lipid profiles. These tests can be part of the yearly physical conducted on athletes.
- Screening of iron deficiency and iron deficiency anemia
- Nutrition education at the training table/food hall that provides nutrition examples and food strategies
- Nutritional information on the dishes and meals offered at the training table
- Diet and nutritional analysis
- Team seminars
- Individual nutritional counseling to provide meal plans for training during the training season, for competition, and in the off-season

- Assistance with on-campus meal choices and strategies at various venues frequented by the athlete
- Nutritional counseling for health-related concerns that can be integrated with the sports nutrition meal plan
- Team seminars on various sports nutrition topics such as fluids and hydration, nutritional recovery strategies, and sports nutrition supplements
- Nutritional protocols for providing foods and fluid for pregame ingestion
- Nutritional protocols for fluids and sports supplement availability at games

Unfortunately, not all of these services and follow-up are available to the collegiate athletes, with the athletic trainer often fielding sports nutrition concerns. If on-campus sports nutrition services are not available, off-campus qualified sports nutritionists can be contacted to provide various services.

Energy and Protein Requirements

Fuel needs of many collegiate winter sport athletes can be high, though this can vary depending on the sport, time of year, and training program. For example, a downhill skier who is in a heavy muscle-building phase of her program can expend many calories, while a cross-country skier can participate on longer extended endurance sessions both on and off the snow. Hockey players can easily burn through a few hundred calories in a demanding practice. Energy needs of winter sports are outlined in Table 3.5. As indicated, the energy burned per hour can vary with body weight and sport.

Protein requirements need to be calculated to encompass any strength-training components for the winter sport athlete and the number of hours spent training. As with younger athletes, the protein needs of collegiate athletes are easily met with an appropriately chosen diet; expensive protein supplements are not needed. For serious weight training, timing of protein intake around the training sessions may significantly enhance muscle building. (More of these strategies are covered in Chapter 5.) Lean protein sources low in saturated fat and prepared with less fat should be emphasized. Adequate caloric consumption also ensures that the protein consumed is used for important protein functions such as maintaining immune function.

Fluids and Hydration

College athletes also need to have workable strategies for maintaining daily hydration. They can carry water bottles and consume other hydrating fluids such as milk and juice to maintain hydration levels. Caffeine intake should be kept to moderate levels. Fluids should also be easily available during training sessions. (More on fluid intake before, during, and after training is covered in Chapters 3 and 4.) Players should be educated on how to monitor fluid status. For example, pale urine reflects adequate hydration, as does four full bladders of urine daily.

Supplements

Athletes should be aware of supplements that are banned by the National Collegiate Athletic Association (NCAA). Over-the-counter nutritional supplements may also contain banned substances due to poor quality control at the time of production of raw materials and product manufacture. Many schools may have a dietary supplement policy designed to prevent ingestion of banned substance, prevent harmful effects of products, keep the athlete from spending money on unnecessary products, and take legal supplements appropriately.

Collegiate athletes may benefit from a daily multivitamin mineral supplement providing 100 percent of the DVs, to augment any marginal intakes of nutrients. Iron supplementation to treat or prevent anemia should be monitored with regular blood work. Any other vitamin and mineral supplement recommendations should be provided under the recommendations of a sports nutritionist.

Food Service

A sports nutritionist can work directly with the food service program and chef to make menu recommendations and suggest recipe modifications. Athletes can be offered a wide variety of menu items and also be educated on appropriate choices and portions to consume for their nutritional plan. Some healthy offerings may include a nutrient-dense salad bar, pasta and potato bars, whole-grain choices, and fresh fruits.

Both high school and collegiate athletes may frequent fast-food establishments. It is important that they make the best choices possible at these establishments not only for performance but also for lifelong good health. (Chapter 6 outlines some fast-food options.)

Team personnel, with the assistance of the sports nutritionist, can also set up healthy meals for the team when traveling for competition. Restaurants can be contacted ahead of time to set up team meals. Athletes should be educated on healthy food choices when eating out for fast food, in airports, and at various types of restaurants and ethnic cuisine, information that will be valuable even when they're not training.

FUEL FOR THE MASTERS ATHLETE

The age at which an athlete is defined as being a master can vary from sport to sport, though 30 to 40 is common. With hundreds of thousands of baby boomers now well into their 40s, it is not unusual to see many masters athletes participating in winter sports. They may have participated in the sport in college and have found a club or league that allows them to participate in their chosen sport for part of the year. Besides training and competing for the love of their sport, they also receive the added bonus of staying fit and healthy. Masters athletes often also participate in a weight-training or resistance-training program to maintain lean body mass and strength.

Plenty of data indicate that these older athletes enjoy better health than nonathletes, as many of the supposed normal age-related health changes could actually result from a sedentary lifestyle. However, masters athletes will experience some physiological changes with aging, such as decreases in heart function, muscle mass, and aerobic capacity. These changes are not as pronounced in masters athletes as they are in their sedentary peers. Compared to younger athletes, masters athletes are more likely to experience sports-related injuries and adjust to training at a slower rate. They also recover from training more slowly.

Nutritional considerations for masters athletes focus both on these physiological changes as well as on the nutritional demands of the training program for their team sport. Masters participation varies from sport to sport, with playing time often limited to two or fewer practices per week.

Performances of world-class athletes tend to decline after ages 30 to 35 years due to a number of physiological age-related factors. Muscle strength peaks at around 25 years of age and levels off from 30 to 35 years, and then declines after ages 35 to 40. This decrease is related to reduced muscle mass, rather than in actual decrease in the capacity of muscle fibers. Training programs that incorporate muscle building can offset some of this muscle loss and help maintain strength. Specific nutrition strategies can also maximize your muscle-building efforts (see Chapter 5).

Aerobic capacity decreases each decade beginning at about 25 years. This age-related rate of decrease is slightly slower in athletes than their sedentary counterparts. However, it is clear that masters athletes benefit from a health perspective and likely have a lower risk of chronic diseases such as cardiovascular disease, hypertension, and diabetes.

Energy and Protein Requirements

Basal metabolic rate declines with aging, and there may also be a decrease in calories burned with exercise, depending on the intensity and duration of the training program. While the energy or calorie needs of masters athletes may decline over the course of their athletic career, they can still consume more than their sedentary counterparts. Adjustments in food intake may be required to prevent unwanted weight gain. Resistance training also increases calorie needs. Masters athletes should continue to consume more protein than their sedentary counterparts, and they likely require the same amounts as younger athletes. Their total protein needs are easily met by making the proper food choices and do not demand any specific protein supplements.

Carbohydrate should continue to be the major source of energy in the masters athlete's diet, though the amount required can vary depending on the training program, specific training session, and time of the season. Fat intake can make up the remainder of the calories consumed, with the emphasis being placed on healthy types of fats as reviewed in Chapter 1.

Vitamins and Minerals

Both male and female masters athletes should pay close attention to optimal bone health and the nutrients that support this important body tissue, particularly calcium and vitamin D. It is important that you meet your calcium needs on a daily basis. From ages 30 to 50, men should obtain at least 1,000 milligrams of calcium daily and supplement as needed if this is not provided in the diet. Calcium needs increase further beyond these ages, with 1,200 milligrams being the recommended amount for men aged 50 to 70. Many experts believe that women should consume at least 1,200 milligrams of calcium daily from ages 30 to 50 and 1,500 milligrams after menopause.

Vitamin D is also crucial for healthy bones, aiding in the optimal absorption of calcium. Aging decreases the capacity of our skin to synthesize vitamin D from sunlight, and less vitamin D is absorbed with age. For these reasons, vitamin D requirements double at age 50, for both men and women, from 200 to 400 IU daily. A standard multivitamin can supplement your food intake of this nutrient, and many formulations for individuals over 50 provide the full daily requirement.

There are several other important nutrients that masters athletes should consider increasing in their diet by choosing good food sources. Vitamin B6, vitamin E, and zinc are important to maintaining optimal immune function, which can decline with age. Folate, vitamin B6, and vitamin B12 are important nutrients that keep levels of homocysteine in the blood down to acceptable levels. High levels of homocysteine are associated with increased risk of developing heart disease. Absorption of B12 also decreases with age due to decreased gastric acid levels. Increasing food sources of these nutrients is one important strategy, but you can also consider a standard-dose multivitamin mineral supplement that provides 100 percent of the Daily Values. Formulations for older individuals that specifically provide higher amounts of these nutrients are also available.

Fluid and Hydration

Masters athletes should pay extra attention to daily fluid intake for a number of reasons related to aging. As we age, thirst sensation decreases, affecting regulation of hydration status. Body water also declines in older people. After age 40, the kidneys require more water to remove waste products from the body.

Not keeping up with sweat losses can impair training, particularly when exercising in the heat. Masters athletes may be more susceptible to overheating and should consume as much fluid as possible before and after training. They should give themselves more time to acclimate to hot weather and pay attention to warning signs of dehydration and heat exhaustion. They should also be aware of how any prescription drug they take can affect body temperature regulation in a hot environment, discussing this with their physician as needed. More specific guidelines on hydration strategies before, during, and after exercise are outlined in Chapters 3 and 4.

SPECIAL CONSIDERATION FOR FEMALE ATHLETES

Female athletes may need to pay special attention to specific nutrients at various stages in their training and in their lives. Bone health is a special concern in females, as they are at greater risk for osteoporosis, and those who develop menstrual irregularities are at even greater risk. Because our society places such value on thinness in women, they are highly susceptible to developing eating disorders.

Body Weight, Amenorrhea, and Bone Density

Bone health is an issue that has received heightened attention over the past two decades due to the increasing rate of osteoporotic fractures and a focus on stress fractures. The athlete at risk for development of compromised bone health should appreciate the influence of exercise, hormone balance, genetics, and nutritional factors such as calcium intake on maintaining appropriate levels of this important body tissue. Calcium balance is maintained by the amount of calcium you both consume and absorb, and how much calcium you lose in your urine.

Bone is a dynamic tissue that is constantly being broken down and rebuilt under the regulation of your body's hormones. When the process of bone breakdown or bone resorption exceeds bone formation, bone loss occurs. If this bone loss is prolonged, osteoporosis, a condition in which low bone mass has developed and bone is fragile, can result, and there is greater risk for fracture.

The hormone estrogen plays a crucial role in maintaining bone in women. When estrogen levels are low, the bone serves as a source of calcium to maintain normal levels of calcium in the blood and perform important physiological functions in the body. Even if physical activity is high, low estrogen levels, as seen in amenorrhea and after menopause, can result in bone loss.

Female athletes seem to have a higher incidence of menstrual irregularities than the general population. The term *athletic amenorrhea* has been used to describe menstrual imbalances in female athletes. A variety of factors have been implicated in the development of amenorrhea in athletes. It appears that the predominant factor is inadequate energy (calorie) intake. An excessive training load or increase in training that is not matched with proper food intake creates a caloric deficiency that can result in amenorrhea. Of course, disordered eating and a full-blown eating disorder can also result from a chronically low intake of calories. Amenorrhea may also be more common in certain sports such as running, gymnastics, and dance, which can place particular emphasis on small frames and light weight, rather than winter sports, but it can occur in any sports under the proper precipitating conditions.

What has been determined is that female athletes with amenorrhea have lower bone mass than athletes who menstruate regularly. Greater incidence of stress fractures has also been reported in athletes with current or past menstrual disturbances. Athletes with the health concerns should see a sports medicine physician for assessment of bone mass, hormonal status, and appropriate medical treatment. This may include hormone replacement, weight gain recommendations, and modifications in training. These female athletes can benefit greatly from guidance from a sports nutritionist regarding appropriate calorie intake and the balance of other nutrients in their diet.

Athletes being treated for amenorrhea should increase their calcium intake to 1,500 milligrams daily. Refer back to Table 1.13 for a list of foods high in calcium. If this amount cannot be achieved through diet, calcium supplements can make up the difference. Doses of 500 milligrams of calcium carbonate or calcium citrate can be taken one to two times daily. Excessive intake protein when combined with inadequate calcium intake, and high intakes of caffeine and sodium can also aggravate calcium absorption. Overall balance in the diet, especially adequate calorie intake, should also be restored. Weight-bearing exercise may also be continued, though not at excessive levels.

The Spectrum of Disordered Eating

For many female athletes, winter sport training and perhaps competition involves moving your body quickly over short or longer distance, often at top speeds, and requires the need to reaccelerate several times during practice or competition. Because of the desire to be quick, having a lower level of body fat is considered to be a mechanical advantage. However, many female athletes do become overly focused on their weight and body fat levels. Because athletes may be obsessive by nature, as well as perfectionistic and very competitive, some of these qualities may manifest in unrealistic weight and body fat goals, placing a high degree of importance on losing a few pounds. Pressure to lose this weight may come from a number of outside sources, including trainers, coaches, and athletic peers. Chapter 6 discusses issues pertinent to the winter sport athlete interested in changing body composition and provides an overview of eating disorders in athletes.

» NUTRITION FOR PREGNANCY AND EXERCISE

Many pregnant female athletes desire to maintain a high degree of fitness during pregnancy and often return to training and competition as quickly as possible. It is no longer unusual for Olympic or professional athletes to have a child and resume training at a high level. Although these athletes may be most concerned about consuming an adequate number of calories for a healthy and appropriate weight gain, the nutrients consumed while planning a pregnancy are also very important.

Often women plan to see their physician before trying to conceive and take a prenatal multivitamin mineral supplement in order to obtain folic acid and other important nutrients. Folate (found from food sources) and folic acid (from supplement sources) deserve serious attention from women athletes even contemplating pregnancy. An adequate intake of folate, both prior to conception and during the first several weeks of pregnancy, can help prevent birth defects such as spina bifida. Folate is used for the synthesis of DNA, the building block of all cells. During the first 28 days of pregnancy, cells divide rapidly and form the neural tubes that become the baby's brain and spine. Many Americans fall short of the recommended 400 micrograms of folate.

Good food sources include asparagus, lentils, spinach and other leafy green vegetables, dried beans such as kidney beans, and orange juice. Grain products such as bread, pasta, rice, and enriched flour have been fortified with folic acid for several years, and a decrease in these types of birth defects has been the result. Many health experts also recommend that any woman who may become pregnant take a multivitamin providing 400 micrograms of folate.

During the first 3 months of pregnancy, it is normal to have no weight gain or up to a 5-pound weight gain. After the first trimester, a weight gain of up to 1 pound weekly is normal. Generally a total weight gain of 25 to 35 pounds is recommended. Underweight or lean women may be advised to gain more weight, at about 28 to 40 pounds. Adequate weight gain comes down to finding the right balance of calories to build your own tissue during pregnancy, to support the growth of the baby, and to meet your energy needs from exercise in order to prevent having a low-birth-weight baby or a premature delivery. Starting in the second trimester, pregnancy requires only an additional 300 calories daily above your usual energy needs and another 10 to 12 grams of protein. These additional nutrient amounts are easily met with an increased food intake—for example, 8 ounces of milk and a small turkey sandwich.

The expectant mother's weight gain comes from growth in her own body tissues, the baby's body weight, and tissues that support the baby's growth. It includes an increased blood volume, body fluid, breast tissue, and weight gain from the placenta, umbilical cord, and amniotic fluid. Body fat stores increase in anticipation of lactation, which requires at least an additional 500 calories or more daily, above normal non-pregnancy requirements. The physician will monitor not only your total weight gain but also the pattern of weight gain to make sure that it is appropriate.

Fluid requirements also increase during pregnancy, and it is critical to maintain proper hydration during exercise and training. Basic fluid requirements are about 2.5 to 3 quarts (slightly less than 2.5 to 3 liters) daily, plus sweat losses

CONTINUED

during exercise. It is essential that exercise begin in the well-hydrated state. Overheating could have serious negative effects on the unborn baby. Plenty of fluids should be consumed several hours before exercise and at least 4 to 8 ounces (120 to 240 milliliters) of fluid consumed every 15 to 20 minutes. Carbohydrates can be consumed several hours before exercise to prevent hypoglycemia. Sports drinks, carbohydrate gels, and energy bars that have no extra vitamin, mineral, or herbal additives can be consumed during exercise to maintain blood glucose levels. Food choices and prenatal vitamin and mineral supplements should be more than adequate to meet these nutrient requirements, and they should not be overconsumed. Herbal products have not been tested in pregnancy and should be avoided.

Other important nutrients to include in the diet during pregnancy are iron and calcium. Iron requirements double due to a pregnant woman's expanded blood volume. Most pregnant women receive adequate iron in their prenatal vitamin and mineral supplement, but some require an additional iron supplement in order to prevent anemia. Anemia can result in fatigue, shortness of breath, and increased delivery risks. The baby also runs the risk of developing anemia if iron stores run too low, and athletes may already have low iron stores. Iron levels should be checked early in pregnancy and at regular intervals afterward. Concentrate on including plenty of high-iron foods in your diet as listed in Table 1.14.

Calcium plays an important role in every woman's health and deserves extra attention during pregnancy. Calcium requirements increase to 1,200 milligrams daily. As the baby builds bone, the mother's bones serve as a calcium source. If her diet is inadequate to replenish this calcium reservoir, the risk of developing osteoporosis later in life increases. High-calcium food sources are listed in Table 1.13. You can also consider taking a separate calcium supplement during pregnancy to meet your elevated requirements.

Certain nutrients and foods should be limited during pregnancy. Excess vitamin A intake from supplementation can increase the risk of birth defects. Intake from a supplement should not exceed 5,000 IU of vitamin A daily. There is also no room for alcohol in the diet as it can produce severe negative effects on the baby such as fetal alcohol syndrome. Caffeine should be restricted to no more than 300 milligrams daily or avoided altogether. Avoid saccharin and limit other artificial sweeteners as much as possible. Limit soft cheese such as Brie, Camembert, blue cheese, and feta cheese because they can increase the risk of bacterial contamination. In general, pregnant women should be careful with food safety, never eat raw fish, and make sure that all meats are well cooked. Avoid any unpasteurized milk products and raw eggs.

Fish can also be contaminated with mercury, which can have adverse effects on the developing baby. Fatty fish such as swordfish, mackerel, shark, bluefish, tilefish, and striped bass should be avoided completely. Other high-mercury fish to avoid include lobster, marlin, red snapper, trout, fresh tuna, and white canned albacore tuna. Canned light tuna should be limited to less than 6 ounces weekly, and keep your total fish intake to 9 to 12 ounces weekly. Lower-mercury fish include sole, tilapia, scallops, shrimp, canned salmon (wild Alaskan), and catfish. Eat low-fat fish and trim excess fat as much as possible. Avoid all herbal supplements and herbal products such as teas, as they have not been tested in pregnancy.

Lactation or breast-feeding increases daily energy requirements 500 calories or more above nonpregnancy requirements. Fat stores accumulated during pregnancy also serve as an important energy source for lactation. Fluid needs are also high during this time. Weight loss can occur gradually with lactation, but it is best to try not to lose more than 1 pound weekly, as an overly restrictive diet will decrease the quantity of milk that you produce. High calcium and iron intakes from pregnancy should be maintained, and the prenatal multi-vitamin mineral supplement can be continued. Limit alcohol and caffeine as they can enter breast milk. It may be best to nurse before exercise due to transient changes that occur in breast milk with exercise. When women train at very high intensities or complete interval training, higher levels of lactic acid in the breast milk may result.

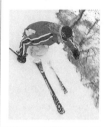

3 Body Fuel: Eating for Training and Recovery

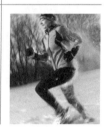

For athletes participating in winter sports, optimal energy output when performance is on the line is everything—whether on the slopes, snow, or ice. At times, participating, training, and perhaps competing in your chosen sport requires tremendous amounts of effort. One very important performance-determining factor is optimal energy production, or power output, over a designated amount of time or distance, while performing the skills and movement specific to your sport. Skiers and snowboarders need to navigate the slopes with speed and dexterity. Cross-country skiers and snowshoers have high aerobic demands for extended periods of time, and hockey players must be able to skate explosively while handling the puck. Skiing and snowboarding rely heavily on short bursts of power, whereas cross-country skiers require a steady power output to perform in their sport.

THE POWER SYSTEMS

Each winter sport has its own unique mix of how body fuel is utilized for energy during various components of an exercise program, during focused training cycles, and during games, competition, and excursions. Appreciating how your body uses fuel for exercise, how your specific training sessions affect energy use and fuel depletion, and how you can best refuel your body to replenish these energy stores is essential to your full nutritional recovery from one training session to the next. Because the way your body uses energy during training directly impacts the nutritional requirements of your sport, winter sport athletes can benefit from a basic review and understanding of energy production and the fuel demands placed on the muscle. Specific nutritional strategies can enhance your body's energy systems and muscle-building efforts, and thus affect your athletic performance.

All of the energy systems use different metabolic pathways to produce energy. How significantly each system will contribute to the energy required for exercise depends on the type of activity performed, which is determined by your sport and training program and how each exercise session is characterized by intensity or the speed at which you train, and how long you train. Obviously, your training sessions can vary in intensity and makeup depending on whether you are building your aerobic system, endurance, or speed, and whether you are training on the slopes, snow, or ice or in the weight room. Some training sessions require quick bursts of activity, some may require steady activity with some periods of faster movement or specific interval training, and other types of training sessions require that your muscles work slowly and continuously. The nutritional needs of the skillful alpine skier, for example, are different from those of the endurance-focused cross-country skier.

The winter sports covered in this book differ in how they utilize these various energy systems during training. The energy to power intense activity is referred to as *anaerobic*, while the energy that powers moderate and steady activity and the recovery process is mainly *aerobic*. Skiing and snowboarding are power and anaerobic sports that benefit from solid aerobic conditioning. Cross-country skiing and snowshoeing are clearly more endurance based and largely depend on a balance between a highly trained aerobic system and specifically trained anaerobic systems. Finally, the team winter sport of hockey requires a combination of high power output for up to 90 seconds, appropriate strength training, and a trained aerobic system for optimal recovery between all-out efforts. Many winter sport athletes are invested in weight training or resistance training to build muscle and strength specific to optimal performance in their sport. While there are some important nutritional principles related to training, performance, and recovery for all winter sport athletes that are to be covered in this part of the book, there are also nutritional strategies specific to each winter sport (covered in Part II).

Your muscles have three energy systems from which to obtain fuel:
• The phosphagen (creatine phosphate) system
• The anaerobic glycolysis (lactic acid) system
• The aerobic system

High-speed activity such as alpine skiing and snowboarding demands the all-out effort of the anaerobic phosphagen system, which may provide energy for up to 10 seconds. This fuel is quickly depleted, but muscles can also use stored carbohydrate or glycogen for fuel, without oxygen or through the anaerobic glycolysis system and at high intensities. There are still limits to this fuel supply, which lasts about 90 seconds or slightly longer, and your muscles will still tap into the aerobic system for energy. Obviously cross-country skiers and snowshoers will train for longer periods due to the nature of these endurance sports and then rely on the aerobic system for fuel, which can burn oxygen for much longer periods of time. The aerobic system only predominates as a fuel source when you are working at low to moderate intensities. Once the pace picks up and your muscles start working faster, oxygen cannot be supplied quickly enough, and it is back to the anaerobic system that predominates. Eventually the anaerobic system runs low on fuel, and you become fatigued. Fuel can also become depleted from use of the lower-intensity aerobic system, but a well-fed athlete should be able to train at lower to moderate levels for several hours.

Well-trained athletes are able to provide plenty of oxygen to their muscles when needed and limit their reliance on the anaerobic system, delaying fatigue. All of these systems, whether aerobic or anaerobic, work best when they have the right fuels available. Some of these fuels are easier to supply than other fuel sources. Fat is in abundant supply, even in the leanest winter sport athletes. Carbohydrates are a much more limited supply and are needed not only as a direct fuel supply but also to allow fat to be burned effectively as a fuel.

ATP: The Ultimate Energy Source

While your muscles contain three different power systems that supply your body with energy for training, ultimately only one source of fuel can be used for muscle contraction: adenosine triphosphate (ATP). You are constantly using ATP for both daily living and training, whether to simply breathe, go to school or work, or practice the skills for your sport. ATP is a high-energy chemical compound found in all muscle cells. When ATP is broken down, the energy released is used for muscle contraction. Because your muscles contain only a small amount of ATP, it must be steadily recharged for training to continue. The rate at which ATP is recharged in your body must meet the demands of the exercise you are performing. Slower-intensity exercise requires a steady supply of ATP, whereas higher-intensity exercise requires a more rapid supply of ATP.

Because your body stores ATP in only small amounts, you require plenty of stored energy to recharge ATP and keep the energy flowing while you train. Body stores of carbohydrate, protein, and fat release varying amounts of ATP at varying rates when they are burned for fuel. Carbohydrate is stored in limited amounts in your blood as glucose and in your muscles and liver as glycogen. Blood glucose is your brain's sole source of energy at rest and during exercise. A steady supply of blood glucose keeps you focused while you traverse across the snow, refine your puck-handling skills, or glide down the slopes.

However, your blood glucose levels can quickly run low to meet the energy demands of training. When this occurs, the liver breaks down its supply of glycogen into glucose and releases it directly into the bloodstream to maintain your blood glucose levels. A well-fed liver can store up to 400 calories' worth of glycogen. But liver glycogen is a relatively short-lived fuel supply that fills up and empties depending on the timing and composition of your last meal. Depending on what you ate and how much you ate, liver glycogen stores generally last from 3 to 5 hours. You have likely experienced hunger and some of the symptoms that come with low blood glucose levels when you have not eaten for several hours. This hunger, which signals the need for fuel, can occur 3 hours after breakfast, in the afternoon before an evening training session, or anytime that your liver stores run low.

Clearly, your liver glycogen and blood glucose levels are a relatively limited supply of fuel. In fact, they can both become depleted fairly quickly during certain types of training sessions and during competition. In contrast to your liver glycogen stores, your muscle glycogen is a much larger storage supply of energy, providing anywhere from 1,400 to 1,800 calories, depending on your body weight and the makeup of your diet. When you train at any intensity from easy to hard, steady or stop-and-go exercise, this glycogen is converted to glucose and used by the muscle fibers for energy. However, when your muscle glycogen stores run low, as can occur during long days and training on the slopes or snow or hard high-intensity and interval training sessions, your muscles can also utilize the glucose in your bloodstream for fuel. You are constantly using your glycogen stores when training at most intensity levels, but how much carbohydrate you actually need, or the rate at which you burn carbohydrate (fast, medium, or slow), depends on how hard and how long you train that day.

Winter sport athletes benefit greatly from ensuring that their muscle glycogen stores are refueled after training sessions that significantly deplete these stores. Even if your training session does not fully deplete muscle glycogen stores, constant partial replacement of stores can drain your performance efforts. Several days of successive training, without adequate glycogen replacement, could ultimately result in poor energy levels and poor training.

Table 3.1 clearly outlines that your body's supply of carbohydrate is relatively limited. These carbohydrate stores are easily depleted during very high-intensity exercise. You have probably experienced the symptoms of low body carbohydrate stores during one training session or another. When your blood glucose levels hit bottom, you may feel dizzy and be unable to focus and concentrate. You may have had to stop exercise altogether or slowed down considerably while consuming carbohydrate to get your blood glucose levels back up. Many winter sport athletes focusing on endurance training have likely experienced

TABLE 3.1 » CALORIES PROVIDED BY BODY FUEL STORES

Carbohydrate Stores	Calories
Blood glucose	80
Liver glycogen	400
Muscle glycogen	1,400–1,800
Fat Stores	
Blood fatty acids	7
Serum triglycerides	75
Muscle triglycerides	2,700
Adipose tissue triglycerides	80,000
Protein Stores	
Muscle protein	30,000

muscle glycogen depletion during which your legs feel heavy and sluggish and normal training seems harder. Winter sport athletes can simply avoid these energy-draining training experiences by starting exercise properly fueled and by consuming enough carbohydrate during exercise to offset body fuel losses.

A quick look at Table 3.1 demonstrates that fat is the body's greatest supply of energy even in the leanest athletes, providing more than 50,000 stored calories depending on body composition. During exercise, when your muscles require fat for fuel, the fat stored within your muscle cells, known as *intramuscular triglycerides*, is used for energy. Just like your muscle glycogen stores, intramuscular triglycerides must be replenished after training, though this fuel is not likely as easily depleted as muscle glycogen. Depending on the intensity and duration of the training session, you will also tap into the fat stored in adipose tissue and convert this fat to fatty acids that are transported to your muscles. It is these more visible body fat stores that provide a relatively unlimited supply of fat for fuel and that are often a focus of the weight management efforts of some winter sport athletes, who may include specific training sessions into their program in order to decrease body fat levels.

Muscle protein stores can also potentially supply several thousand calories worth of energy. However, breaking down your muscle protein for fuel is not ideal for both your recovery and health, and this process could be detrimental to your health and performance. Muscle tissue maintains strength, and constant excess breakdown of this tissue places undue stress on your body and your immune system. Preventing muscle tissue breakdown can best be avoided by maintaining optimal carbohydrate and calorie consumption.

Essentially, fat and glycogen are the major fuels that the body uses for energy during training. Exercise intensity, which can be measured as a percentage of your heart rate, or VO$_2$max, is particularly important in determining which of these two fuels your body prefers. Generally, the harder you train, the more carbohydrate you burn. Interval training or intermittent high-intensity training, in which you take your heart rate to higher intensities repeatedly, burns a significant amount of carbohydrate. Training simply activates the energy system that can best meet the fuel demands of your training session. It is your job to ensure that this energy system is well supplied.

The three energy systems in your body are activated to supply the most appropriate type and amount of fuel that can best meet the energy demands of your training session. If your body needs carbohydrate quickly, then the lactic acid system is activated. If your body requires a steady supply of fat, the aerobic system is activated. The ATP-CP system can be activated for an all-out sprint effort. Table 3.2 summarizes the characteristics of these energy systems. Figure 3.1 illustrates the duration of exercise that is possible when maximizing the use of one energy system.

TABLE 3.2 » THE BODY'S ENERGY SYSTEMS

Anaerobic Systems

ATP-CP System	Anaerobic Glycolysis (Lactic Acid System)
Anaerobic	High rate ATP production
Highest rate of ATP production	Limited supply ATP lasting 1.5-2 minutes
Very limited supply of ATP lasting 6-8 seconds	High power output and intensity level
Highest power output and intensity level	Uses ATP, creatine phosphate, and muscle
Uses ATP and creatine phosphate stored in body	glycogen for fuel
Development of explosive power	Development of lactate tolerance

The Aerobic System

Glycolytic (Aerobic Glycolysis)	Glycolytic and Lipolytic
15-90 minutes of exercise	Greater than 90 minutes of exercise
Low rate of ATP production	Lowest rate of ATP production
High supply ATP	High supply ATP
Low power production	Lowest power output
Lower intensity	Lowest intensity level
15-30 minutes of exercise: use muscle glycogen and blood glucose for energy	Longer than 90 minutes of exercise: use muscle glycogen, blood glucose, intramuscular fat, and adipose tissue fat
60-90 minutes of exercise: use muscle glycogen, blood glucose, and intramuscular fat for energy	for energy

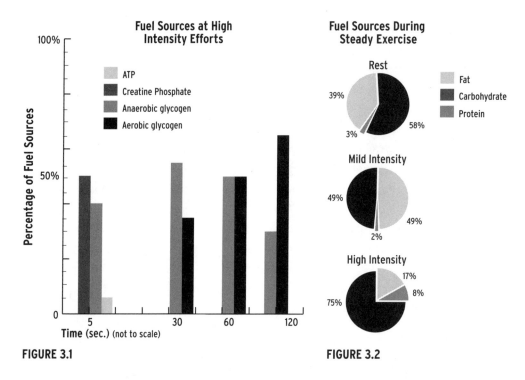

FIGURE 3.1   **FIGURE 3.2**

NOTE: The duration and intensity of exercise determines the fuel sources utilized.

It's also important for you to realize that although you may specifically train a selected energy system, the majority of the time neither aerobic nor anaerobic metabolism works exclusively to provide energy during practice and competition, though one energy system may predominate during various types of training sessions. While one system may predominate during a training session, these two metabolic pathways can work together and complement one another to meet the body's energy demands.

The Phosphagen System (The ATP-CP System)

As its name indicates, the ATP-CP system consists of both ATP and another high-energy compound called creatine phosphate (CP). Because ATP is in such short supply, it must be continuously and rapidly resynthesized to provide energy. Like ATP, CP is an energy-rich compound. When it is broken down, it, too, supplies energy. However, CP's released energy does not directly fuel muscle contraction. Rather, the energy released by CP resynthesizes ATP. Like ATP and the energy released from it, CP is in short supply. Energy from the ATP-CP system can fuel high-intensity efforts for only 6 to 8 seconds. Even at 6 seconds' duration, only half of your energy needs come from ATP-CP. Fast-twitch muscle fibers use the ATP-CP system rapidly. This system fuels the initial seconds of sprint events and other events where maximal force is required. It is an important fuel source for downhill skiers and snowboarders where single bursts of sustained high-intensity activity are utilized during runs. For hockey players, cross-country skiers, and snowshoers, any type of workout that involves successive bursts of high-intensity activity intermingled with lower-intensity activity will also rely on the phosphagen system for fuel.

The winter sport athlete who has the ability to store more creatine would have an advantage during this type of training. With enhanced storage of this important fuel, you can maintain a higher power output on the successive bouts of very high-intensity activity. To improve the storage of creatine in your muscle, you must perform activities that focus on this energy system, by performing high-intensity movements that are repeated multiple times during an exercise session. Also consuming enough calories, carbohydrate, and protein for recovery improves your short-duration, high-intensity performance.

Anaerobic Glycolysis

Glycolysis is the second metabolic pathway within your muscle cells that is capable of rapidly producing ATP. As its name indicates, this occurs through the breakdown of glycogen or carbohydrate, without oxygen being present. In glycolysis, a single glucose molecule is broken down from muscle glycogen to produce ATP. Anaerobic glycolysis provides energy for short-duration, high-intensity exercise, lasting 10 seconds to several minutes. As exercise continues beyond 1 to 2 minutes, this system provides less than half of your energy needs. Anaerobic glycolysis fuels activities such as skating across the ice or navigating a slope or high-intensity interval training sessions. At the onset of intense exercise when oxygen cannot be delivered to your muscles quickly enough, this energy system is rapidly ignited to supply ATP.

The predominant source of energy during this type of activity is stored muscle glycogen. When this fuel runs out, your muscles cannot continue to perform at the same intensity, and you become fatigued. This anaerobic energy source runs out quickly (90 seconds) and must be followed by a period of rest, about 3 to 5 minutes, for your muscles to become replenished with energy. This rest and recovery time is just as important as the high-intensity training time. For hockey players going at full effort at various moments in a game, this anaerobic pathway is crucial.

For the power sports of skiing and snowboarding, fat is less likely to be metabolized as a fuel, while creatine phosphate and muscle glycogen are mainly used for energy. Because of this low reliance on fat for fuel and the nature of multiple periods of rest when training (going back up the mountain) skiers and snowboarders generally compete at higher levels of body fat than competitive endurance winter athletes. Another important aspect of these two sports is that there is an off-season during which the athlete's training program may change dramatically. Often weight and body fat can be gained during the off-season. However, due to heavy training schedules and weight-training programs, many winter sport athletes such as cross-country skiers may actually have fairly high energy needs due to their large level of muscle mass and the high amount of energy required for training, which can include several practices a day and often a weight-training program. Nutrition programs need to be adjusted for various times of the season to prevent extremes in weight gain or weight cycling. Since weight training is often a large part of the winter sport athlete's diet, Chapter 5 is devoted to nutritional strategies for maximizing muscle building.

Aerobic Metabolism

The aerobic pathway is the primary energy source for lower-intensity, prolonged exercise. This system is glycolytic and lipolytic as it derives energy from both carbohydrates and fat, respectively. This pathway provides half of the energy for exercise lasting longer than 1 minute and the majority of the energy for exercise lasting longer than 2 minutes. When you begin exercise, you initially use the anaerobic pathways for energy but then switch to a predominantly aerobic pathway. An adequate supply of oxygen must be delivered to the muscles in order for the oxygen system to release the energy stored in carbohydrates and fats. Protein is not normally used for energy production, but under certain conditions it may become a significant source of energy for the oxygen system.

While the aerobic system cannot produce ATP as rapidly as the two anaerobic systems, it can produce much greater quantities at a slower rate. The rate at which the oxygen system produces ATP also depends on whether aerobic glycolysis (carbohydrate) or aerobic lipolysis (fat) is burned for fuel. Carbohydrate is a more efficient fuel than fat and is the predominant fuel for steady exercise lasting more than 2 minutes and up to 3 hours. But your storage capacity for carbohydrates in the muscles and liver is inadequate for certain endurance events, whereas fat stores are extensive. For the winter sport athlete, however, glycogen depletion can occur when combining aerobic training with anaerobic training, eventually depleting muscle glycogen stores. For longer and lower-intensity ultraendurance events, lasting 4 to 6 hours, fat is primarily burned for energy, though this aspect of fuel burning is less applicable to many winter sport athletes but could be relevant to ultraendurance cross-country skiing.

The endurance power/middle-distance sport of hockey does utilize the aerobic system as training combines periods of steady, continuous movement with occasional fast bursts of movement. Cross-country skiing and snowshoeing are endurance sports that require good fuel reserves for continuous and steady movement. For any winter sport, having adequate fuel stores for various types of training is crucial, and running low on fuel leads to fatigue and poor-quality training sessions. These types of training sessions benefit not only from the right nutrient mix in the daily diet but also proper nutrient intake immediately before, during, and after training.

MUSCLE FIBER TYPES

There is also a link between exercise performance and the composition of muscle fibers. The three major fiber types, Type I, IIa, and IIb, all have specific training properties. Type I fibers are slow-twitch fibers that predominate in endurance activities such as cross-country skiing and snowshoeing. These fibers have a high capacity to produce aerobic energy and store fat for fuel. Both Type IIa and IIb fibers are fast-twitch fibers that can produce anaerobic energy but differ in some of their characteristics. Type IIa fibers are more of an intermediate fast-twitch fiber and also have the ability to produce energy aerobically. The type of training that you perform affects the aerobic capacity of this fiber, which can behave more like an endurance fiber with aerobic training. The IIb muscle fiber is purely fast-twitch and anaerobic and has a high capacity to produce power and store and burn muscle glycogen.

The fat-burning, slow-twitch Type I fibers are larger and predominate in the larger muscle groups. Type II fibers are narrow and create speed. Not surprisingly, cross-country skiers have been measured to have a higher percentage of Type I fibers than other types of skiers, while alpine skiers have a greater percentage of Type II fibers in their lower extremities.

TABLE 3.3 » PHYSIOLOGICAL PROFILE OF WINTER SPORTS

Sport	Physiological Characteristics
POWER SPORTS	
Alpine skiing	Primarily uses the phosphagen and anaerobic glycolysis systems
	Training specific muscle groups for motor skills takes precedence over aerobic training.
	Requires muscular strength, anaerobic power, coordination, agility, balance, and flexibility
	Moderate aerobic power should be developed to allow for quicker recovery between repeated bouts of anaerobic exercise.
	Some downhill events (slalom, giant slalom) derive energy from both aerobic and anaerobic fuel systems.
	Speed events or longer runs may derive a greater contribution from the aerobic system, up to 50 percent.
	Weight-training programs should be specific to skiing movement.
	There is a high rate of muscle glycogen use that can result in significant depletion of these fuel stores by the end of the day.

CONTINUED

TABLE 3.3 continued

Sport	Physiological Characteristics
POWER SPORTS	
Snowboarding	Primarily uses the phosphagen and anaerobic glycolysis system
	Requires muscular strength, anaerobic power, coordination, agility, balance, and flexibility
	Moderate to high aerobic power and conditioning should be developed to allow for quicker recovery between repeated bouts of anaerobic exercise and qualifying rounds for competition.
	Weight-training programs should be specific to snowboarding movement.
	Uses greater amount of upper-body strength than alpine skiing
	Freestyle snowboarders require high aerobic conditioning to "hike the pike" and return to the top.
	Long training days can result in significant amounts of glycogen depletion.
ENDURANCE SPORTS	
Cross-country skiing	Heavy reliance on the aerobic system
	Also uses anaerobic glycolysis
	Very high energy demands
	Complete sport that utilizes total body fitness
	Top skiers have a high VO_2max.
	Top elite skiers are lean.
Snowshoeing	Utilizes the aerobic and anaerobic systems
	When using poles, requires both upper- and lower-body strength
	Requires coordination over varying terrain
	Utilizes mainly the hip flexors, upper leg muscles, and calf muscles
	Requires flexibility and balance
	High energy demands that vary with snow conditions
TEAM SPORTS	
Hockey	Power sport
	Middle-distance sport depending on practice and playing time
	Heavy reliance on phosphagen system, moderate reliance on anaerobic glycolysis, and some reliance on aerobic
	Trained aerobic system improves recovery
	Requires variety of skills including skating at high speeds, turning and maneuvering, and racing for the puck
	Requires strength endurance, agility, and balance

Summary

Although winter sports have distinct differences in terms of their physiological profiles, training programs, and ultimately nutritional requirements, some basic nutrition concepts apply to all of these winter sports. The unique nutritional demands for each sport will be addressed in more detail in Part II, but we can summarize the following about winter sports:

- Winter sport athletes need to start training, day excursions, and competition with adequate fuel stores.
- Winter sport athletes all need to pay attention to the principles of hydration and can become dehydrated during any type of exercise.
- The majority of fuel that supplies energy for athletes participating in winter sports is stored within the muscle.
- Winter sports all require a high level of skill and technique development unique to that particular sport.
- The proper nutrient diet mix and energy intake maximizes recovery of fuel stores and supports development of optimal body composition.
- Adequate amounts of carbohydrate are required to replenish muscle glycogen stores.
- Winter sport athletes frequently include resistance training in their program to varying degrees during the season and require the proper nutritional program to support these efforts.
- Timing of nutrient intake before, during, and after exercise can improve the quality of training.
- Optimal fluid, electrolyte, and carbohydrate intake during training and competition can improve performance.

Power Sports

- The power winter sport athletes rely heavily on the short-lived phosphagen with ATP and creatine phosphate as fuel sources, and the anaerobic glycolytic systems with muscle glycogen as a fuel source.
- These power sports rely to varying degrees on the aerobic system, but mainly through carbohydrate as a fuel source, with limited use of intramuscular fat as a fuel source.
- The power downhill sports and hockey benefit from the development of moderate to high aerobic power for moderate-intensity activity and improved recovery.

Endurance Sports

- The endurance winter sports rely mainly on the aerobic system and anaerobic glycolysis for fuel sources.
- Extended training sessions for these endurance sports increase reliance on intramuscular triglycerides for a fuel source.
- These sports have high energy demands depending on the distance and intensity of the training session.

Team Sports

- Hockey players rely on all three fuel systems, but mainly the short-lived phosphagen system and heavily on the anaerobic glycolysis system with muscle glycogen as a fuel source.
- A trained aerobic system improves recovery between all-out efforts on the ice.

FOODS AND FLUIDS FOR REFUELING AND RECOVERY

Several essential nutrition practices transform your diet from one designed for good health based on consuming a variety of nutritious foods (as outlined in Chapter 1), to a sports diet that is designed to provide fuel for your chosen winter sport. High-performance training nutrition is a direct result of choosing the right portions of various types of foods and nutrients at the right times. Portions and timing of food intake should match your training session and current training cycle. Because winter sports are highly seasonal, often only the most serious and elite competitors train on the slopes, snow, and ice year-round. Training nutrition must also match with your current training cycle, whether it is serious training for another sport in the warmer months, or off-season and preseason training specific to your winter sport.

This chapter focuses on the big picture of your recovery diet—the food and fluid strategies that replenish your body stores after training and up to the next training session, including meals and snacks throughout the day:

- Consuming optimal energy or balance of calories for recovery from training, tissue building, and growth for younger athletes
- Consuming enough grams of carbohydrate to match that day's level of glycogen depletion and to be adequately fueled before the next training session
- Timing your intake of carbohydrate to expedite the process of muscle glycogen recovery resynthesis
- Consuming optimal amounts of protein for muscle recovery, muscle tissue repair, and maintaining a strong immune system

- Consuming healthy fats and good sources of essential fatty acids to balance out the diet and calorie intake after meeting carbohydrate and protein requirements
- Consuming adequate amounts of fluids and electrolytes, particularly sodium after training to rehydrate and replenish body fluids
- Timing your postexercise meals and snacks to maximize recovery until the next training session, particularly immediate postexercise nutrition recovery guidelines

Remember that your nutritional recovery can vary depending on the time of training season, where you are specifically in your winter season training program, and the time of day in relation to your training session. So your nutritional needs can vary with the season, month, week, day, and hour.

The Phases of Glycogen Replenishment

Because muscle glycogen is the fuel source most likely to be depleted with winter sport exercise and training, it is the fuel that receives the most attention in regard to recovery nutrition. Initially there is a very rapid phase of muscle glycogen repletion that lasts 30 to 60 minutes. This rapid phase occurs without the use of insulin and when your muscle glycogen stores are very low after exercise. After this 60-minute post-training period, insulin is needed to make muscle glycogen, and the rate at which you can make muscle glycogen slows down. However, during the 6 hours after training, providing your body with adequate amounts of carbohydrate at regular intervals is one of the most important strategies for muscle glycogen recovery. Taking advantage of this carbohydrate timing is very important if your next training session takes place in less than 12 hours. If you do not train for another 24 hours, the hours after training remain important, but muscle glycogen replenishment is possible over the 24-hour period if you consume enough carbohydrates.

PERIODIZING YOUR RECOVERY NUTRITION PLAN

As a winter sport athlete, it is very likely that your training program changes throughout the year depending on your level of competition and participation in your sport. You may approach your winter sport from a recreational perspective, while training very seriously for an endurance sport or team sport during other times of the year. It is very likely that you have a lot to accomplish in your yearly training program, including aerobic conditioning, anaerobic conditioning, developing strength and power, building muscular endurance, and developing quickness, agility, speed, and flexibility. All of these components of your training program complement one another to ultimately improve your performance. At specific times of the year, you may highlight a particular component of your program. Certain components of your program need to be built before others, while others are emphasized when specific training components of your program are de-emphasized. The year-round schedule and cycling of your training program is called periodization, and it is designed to optimize performance results and prevent overtraining.

An entire year of conditioning and training is referred to as the *macrocycle*, which is broken down into smaller *mesocycles*, generally off-season, preseason, in-season, and post-season. Each mesocycle is further broken down into *microcycles* around which the athlete's weekly schedule is planned.

How you plan your off-season, preseason, in-season, and postseason program depends on your sport, level of training and perhaps competition, and participation in other sports during the warmer months. Generally the off-season is time to build a base for both aerobic fitness and strength. In the preseason, training shifts to more sport-specific activity and more high-intensity training, speed work, and intervals. During the season, you focus on preparing for competition, maintaining fitness and developing any weaker areas. Depending on your sport and whether you are a high school, collegiate, masters, or professional athlete, you may compete several times a week, in weekend tournaments, or only once weekly or monthly during the season, all of which affects your training program and recovery time. Postseason is a rest period and varies in length for each sport and athlete.

These cycles in your training program all require adjustments in your diet composition and meal timing. Changes in your diet can occur in a number of ways, depending on your specific program. For example, you may need to adjust your total caloric intake for decreases in intensity of training. During the off-season, the overall intensity of your program may decrease and be focused on aerobic conditioning. Your energy needs for training may lessen without the intensity of preseason training and competition. Volume may also build with low-intensity aerobic base building and affect your carbohydrate and energy requirements as this training cycle progresses.

As you build a strength base, you may require a heavy focus on the nutritional strategies required for muscle building. (These guidelines are reviewed in Chapter 5.) Depending on your program, your energy and carbohydrate needs may still be quite high, with a different focus on the timing of your meals and snacks and a modification in the timing of your protein and carbohydrate intake.

Meal-timing adjustments can be made depending on your training schedule. After high-intensity, shorter duration, and interval training, you should still focus on recovery nutrition and beginning the glycogen resynthesis process. After more moderate training, continue to focus on rehydration, even for workouts that are only mildly dehydrating.

Refer to the guidelines for calories, carbohydrates, and protein provided in this chapter that are based on the volume and intensity of training to determine how these nutrient requirements can change during the season and for each training cycle. Carbohydrate requirements can decrease when volume and intensity drop off and there is less training time. The breakdown of your diet may change, with less emphasis on carbohydrates and a slight shift to increased protein in the strength-building phase and during the preseason.

How nutritional needs cycle throughout the season is unique to each athlete. These requirements can vary with your body composition goals, individual training program, development of skills, and both aerobic and anaerobic conditioning as you fine-tune the program that best fits your sport and specific goals. Table 3.4 outlines how various types of training sessions can affect your daily nutritional needs and ultimately recovery. If you train for an endurance sport in the nonwinter months, please refer to *Sports Nutrition for Endurance Athletes* (VeloPress) for a nutrition program. Winter sport athletes who participate in a team sport during the nonwinter months can refer to *Performance Nutrition for Team Sports* (Peak Sports Press) for their sport-specific nutritional advice.

Daily Nutritional Recovery

Recovery for the winter sport athlete starts when training finishes and takes place until the next training session begins. Depending on your training schedule and training cycle, your recovery nutrition strategies may focus on the next 24, 12, 8, or even 4 hours to restore adequate amounts of fuel before exercise begins again. Your daily diet is your recovery diet, and you must appreciate the amount and types of fuel burned during various training efforts in order to time and portion your meals and snacks properly. Daily recovery results in solid training and sustains you from week to week during your training program (Table 3.4).

Energy for Training

As a winter sport athlete who wants to excel and enjoy your sport, you must consume the amount of energy or daily calories that your body requires for both everyday life and training. At times your training can be tough and tiring, and eating enough food is essential to completing demanding training programs that test your endurance, power, and skill.

Many athletes speculate on the calorie intake that they should consume for both their training and body composition goals. Estimating energy needs is not a precise science, and although many formulas work fairly well, every athlete has a unique energy system with its own tally of energy burning throughout the day. Your daily energy requirements are made up of the following components:

Resting metabolic rate (RMR), which is the amount of energy required to keep your body functioning metabolically at rest, such as basic brain function, breathing, and keeping your heart beating. You also burn a little bit of energy when you digest food, but this

TABLE 3.4 » DAILY NUTRITIONAL RECOVERY FOR TRAINING SESSIONS

Type of Training Session	Recovery Requirements
AEROBIC CONDITIONING, <60 MINUTES Example: Cardiovascular gym workout on various machines	Rehydrate as needed based on weight changes before and after exercise. Drink fluids until urine is clear. Follow with moderate amount of carbohydrate snack or consume carbohydrate-containing meal within 1 hour of training. Calorie requirements for the day are generally lower with shorter training time. Carbohydrate requirements can increase with higher-intensity training. Moderate protein requirements. Low-fat requirements.
INTERVAL TRAINING, 60–90 MINUTES Examples: Intense hockey practice Off-season running or cycling training Higher-intensity endurance training on the snow	Replenish with fluids and carbohydrates within 30 minutes of training. Consume 0.5 g carbohydrate per pound body weight (1 g/kg). Can consume 10 to 15 g of high-quality protein. Consume 24 oz. fluid for every pound (0.5 kg) of body weight lost during training. Consume a snack or meal containing carbohydrate and protein within 2 hours of initial recovery fuel intake. Calorie requirements are higher with high-intensity training and increased duration of training. Require moderate to high amount of carbohydrates due to intensity and duration of training session.
ENDURANCE TRAINING, >90 MINUTES Example: Steady snowshoeing and cross-country ski snow training	Consume 0.5 g carbohydrate per pound of body weight (1 g/kg weight) within 30 minutes of training. Consume 24 oz. fluid for pound (0.5 kg) of body weight lost during training. Consume a snack or meal containing carbohydrate and protein within 2 hours of initial recovery fuel. Calorie requirements are high due to duration of training. Moderate to high carbohydrate needs as training sessions increase in duration. Moderate to high protein requirements. Need to meet fat requirements with very long training sessions.
RESISTANCE TRAINING Example: Both low-weight/ endurance work and high-weight/power-building work	Within 1 hour after training consume 10-20 g high-quality protein and 50-75 g of carbohydrate. Drink fluids as needed to rehydrate. Consume protein and carbohydrate mix within 3 hours after training. Require additional calories for optimal muscle building. Need moderate to high amounts of protein. Meet daily fat requirements.
SUSTAINED BURSTS OF HIGH-INTENSITY TRAINING WITH REST PERIODS Example: Alpine skiing and snow-board training on the mountain	Emphasize recovery nutrition strategies after runs. Replenish with carbohydrate and fluid. Consume 8 to 16 oz. of a sports drink at regular intervals. Replenish fuel stores with a midday meal high in carbohydrate and containing moderate amounts of protein. Rehydrate so that urine is clear. Follow similar guidelines for an evening meal.

is not a large factor in your energy balance equation. For many North Americans, your RMR accounts for 60 to 75 percent of your total energy expenditure for the day. However, this percentage can be far lower for many athletes who burn a significant number of calories when training. Metabolic rate can be measured now outside strict laboratory conditions with a decent degree of accuracy, allowing you to more accurately predict your energy needs. RMR can vary greatly from athlete to athlete. RMR decreases with age, is greater in individuals with greater body mass, increases with greater muscle mass, and decreases with greater body fat stores. These are only some of the factors that affect your RMR.

Growth, which refers to children and adolescent athletes who are experiencing the high energy needs of growth, as well as the energy demands of being active and involved in a winter sport. Pregnant and breast-feeding female athletes are also going though a period where their energy needs increase (see the sidebar in Chapter 2), with an additional 350 calories above normal required in the second trimester of pregnancy and an additional 500 calories above normal required in the third trimester of pregnancy.

Daily physical activity, which includes the small amount of calories burned when you work (unless you have a very physically active job) or go to school. For many individuals, activity may only comprise 15 percent of their energy requirements.

Training expenditure, or the amount of calories that you burn with exercise. This can be a large or small variable for the winter sport athlete depending on that day's training intensity and duration. A cross-country skier burns through thousands of calories with several hours of outdoor skiing, while a 60-minute gym workout in the evening after work burns significantly fewer calories.

Estimating Energy Needs

While determining energy needs is not a precise science, some general indicators can give you an appreciation of just how low, moderate, or high your calorie needs may be for daily recovery from one training session to the next. Of course, many athletes want to consider the proper calorie adjustments to be made for their body composition goals, whether for muscle building, fat loss, or both. More specific nutritional information on changing body composition is provided in Chapter 5.

One method for estimating daily calorie needs is based on the amount of calories you require per pound of body weight as directly related to the amount of training you complete that day. When in serious training mode and preparing for an important day of exercise on the slopes, a long training session, or competition, it is best not to fall short on your calorie requirements. Several days in a row of not recharging your batteries fully may result in some unplanned rest days, days off, or poor-quality training sessions, all of which can hamper your athletic goals.

The calorie descriptions listed here explain how your activity can affect your total calorie needs for that day. Clearly energy needs are not consistent every day. A 160-pound (73-kilogram) adult who trains for 90 minutes one day would require 18 to 24 calories per pound (40 to 53 kilocalories per kilogram) of body weight, or 2,880 to 3,840 calories to meet their energy needs, while that same adult completing 3 hours of training would require 24 to 29 calories per pound (52 to 63 kilocalories per kilogram) of body weight, or up to 4,640 calories for training.

Mild activity, with no purposeful exercise or training: 12 to 14 calories per pound (26 to 31 kilocalories per kilogram) body weight

Moderate activity, with up to 1 hour of moderate intensity exercise: 15 to 17 calories per pound (33 to 37 kilocalories per kilogram) body weight

High activity, with 1 to 2 hours daily of moderate intensity exercise: 18 to 24 calories per pound (40 to 53 kilocalories per kilogram) body weight

Very high activity, with several hours of training daily: 24 to 29 calories per pound (53 to 63 kilocalories per kilogram) body weight

Calories burned for a particular day of training can also be estimated based on your estimated or measured RMR, daily activity when not training, and the amount of calories that you burn specific to your sport or activity and the amount of time that you train. RMR is generally estimated at 11 to 12 calories per pound (24 to 26 kilocalories per kilogram) of body weight, but it can be lower or higher in some individuals. You can also have your RMR tested now at various health and training centers with the newer, portable versions of testing equipment. Daily expenditure outside of training may add another few hundred calories daily. But clearly the amount of calories you burn can add up depending on your training. Table 3.5 outlines the amount of calories burned per minute for various body weights.

For example, a cross-country skier who weighs 140 pounds (64 kilograms) could estimate her RMR at 1,540 calories. She has a desk job and drives to work and may burn another 150 to 200 calories daily. When she trains on the snow for 2 hours at a pace of 4 miles per hour, she burns a total of about 1,300 calories. On this training day her total energy needs run from 2,990 to 3,040 calories. If she spends one day of the week training indoors and does about 1 hour of moderate aerobic conditioning, she may burn 400 calories and require 2,090 to 2,140 calories for the day. Clearly adjustments need to be made in energy intake based on that day's training.

The calorie expenditure in Table 3.5 is listed per minute of activity. For the endurance sports of cross-country skiing and snowshoeing, estimating the expenditure of your training is fairly straightforward because your activity is often steady with some higher-intensity efforts. Hockey players should estimate the energy burned based on actual time

TABLE 3.5 » CALORIE EXPENDITURE PER MINUTE OF WINTER SPORTS AND TRAINING ACTIVITIES

	Weight in pounds (kg)										
	100 (45)	110 (50)	120 (55)	130 (59)	140 (64)	150 (68)	160 (73)	170 (77)	180 (82)	190 (86)	200 (91)
DOWNHILL SPORTS											
Alpine skiing	6.5	7.2	7.8	8.5	9.5	9.9	10.5	11.2	11.9	12.5	13.2
Leisure alpine skiing (males)	5.1	5.6	6	6.5	7	7.5	8	8.5	9	9.5	10
Leisure alpine skiing (females)	4.5	4.9	5.3	5.8	7.1	7.5	7.2	7.5	8	8.4	8.9
Alpine snowboarding	No published data. Use values for alpine skiing to estimate energy requirements.										
ENDURANCE SPORTS											
Cross-country skiing 4 mph (6.5 km/hr)	6.5	7.2	7.8	8.5	9.2	9.9	10.5	8.5	9	9.5	10
Cross-country skiing 5 mph (8 km/hr)	7.7	8.4	9.2	10	10.8	11.5	12.3	13.1	13.9	14.7	15.4
Snow-shoeing 3 mph (5.6 km/hr) on fresh unpacked powder	7.7	8.5	9.2	10	10.8	11.5	12.3	13.1	13.9	14.7	15.4
HOCKEY	6.6	7.3	8	8.7	9.4	10	10.7	11.4	12.1	12.7	13.4
WEIGHT TRAINING	5.2	5.7	6.2	6.8	7.3	7.8	8.3	8.9	9.4	9.9	10.5
AEROBIC CONDITIONING (MODERATE INTENSITY)	4.7	5.2	5.7	6.1	6.5	7	7.5	7.9	8.3	8.9	9.4

of practice. Skiers and snowboarders need to note that calories are burned down the slopes, with far fewer calories burned during time spent going up the mountain after each run. Resistance training is often part of an exercise program for many winter sport athletes and can contribute significant calorie burning to the entire training program.

Seasoned athletes can also become much more efficient in the movement they create when training for their sport. This can result in fewer calories burned when training. Newer athletes who are not as efficient in their movement can also burn more calories when training. Many athletes now train with a heart rate monitor that can provide reading for calorie burning.

Carbohydrate—The Recovery Fuel

While you may or may not have experienced the symptoms of glycogen depletion during a single training team session, the symptoms of gradual glycogen depletion due to inadequate carbohydrate recovery can occur over successive days of training and be much more subtle. Symptoms of glycogen depletion can creep up over a week's time or longer, producing feelings of sluggishness or heaviness. Besides general lethargy, you may put out an increased or even normal effort during training and find it difficult to maintain your usual intensity and duration of training. The more muscle glycogen stores in your body, the faster you skate across the ice, the longer you can skillfully complete one ski run after another, or the faster you can ski to run across the snow. Figure 3.3 illustrates how gradual glycogen depletion due to training and inadequate carbohydrate intake can occur.

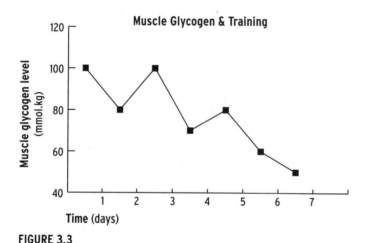

FIGURE 3.3

NOTE: Glycogen depletion is directly related to the exercise intensity and duration and the amount of carbohydrate consumed between exercise sessions.

Numerous scientifi   ）ohydrate is
superior in building, m   The amount
of carbohydrate you co   gen you store
in your muscles and 1   l to partial replenishment of mus   ccurs from one
day to the next, gly   : time, and your
training will suffe   raining session,
whether it is 4, 8   .e exercise at the
desired duration

Daily Carboh   ıg

Carbohydrate   total calories. This
is appropriat   :n the goal is to decrease unwa   :s from whole grains
and fruits   more appropriate to
express ca   :ight based on the intensity an   day. Regardless of the
type of tra   t of carbohydrate to recover sufficiei..,,.   : are endurance based or
that include plenty of high-intensit, _   lete carbohydrate stores.

The ceiling for daily carbohydrate consumption, aι w.. ＿point your muscle storage capacity has been reached, is 4.5 to 5.5 grams of carbohydrate for every pound (10 to 12 grams per kilogram) of weight. Depending on the size of the athlete, this translates to anywhere from 500 to 700 grams of carbohydrate daily, and higher levels than these absolute amounts may not resynthesize muscle glycogen stores faster. Most winter sport athletes who meet both their energy and carbohydrate needs can average about 50 to 60 percent carbohydrate calories in their training diet. But depending on whether you are restricting calories for weight management or have very high energy needs, the percentage of carbohydrate consumed may vary. Typically, as an athlete, you will have to consume greater quantities of carbohydrate than most people, including athletes participating in sports that do not have as high a fuel demand as many winter sport training sessions (see Table 3.6).

Practical Carbohydrate Issues

As an athlete, you must make a concerted effort to obtain adequate amounts of carbohydrate at specific times in portions that allow you to prepare for training, recovery from training, and competition. While one of the significant challenges in the North American food environment is obtaining wholesome carbohydrates conveniently, consuming the

TABLE 3.6 » DAILY CARBOHYDRATE REQUIREMENTS FOR TRAINING

Grams per Pound of Weight (g/kg weight)	Training Regimen	Example
4.5-5.5 (10-12)	Duration 3-4 hours daily at moderate/ high intensity	Long cross-country and snowshoeing excursions. Extended alpine skiing time on slopes with runs totaling over 3 hours. Extended hockey practice.
3.0-4.5 (7-10)	Duration 90 minutes to 3 hours daily at moderate/high intensity	Weight training and aerobic conditioning reaching 90 minutes.
2.25-3.0 (5-7)	Moderate intensity under 1 hour daily or low intensity for several hours daily	Indoor aerobic conditioning workout or light resistance training session

proper amounts at the right times also requires focus. Some winter sport athletes can easily meet their carbohydrate requirements on specific training days with plenty of well-chosen wholesome carbohydrates. However, on specific training days for many team sport athletes, the amounts required for fuel may exceed appetite and hunger levels and even exceed the portions that are typically provided in the North American diet. While wholesome carbohydrates are appreciated for their nutritional content and health benefits, for specific times around training, you may need to focus on carbohydrate-rich foods that are appealing, convenient, and carbohydrate-dense for a given serving in order to maximize your nutritional recovery.

Food tables that provide carbohydrate portions for 30-gram servings are provided in Chapter 6, which covers meal planning and provides practical guidelines for putting together a top winter sport diet. You can match up these carbohydrate amounts to provide you with the total grams of carbohydrate required for training on a given day. A 180-pound snowshoer training for 3 hours one day may require a full 700 grams of carbohydrate, while a snowboarder of the same weight practicing skills on the slopes for several hours may require only 400 grams of carbohydrate daily. Consuming 400 grams of carbohydrate in a given training day is much simpler than consuming 700 grams, as attaining the higher carbohydrate amount would likely require more structure and planning.

The food system outlined in Chapter 6 provides you with the flexibility to emphasize various carbohydrate sources from one day to the next, depending on your food preferences, fuel needs, training schedule, and training cycle. However, for those very high-carbohydrate days with a full and intense day on the slopes, during the height of hockey season, and for the endurance winter sports, you may want to consider the suggestions described in the following paragraphs.

Sports bars or energy bars are a concentrated and convenient source of carbohydrate, supplying up to 50 grams per serving. They travel well and can be consumed quickly between training sessions or on the way back to class or work. But do keep in mind that these bars are often vitamin and mineral fortified. Make sure that you do not consume too high doses of these nutrients simply by overconsuming sports bars. Energy bars should not replace fruits, vegetables, and whole grains in your diet but simply add to a high-energy, high-carbohydrate diet.

Low-fiber carbohydrate foods may be more practical when carbohydrate needs to be consumed in very large amounts on hard and intense training days. They can be consumed in combination with higher-fiber items and still be part of a diet that is adequate in fiber, vitamins, and minerals. Choices include large bagels, calorically dense cereals, fruit juices, jams, honey, and syrup.

A well-timed snack of yogurt with fruit, a low-fat milkshake, or fruit smoothie can up your carbohydrate intake considerably and provide needed fluid as well. They also taste good! High-carbohydrate supplement drinks or meal replacements may also be a convenient source of carbohydrate and are easy to carry and quickly consumed. These products should not replace wholesome foods. Desserts can be part of a nutritious diet in reasonable amounts. Some carbohydrate-dense choices include sherbet, sorbet, and frozen yogurt topped with fruit.

Meeting your daily carbohydrate intake often requires consuming between-meal snacks and "grazing" throughout the day. Carbohydrate-rich foods should comprise at least half of your meals and snacks. Low-fiber choices may be best tolerated when food is consumed close to the start of exercise.

Keep an eye out for carbohydrate foods that are also high in fat (often unhealthy fats), such as croissants, creamed or deep-fried vegetables, doughnuts, French toast, fried rice, muffins, pancakes, pastry, potato chips, snack crackers, and popcorn popped with oil.

Obtaining the total grams of carbohydrate that you require to match your training may be your biggest nutritional challenge on specific training days, particularly on hard training days. While you want to emphasize fruits, vegetables, and whole grains, higher carbohydrate needs for more intense and longer training may require that you incorporate less filling but carbohydrate-dense foods into your diet. Meeting these higher carbohydrate amounts requires planning and a good appetite.

Protein and Your Daily Recovery Requirements

While carbohydrate intake is clearly emphasized in your winter sport diet, your training program and training for power and strength also increase your need for protein. Protein needs are higher in winter sport athletes who incorporate resistance training into their program and who benefit from increased muscle mass for athletic performance (see Table 3.7). Team sports such as hockey can also have a significant wear and tear on the muscles and ligaments, requiring protein for repair. Winter sport athletes who engage in strength training can rely on glycogen for fuel during this mode of exercise and, most important, should consume enough adequate carbohydrate so that protein is not utilized for fuel during training.

What is most important for you to appreciate is that your elevated protein requirements are easily met by a well-planned sports diet. What distinguishes a sports diet is how you time your protein intake, particularly around resistance training (see Chapter 5). Often the higher calorie intake of your sports nutrition plan simply results in more total protein being consumed. Most North Americans consume a diet that easily meets the protein needs of an athlete participating in a demanding training program. Inadequate protein

TABLE 3.7 » PROTEIN REQUIREMENTS

Exercise Profile	Protein Requirements per Weight
Endurance and team sport training	Moderate training: 0.45 g/lb. (1 g/kg) Heavy training: 0.50-0.75 g/lb. (1.1-1.6 g/kg) Very intense training: 0.8-0.9 g/lb. (1.8-2.0 g/kg)
Growing teenage athlete	0.8-0.9 g/lb. (1.8-2.0 g/kg)
Athlete restricting calories	0.8-0.9 g/lb. (1.8-2.0 g/kg)
Strength training phase of training	Experienced: 0.5-0.7 g/lb. (1-1.5 g/kg) Novice: 0.8 g/lb. (1.8 g/kg)
Maximum recommended amount for extreme exercise loads	1.0 g/lb. (2.2 g/kg)

intake may only be a concern for a poorly planned vegetarian diet or athletes following a calorie restriction. Consider how easy it is to meet your daily protein requirements. Having some peanut butter and cereal with milk for breakfast, followed by a turkey sandwich for lunch and a stir-fry of lean red meat and rice for dinner, will supply about 90 grams of protein. You will obtain additional protein from between-meal snacks. Foods such as whole grains and vegetables, which are not as concentrated in protein, still contribute to your total protein intake and can provide moderate amounts over the course of a day and supplement your intake of more concentrated protein foods.

Healthy Proteins in the Right Amounts

A well-balanced diet with adequate calories and up to 15 to 20 or more percent protein calories provides enough total grams of protein for the muscle growth and repair required for winter sport athletes engaged in hard training who also strength train. Protein consumed in excess of your requirements is simply excess calories and then either burned for energy or stored as fat. Converting protein to fuel for exercise is inefficient when compared to carbohydrates, which are much more easily burned for energy.

Consuming excess protein can result in other negative effects. Protein from both food and supplements increases your need for fluid, as your kidneys require more water to eliminate the end products of protein metabolism. A high protein intake should be accompanied with a high fluid intake. Individuals with liver or kidney problems are also susceptible to negative effects of very excessive dietary protein. Excess dietary protein leads to a short-lived increased urinary excretion of calcium, an important mineral for building healthy bone tissue. Daily high protein intakes should be accompanied with adequate amounts of calcium. While food sources of protein are best, they can also contribute substantial amounts of fat and cholesterol to the diet. Consuming excess protein can mean taking in excess fat and cholesterol and increasing your risk of heart disease and other health problems. You should be selective regarding the type of protein foods you eat. There are plenty of low-fat animal protein food sources to choose from and plenty of healthy plant proteins as well.

Your protein needs for your training program, and for muscle repair and other important protein functions, are easily met through a well-planned diet adequate in calories. The key is to obtain adequate amounts of quality lean or low-fat protein sources throughout the day and to consume enough calories so that protein is not burned for energy.

Fat Requirements

Winter sport athletes have total fat requirements at about 0.5 gram per pound (1 gram per kilogram) of body weight to obtain adequate amounts of essential fatty acids. Fat can provide from 15 to 30 percent of the day's calories depending on the carbohydrate, protein, and especially energy needs for that day's training. Once carbohydrate and protein requirements are met for your training program and recovery, fat can make up the remainder of the calories appropriate for your weight and body composition goals

The most important strategy regarding fat intake is to consume enough healthy fats high in essential fatty acids as outlined in Chapter 1. For athletes who may need to monitor their weight closely and prevent unwanted weight gain, as may happen for winter sport athletes with lower energy needs, there may be a problem of too much fat in their diet, especially when away at training camps or traveling for competition. Some athletes may be accustomed to eating out and frequenting fast-food establishments. A high-fat diet is often very calorie-dense and leaves less room for quality carbohydrates. Weight-conscious athletes should keep fat calories at 20 to 25 percent of total intake. (More on body composition strategies is covered in Chapter 5.)

For the cross-country skier and snowshoer who participate in ultraendurance exercise, the amount of fat in your diet could have an important impact on your recovery. While research regarding the fat requirements of ultraendurance athletes is still developing, it is speculated that a diet too low in fat could lead to inadequate replenishment of intramuscular triglycerides. Just how much fat is needed for these long training sessions has not been definitely determined. But a diet at less than 20 percent fat calories or under 0.5 gram per pound (1 gram per kilogram) of body weight could be too low.

Fluid Requirements

As reviewed in Chapter 1, water and fluid are essential parts of your diet. Thirst is not a good indicator of when you need to drink; it only signals that you have become dehydrated. (More specifics on fluid intake during exercise are covered in Chapter 4.) If you are not attempting to lose body weight or body fat, chronic weight loss on the scale could signal inadequate daily hydration and poor rehydration efforts when not training. In many instances your fluid losses may be much greater during training than during competition, though not always. Drink steadily throughout the day and consume both cold and warm hydrating fluids. Specific rehydration steps immediately after training are covered later in this chapter. The color of your urine should indicate the success of your daily hydration efforts: Clear or lemonade-colored urine indicates adequate hydration; darker urine indicates that you need to increase your fluid intake.

Daily Recovery Picture

Overall, your daily recovery hinges on obtaining the appropriate amount of calories for your training, with the proper amounts of carbohydrate, proteins, and fat in your diet to replace the fuels you burned in training and to maximize your strength and power-building efforts. Because of the relatively limited supply of glycogen in the body and the integral role of glycogen in supplying some amount of fuel during all types of training, carbohydrate is an important nutrient for the winter sport athlete. Carbohydrates are needed to synthesize glycogen, and you must consume enough total grams of carbohydrate to fully replenish stores, whatever the level of depletion, to continue to participate in high-quality training sessions. It is also important that the amount of carbohydrate you consume match your training for that day.

Protein is needed to build and repair muscle tissue. Adequate protein in your diet will also maintain a strong immune system. Your higher protein requirements are easily met through a well-planned diet that is adequate in calories.

Fat can provide the remainder of calories, and levels can be adjusted whether the athlete is trying to meet high energy needs or control calories as desired.

IMMEDIATE NUTRITIONAL RECOVERY

What you drink and eat during the day from one training session to the next has a very significant impact on your nutritional recovery. Consuming the fluid, carbohydrate, protein, and fat that you require for nutritional recovery is essential. But in the 4 to 6 hours after moderate to hard training, you can actually make the most of the nutritional recovery, because the rate of nutritional recovery in the few hours after training is accelerated.

Carbohydrate and Immediate Recovery

Consuming carbohydrate immediately after exercise is one of the most important nutritional recovery steps that you can take. Even delaying your carbohydrate intake after a tough training session by 2 hours can slow down the process. Several scientific studies have resulted in the recommendation to consume anywhere from 0.5 to 0.7 gram of carbohydrate per pound (1 to 1.5 grams per kilogram) of body weight within 30 minutes after completing intense exercise, the time when a significant depletion of muscle glycogen occurs. One study demonstrated that subjects fed carbohydrate a full 2 hours after exercise synthesized the carbohydrate into glycogen 45 percent more slowly than subjects fed carbohydrate immediately after exercise. It appears that muscle glycogen storage is slightly enhanced for up to 2 hours after exercise, during which time the muscle has a greater capacity to take up blood glucose.

Studies have shown that both liquid and solid carbohydrates are adequate in refueling the body after hard exercise. However, emphasizing higher glycemic carbohydrate foods that elicit a higher insulin response, such as sports nutrition supplements and breads and cereals, may enhance glycogen resynthesis. A list of high-glycemic foods is provided in Appendix A.

Besides consuming carbohydrate immediately after hard training, you should consume the same recommended carbohydrate amount again in 2 hours. This allows you to continue to take advantage of the recovery process and stimulate the muscle glycogen resynthesis process.

For the rest of the day, carbohydrate can be consumed as a series of snacks, or a few larger meals, depending on your training schedule, food preferences, and total daily carbohydrate requirements. Both eating styles will sufficiently promote glycogen recovery if the total amount of carbohydrate consumed is adequate. Eating a balanced mix of low-, moderate-, and high-glycemic carbohydrates throughout the day will support the glycogen recovery process. But consuming an adequate amount of total carbohydrate grams over the 24-hour period is a very important carbohydrate recovery strategy.

Recovery products concentrated in carbohydrate, providing anywhere from 50 to 100 grams per 16-ounce (480-millimeter) serving, are available. Some of these products also provide up to 25 grams of protein per serving. Sports tubes that provide only protein are also available and can be consumed with a high-carbohydrate food or fluid source. Aim for recovery products that have a higher sodium content.

Protein and Immediate Recovery

A fair amount of debate has focused on the benefits of adding protein to the recovery carbohydrate snack immediately after exercise. Study results have varied depending on whether the protein provided additional calories or whether researchers provided the same amount of calories when comparing a carbohydrate-only dose to a carbohydrate-and-protein combination dose. What is certain is that having protein comprise about one-fourth of your recovery snack will not compromise your muscle glycogen recovery, and it could facilitate muscle glycogen recovery. Consuming some protein immediately after exercise may also speed up the repair of muscle tissue and provide important nutrients for your immune system. It will also send you on your way to optimizing your protein intake until the next training session when you have a tough training schedule or perhaps even another training session that day.

Often, whether you consume carbohydrate alone or a carbohydrate and protein combination is a matter of convenience. Transporting and packing high-carbohydrate items may be easier than also packing items containing protein. Recovery protein should be from high-quality sources such as dairy and soy milk, yogurt, and lean animal proteins. A variety of commercial recovery products, while not necessary for immediate recovery eating, can be very convenient for replenishing immediately after training. Experiment with your own low-fat shake and smoothie recipes made from dairy milk, yogurt, soy milk, or juice and fresh or frozen fruit for a hydrating carbohydrate-and-protein combination.

Fluid and Immediate Recovery

Rehydration is also a top priority after moderate to hard training, as athletes typically replace only three-fourths of their sweat losses during exercise by drinking fluids during exercise. Your goal is to fully restore fluid losses from one training session to the next, while keeping in mind that thirst is not a reliable indicator of fluid losses. You are already dehydrated when you are thirsty, and the thirst mechanism will shut down before you have sufficiently replaced all your fluid losses. Try to consume 20 to 24 ounces (600 to 720 milliliters) of fluid for every pound (0.5 kilogram) of weight lost after training. Sixteen ounces (480 milliliters) actually replaces a fluid loss of 1 pound (0.5 kilogram), but the higher volume of 24 ounces (720 milliliters) will replace both sweat and urine losses.

Pay attention to what stimulates your desire to drink. You may prefer a sweeter product or something a bit salty. The temperature of the drink may also affect the volume of fluid you consume. It makes sense that a cool drink would be more palatable, particularly in hot weather, while it may be difficult to drink large amounts of a cold beverage.

Some athletes may feel reluctant to weigh themselves before and after every training session. You may also not have a scale available every time you train or would prefer not to get overly focused on a weight number. What you can do is obtain pre- and postexercise weights after specific types of training sessions. For example, you may determine that you replace only 50 percent of your fluid needs during hard training sessions, whereas you meet 80 percent of your fluid requirements during less demanding exercise when it may be easier to consume fluid. Once you have established the replenishment levels of your best drinking efforts, you can then develop a system for rehydrating after exercise. You may want to determine what your typical fluid losses are for specific types of environmental conditions, both indoor and outdoor cold-weather training. You can also check the color of your urine to evaluate your hydration efforts.

On days when you know you are to train or compete in more extreme conditions, you may want to check your weight before and after exercise carefully. During intense training times and in hot-weather training, you can perform a daily check on your hydration status. After urinating in the morning, check your weight. If your usual weight is down by more than 1 pound (0.5 kilogram), you may not be keeping up with your usual fluid requirements.

Limit caffeine-containing beverages after exercise to optimize fluid replacement. Consume alcohol only after fluid balance has been restored, if at all.

Sodium and Immediate Recovery

Sodium or salt not only may stimulate your drive to drink but also can enhance the rehydration process. Generally, in most athletes, sweating results in large fluid losses and relatively small sodium losses. When you finish exercise, your blood volume and total body water are reduced, while there is a mild increase in blood concentration and its sodium content. When you consume large amounts of plain water after exercise, you will dilute your blood before your full blood volume has been restored. This dilutional effect will shut down the thirst mechanism, and you will urinate to bring the concentration of the blood to a normal level. The end result is that you have produced a large amount of dilute urine before you are fully rehydrated.

You can offset this negative effect by consuming some sodium or salt after exercise. A series of studies determined that rehydrating with drinks higher in sodium produced significantly lower urine losses than low-sodium drinks, indicating that more of the fluid consumed was retained and therefore hydrating. Therefore, it is recommended that when your fluid losses are significant, you replace sodium losses as well. It also appears that some individuals may have greater sodium sweat losses than others, so consuming sodium after exercise may be prudent unless medically contraindicated. Some athletes may actually require up to several grams of sodium over the course of the day, especially when training in more extreme conditions.

If your fluid losses exceed 1 to 2 pounds (0.5 to 1 kilogram) during exercise, you should make a focused effort to drink fluids on schedule and incorporate fluids into your recovery nutrition strategies. Products that contain sodium can also be integrated into your food and fluid choices to facilitate rehydration. If your recovery time is short, and the next training session is to take place in several hours, it makes sense to actively include sodium into your fluid and food choices.

Sports drinks are formulated for tolerable consumption during exercise, not after exercise. Postexercise, a 150-pound (68-kilogram) athlete requires 75 grams of carbohydrate, which translates to 40 ounces (1,200 milliliters) of a sports drink.

Sports drinks are relatively low in sodium, though higher-sodium formulas are available. You may consider adding 0.25 to 0.5 teaspoon of salt to your total fluid intake. However, consuming a sports drinks rather than a recovery drink may not be your most effective recovery fluid choice, though it is preferable to plain water when rehydration is important.

While the recovery process is a continual effort that takes place after one training session and until the next, you can get off to a good start by paying close attention to what you consume immediately and within the 2 hours after exercise. Then follow these post-exercise nutrition practices with food and fluid choices that match your daily training requirements. Table 3.8 outlines the principles of immediate nutritional recovery.

TABLE 3.8 » PRINCIPLES OF NUTRITIONAL RECOVERY

Training Program	Post-training (30–60 minutes after workout)	Ongoing Recovery Strategies
High-intensity training greater than 60 minutes	Consume 50-75 g carbohydrates. Choose high-glycemic carbohydrates. Can have 10-15 g high-quality proteins. Drink 20-24 oz. (600-720 ml) for every pound of weight lost. Consume sodium-containing fluids in hot weather.	Consume another 50-75 g carbohydrate in 2-3 hours. Continue rehydrating to baseline weight. Include sodium in meals and snacks in hot weather.
Moderate-/high-intensity training greater than 90 minutes	Consume 50-75 g carbohydrates. Choose high-glycemic carbohydrates. Consume 10-15 g high-quality proteins. Drink 20-24 oz. (600-720 ml) fluid for every pound of weight lost. Consume 250 mg sodium with rehydration.	Consume another 50-75 g. carbohydrate in 2-3 hours. Continue rehydrating to baseline weight. Include sodium in meals and snacks.
Aerobic conditioning less than 60 minutes	Rehydrate with liquid supplement containing carbohydrate and sodium. Light carbohydrate snack of up to 50 g.	Monitor weight and return to baseline with fluid intake. Regular intake of meals and snacks to meet nutritional needs.

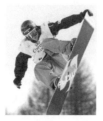

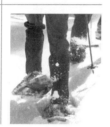

4

Eating for Performance and Competition

Nutritional recovery for your winter sport training is directly linked to the daily training diet. Quality foods and fluids, consumed in the proper quantities from one training session to the next, replenish body fuel stores, hydrate your body, and provide high-quality nutrients. Focusing on the big picture of your training diet is crucial, but the foods and fluids that you consume in the hours before and during training sessions can also have a positive, significant impact on your performance. Proper nutritional training makes it clear that exercising with a full fuel tank and hydrated body results in optimal energy levels and top-quality workouts. Research has shown that there are very specific nutritional strategies that benefit your performance in the hours leading up to a training session and during training.

NUTRITION BEFORE TRAINING AND COMPETITION

Ideally, you will consume a diet for training and recovery designed to take you in top nutritional form from one training session to the next. However, real life can sometimes (or perhaps often) get in the way of recharging your fuel stores to the optimal levels required for quality training. A hectic training schedule, especially when combined with work or school, often leaves little leftover time for eating, let alone meal preparation. For some winter sport athletes, one or two training sessions daily and other life commitments often result in brief windows of time during which the recommended amounts of fuel must be consumed. Even the winter sport athlete with the most optimal daily training diet can obtain a clear performance boost from paying attention to the foods and fluids consumed sometime in the 4-hour period before training. You can also prepare nutritionally for competition and daylong events and excursions with specific nutrition strategies. Focusing on the fuel consumed in the several days or 24 hours before competition can impact the quality of your time on the snow, slopes, and ice.

When training for your winter sport, the longer and harder your training session, the greater the risk of developing glycogen depletion and dehydration. Remember that your full supply of glycogen stores provide anywhere from 1,400 to 1,800 calories' worth of fuel. During steady exercise at moderate to high intensities, you burn through this fuel in less than 90 minutes. During intermittent training at high intensities, you can burn through fuel quickly as well and experience significant glycogen depletion after a day on the slopes. Once you experience muscle glycogen depletion, fatigue sets in as you cannot respond to the demands of training. Even with plenty of fat stores remaining, you may need to decrease your exercise intensity, or you may not even be able to complete the training session. Your fat stores cannot supply fuel quickly enough to sustain the high intensities seen for some winter sport training, and consequently your muscle fibers don't receive the fuel needed to contract during exercise.

How quickly you deplete your body fuel stores depends on the nature of your training. Cross-country skiers and snowshoers completing a long, steady endurance workout burn a combination of fat and carbohydrate, eventually depleting their more limited muscle glycogen stores. Hockey players completing a strenuous practice on the ice can also quickly deplete their muscle fibers of glycogen. Skiers and snowboarders also deplete their muscle glycogen stores during practice runs, and they can eventually deplete muscle glycogen stores after multiple runs. Indoor gym workouts that incorporate cardiovascular work and resistance training are also glycogen depleting. Glycogen depletion from one training session can be significant or it can occur gradually over several days' time or even one or several weeks' time.

Blood glucose provides a very limited amount of fuel during exercise. It is your brain's only fuel source and is maintained by your liver glycogen stores. When you run low on blood glucose, you cannot focus on the exercise task at hand. You may experience light-headedness, poor concentration, and irritability and not perform the skills for your sport as easily. Exercise will seem much harder, and coordination will suffer. Your judgment can also become impaired and affect your technique, an all-important consideration for many winter sports. You may also have to slow down considerably or stop exercise altogether as the blood glucose supplied by your liver is also an important fuel source for your muscles when they become depleted of glycogen.

While glycogen depletion can be come a significant factor limiting performance during a day on the snow or training on the ice, other body nutrient stores can also become depleted. Fluid depletion or dehydration is also an important concern and can impede your training efforts. Dehydration can slow down high-intensity efforts, impair your mental concentration, decrease muscular endurance, and result in overheating, possibly to dangerous levels in hotter weather. Depending on the environmental conditions, the nature of the training session, and the individual athletes, significant electrolyte depletion can also occur, though this is more likely during hot-weather training.

Winter sport athletes who want to complete their training program or compete at their best benefit from several pre-exercise nutrition strategies designed to minimize the fuel, fluid, and electrolyte depletion that can occur during training. Making the most of specific food and fluid choices before training or competition offers several important performance advantages:

- Starting training or competition with optimal fluid levels to help delay or minimize dehydration
- Refilling liver glycogen stores and decreasing risk of developing hypoglycemia during exercise
- Topping off muscle glycogen stores and delaying glycogen depletion while training and competing
- Providing fuel and fluid during the early part of exercise
- Settling your stomach and preventing hunger pains during exercise
- Providing a psychological edge and comfort level regarding your pre-exercise meal

Fueling Up Before Exercise

Clearly, stocking your liver and muscle glycogen stores before exercise is essential prior to demanding training sessions. Nutritional strategies recommended before exercise vary depending on how close to training you need or have to eat. You may want to carefully time your meals prior to exercise, yet your work, school, or practice schedule may dictate when you can actually eat before training. Often an appropriately portioned and timed pre-exercise meal is just what a winter sport athlete requires to fuel their training session, replete fuel depleted from a previous training session, and replenish fuel stores after the overnight fast that takes place during sleep. Recommended portions and foods and fluids to be consumed are directly related to the timing of your pre-exercise meal. Metabolically speaking, there are two distinct time periods for pre-exercise eating: the 2 to 4 hours before exercise, and the 30 to 60 minutes before exercise. When you eat is often a matter of practicality and scheduling. What you eat is truly a matter of metabolic and personal tolerances.

3 to 4 Hours Before Exercise

Depending on your training start time, personal tolerances, and schedule, you should consume a moderate to larger meal in the 3 to 4 hours before training. Many seasoned athletes have identified this time interval as optimal for pretraining eating, as you can achieve a good balance between adequate food consumption and plenty of digestion time. The main focus of this pre-exercise meal should be to replenish your liver glycogen stores and to store fuel in your gastrointestinal (GI) tract for later release. With the right timing and portions, eating 3 to 4 hours before exercise will provide the following benefits:

- Restore liver glycogen to normal levels
- Store carbohydrate in the muscle as needed if portions are large enough
- Have some carbohydrate stored in the gut for absorption and released during exercise
- Avoid feeling hungry during training

Metabolically you can consume a substantial amount of carbohydrate in the 3- to 4-hour period prior to training. Consuming carbohydrate within this time frame does elevate blood insulin levels and favor the use of carbohydrate as a fuel. But because you can consume a good amount of carbohydrate during this time, blood glucose levels remain nice and steady. Research indicates that eating during this period enhances performance.

Pre-exercise eating portions should be appropriate for your tolerances, but try to consume the upper limits for a fuel and performance benefit. For every hour that you allow yourself some digestion time, consume just under half a gram of carbohydrate for every pound you weigh (approximately 1 gram per kilogram weight). Using this formula, you can safely consume 2 grams per pound (4 grams per kilogram) of carbohydrates 4 hours before exercise, and 1.5 grams per pound (3 grams per kilogram) 3 hours before exercise.

For example, if you decide to eat a larger meal 4 hours before an endurance cross-country skiing or snowshoeing workout, 2 grams of carbohydrate per pound (4 grams per kilogram) of weight for a 160-pound (73-kilogram) athlete would translate to 320 grams of carbohydrate. It would probably be easiest on your stomach if a portion of this fairly substantial meal consisted of dense, low-fiber foods, and even some liquid carbohydrate sources. The more intense the workout, the more carefully you want to pay attention to specific food tolerances. For easy digestion, you can obtain 300 grams of carbohydrate by consuming one large bagel topped with 2 tablespoons of jam, followed by a fruited yogurt and 32 ounces of a sports drink. With the full 4 hours of digestion time, you may also find that 1 cup of granola, 8 ounces of skim milk, one large banana, and 12 ounces of juice accompanied by two slices of toast and 2 tablespoons of jam, all providing 200 grams of carbohydrate, is well tolerated. This pre-exercise meal could be topped off with 12 ounces of a high-carbohydrate energy drink, which would provide close to 300 grams of carbohydrate. Of course, some athletes can only tolerate smaller meals even with 4 hours of digestion time. Every athlete needs to iron out their individual tolerances in regard to foods and portions when eating in the 3- to 4-hour period before training.

Eating a few hours beforehand can be ideal for several exercise start times. An early-morning breakfast can be consumed at 6:00 to 7:00 for a 9:00 to 10:00 a.m. start time. For a later start time, such as 2:00 p.m., you may want to consume a larger breakfast of easily digested foods at 10:00. An evening workout at 6:00 could easily be preceded by a large afternoon snack at 2:00 to 3:00.

2 Hours Before Exercise

Consuming food 3 to 4 hours before training may not always be possible due to scheduling and very early start times (rising at 5:00 a.m. to eat prior to an 8:00 a.m. practice does not sound very appealing). Because of timing constraints, eating 2 hours before training may be your preferred or best timing choice. One good rule for pre-exercise eating is that the closer to exercise you plan to eat, the smaller the meal consumed. Try to keep your intake of carbohydrate to 1 gram per pound of body weight (2 grams per kilogram) in this time interval. A 150-pound athlete could consume 160 grams of carbohydrate or less.

With this close meal timing, it likely is even more important that liquid carbohydrate choices are part of your meal. Breakfast shakes, liquid meal replacements, smoothies, and sports supplements often provide more than 50 grams of carbohydrate per serving. A juice smoothie may work well, as do easily digested energy bars.

Eating 2 hours prior to exercise could be the best timing for an early or midmorning training start time. It can also work well for tricky early-afternoon training times. Following a large breakfast that is well digested, with a small to moderate snack 2 hours before training works well for many athletes who plan ahead for afternoon or evening start times.

Eating an Hour Before Exercise

A variety of scenarios could necessitate the need for food 30 to 60 minutes prior to exercise. Rising in the extremely early hours of the morning simply to eat food and fuel up for an early training time may not be feasible or desirable. Scheduling can also often result in a large time gap between the last meal and the start of a training session, and hunger and limited fuel during training can become a significant issue. You may also find it helpful to eat closer to longer training sessions in which the added fuel provides a performance benefit.

From an athlete's perspective, whether or not you consume carbohydrate 30 to 60 minutes prior to exercise needs to be individualized to your tolerances and training schedule. You are most likely to derive a benefit from ingesting fuel 30 to 60 minutes prior to exercise when the carbohydrate you consume replenishes compromised fuel stores. So consider consuming carbohydrate within an hour before exercise if you have not eaten for 4 hours or more or prior to early-morning training when liver glycogen is low. Eating an hour before intense training sessions can also prevent hunger and would provide extra calories for winter sport athletes who have very high energy requirements.

Consuming carbohydrate in the 30 to 60 minutes prior to exercise is different metabolically to consuming carbohydrate several hours prior to exercise. When you eat at this time, there is a marked increase in blood glucose and blood insulin levels prior to training. These increases are then followed by a decline in blood glucose during training, and your liver also decreases the amount of glucose it sends into your bloodstream.

Due to these metabolic effects, some controversy has surfaced over the years in athletic circles regarding carbohydrate consumption in the hour before exercise. The concern has been that carbohydrate consumption in the hour before exercise can result in hypoglycemia or a decrease in blood glucose levels during exercise that produces some negative symptoms and have an adverse effect on performance. In fact, many studies have confirmed that consuming carbohydrate in the hour before exercise does *not* impair performance and can actually help performance. These studies did use exercise test protocols that mimicked steady-state endurance training, and not the high-intensity, moderate-intensity mix often seen with some winter sport training. What was also interesting about these studies was the variation in individual blood glucose responses seen in the study subjects. Although blood glucose may drop during the early part of training, it quickly corrects itself to normal levels, and the majority of athletes experience no adverse symptoms or performance effects. A small number of subjects, however, did experience some hypoglycemia and a negative effect on performance.

If you are concerned that you are a carbohydrate-sensitive athlete during the hour prior to training, you may find a few sensible strategies useful. Consuming a high enough carbohydrate amount may simply offset any lowered blood glucose levels and hypoglycemic symptoms. Amounts of 70 grams or more seem to maintain blood glucose levels in individuals susceptible to exercise hypoglycemia. Individuals not susceptible to hypoglycemia can consume only 50 grams of carbohydrate and still obtain a performance benefit, but they can consume over 70 grams as well if tolerated. Athletes often tolerate up to 100 grams of carbohydrate in the hour prior to training. Choices and amounts are a matter of preference and GI comfort. Practical choices are carbohydrate gels, energy bars, and carbohydrate or sports drinks, which often provide 30 to 50 grams of carbohydrate per serving.

Winter sport athletes can choose one of the items or any combination of them in portions that are tolerated.

Regardless of your training schedule, a pretraining meal or snack can provide some performance benefit. While the main part of your nutritional intake will be carbohydrate, small amounts of protein, and perhaps fat, may be tolerated if appropriately timed. Determine your optimal pre-exercise meal through experimentation during training. Table 4.1 summarizes the recommended carbohydrate amounts for various pre-exercise meal timings.

The Glycemic Index

Some winter sport athletes can choose to incorporate low- to moderate-glycemic index foods into their pretraining meal in order to maintain steady blood glucose levels over the next few hours and through training. While research regarding pre-exercise eating and low-glycemic foods does not fully back this strategy, choosing low-glycemic foods in the several hours before training certainly does not hurt performance. Often the decision to choose these lower glycemic foods is a matter of personal preferences and tolerances, and what athletes have found works best for them through experimentation. Athletes who feel that they perform better when consuming low- to moderate-glycemic index carbohydrate can incorporate these foods into their pre-exercise meal.

As discussed in Chapter 1, adding protein and a small amount of fat to a meal can also blunt the glycemic effect of the meal. Small amounts of lean protein and easily digested sources of fat can help to maintain steady blood glucose levels and prevent hunger during

TABLE 4.1 » PRE-EXERCISE MEAL TIMING AND PORTIONS

Meal Timing	Recommended Nutrients
3-4 hours prior to training	1.5-2 g carbohydrate per pound weight (3-4 g/kg) Moderate amounts of low-fat protein, such as 3-4 oz. of poultry or fish or an 8-oz. serving of milk or yogurt Low to moderate amounts of easily digested fats
2 hours prior to training	Up to 1 g carbohydrate per pound weight (2 g/kg) Very small amounts of low-fat protein or skim milk products and soy products as tolerated Keep fat intake to a minimum
1 hour prior to training	0.5 g carbohydrate per pound weight (1 g/kg) 50-100 g of easily digested carbohydrate source in the form of liquid or gel, and solid if tolerated

exercise, and these foods are often well tolerated when consumed 2 to 4 hours prior to training. Many low-glycemic carbohydrate options are often good sources of fiber such as unprocessed grains and fruits, and timing can be an important issue for these foods before training. However, in the 30 to 60 minutes prior to training, many well-tolerated options are not likely to be whole, unprocessed foods but rather sports nutrition supplements. Many of these products have a higher glycemic index, though there continue to be newer products available all the time that may have more moderate glycemic index levels.

Athletes should also consider that consuming a carbohydrate source during training (more later on that strategy in this chapter) can easily offset any drop in blood glucose, making the types of carbohydrates that you consume before exercise less important.

The bottom line is that you should focus on pretraining nutrition strategies that are appropriate for your training times, schedule, and tolerances and that are based on smart experimentation. Table 4.2 offers some pre-exercise meal suggestions in various carbohydrate amounts.

Hydration Before Training

Dehydration is one of the most significant performance-related problems that can occur during training (and competition). It can put a halt to your training long before you feel

TABLE 4.2 » PRE-EXERCISE, HIGH-CARBOHYDRATE, LOW-FAT MEALS

Toast or small bagel, 2 slices (60 g) Banana, 1 large Jelly, 2 tbsp. (40 ml) juice, 8 oz. (240 ml) **120 g carbohydrate** **520 calories**	Concentrated carbohydrate beverage, 1 ½ cups (360 ml) Toast, 1 slice (30 g) **90 g carbohydrate** **380 calories**	Carbohydrate gel, 1 packet Sports drink, 24 oz. (720 ml) **95 g carbohydrate** **380 calories**
Chicken, 2 oz. (60 g) Bread, 2 slices (60 g) Fruit juice, 16 oz. (480 ml) Pretzels, 2 oz. (60 g) Carbohydrate supplement, 16 oz. (480 ml) **220 g carbohydrate** **1,030 calories**	Pasta, 2 c. cooked (480 ml) Marinara sauce, 1 c. (240 ml) Bread, 2 slices (60 g) Frozen yogurt, 12 oz. (360 ml) Fruit juice, 8 oz. (240 ml) Margarine, 2 t. (24 ml) **235 g carbohydrate** **986 calories**	Pancakes, 4 medium Fruit topping, ½ c. (120 ml) Syrup, ½ c. (120 ml) Fruit juice, 8 oz. (240 ml) **270 g carbohydrate** **1,200 calories**

CONTINUED

TABLE 4.2 continued

Cooked cereal, 2 c. (480 ml)	Rice, 3 c. cooked (720 ml)	Fruit smoothie:
Instant breakfast drink,	Cooked vegetables, 1 c.	Yogurt, 8 oz. (240 ml)
1 serving	Shrimp, 4 oz. (120 g)	Milk, 8 oz. (240 ml)
Banana, 1 large	Sorbet, 1 c. (240 ml)	Juice, 8 oz. (240 ml)
Orange juice, 8 oz. (240 ml)	Soft drink, 12 oz. (360 ml)	1 c. fruit
Carbohydrate beverage,	Oil, 2 t. (14 ml)	
24 oz. (720 ml)	Carbohydrate beverage,	Bagel, 1 large
	16 oz. (480 ml)	Jam, 2 tbsp. (40 ml)
300 g carbohydrate		Energy bar, 1 whole
1,410 calories	**300 g carbohydrate**	
	1,600 calories	**225 g carbohydrate**
		1,185 calories

the effects of fuel depletion. Despite your best attempts to keep up with your sweat losses during training, it is possible that you are not going to match 100 percent of your fluid losses. Depending on the type of training session and weather conditions, you may have ample or limited opportunity to drink during winter training.

Just as strategies to maximize muscle and liver glycogen stores offer a performance advantage, so do techniques for maximizing fluid stores before training. But prehydrating is not considered to be as optimal as drinking during exercise to offset dehydration and its detrimental performance effects. However, if you anticipate that it will be difficult to drink during training due to limited fluid availability, challenges with carrying and drinking fluid in the cold weather, and lack of opportunities to drink during the training session, pre-hydrating could be a very important and practical strategy. Even when training sessions allow time and opportunities for replenishing fluids and replacing sweat losses, and an athlete is consciously making an effort to hydrate during exercise, only up to 80 percent of sweat losses are usually replaced.

At all costs, avoid starting training in a dehydrated state. Your goal during training is to keep up with sweat losses as much as possible, so starting out dehydrated already puts you behind on your fluid intake efforts. It is important to plan ahead and begin your next training session as well hydrated as possible. To prepare for the next day's training, consume 16 ounces (480 milliliters) of fluid before bedtime. Your early-morning intake should then consist of 16 to 24 ounces (480 to 720 milliliters) of fluid. Prior to training, you should attempt to consume 8 to 10 ounces (240 to 300 milliliters) of fluid every hour during the day. About 1 hour before training, you can also prehydrate by consuming 16 to 32 ounces (480 to 960 milliliters) of fluid. At this time, fluids providing carbohydrates and small amounts of sodium, such as sports drinks, are likely to be the best choice and may have some hydration advantages over water. You can fill your fluid stores further by drinking another 8 to 16 ounces (240 to 480 milliliters), 20 minutes prior to training.

In summary, you should be adequately hydrated in preparation for training if you focus on these simple guidelines:

- Consume 16 ounces (480 milliliters) of fluid before bedtime.
- Consume 8 to 10 ounces (240 to 300 milliliters) of fluid every 1 to 2 hours during the day.
- Prehydrate 1 hour before training by consuming 16 to 32 ounces (480 to 960 milliliters) of fluid. A sports drink can be consumed during this time.
- Consume another 8 to 16 ounces (240 to 480 milliliters) of fluid, such as a sports drink 20 minutes prior to exercise if possible.

NUTRITION DURING TRAINING

During training and competition, athletes participating in winter sports can significantly drain fluid stores, carbohydrates, and even electrolytes during moderate to high-intensity training. That's why consuming adequate fluid, carbohydrates, and electrolytes during training and competition is beneficial. This practice can bring you these benefits:

- Delay and minimize dehydration
- Maintain blood glucose levels
- Offset muscle and liver glycogen depletion
- Fuel your brain
- Offset electrolyte losses, particularly sodium

Fluid Requirements During Exercise

As an athlete participating in winter sports, your performance during both training and competition is greatly affected by your hydration levels. Dehydration can develop when you train, both indoors and outdoors, and negatively affect your performance long before fuel depletion drains your efforts. Dehydration can have a negative effect on exercise in cold weather just as it can when athletes train in the heat. Dehydration can also easily develop when you train indoors when preparing for your winter sport. Hockey players can also develop significant levels of dehydration during intense training on the ice.

When you train, heat is a major by-product of your working muscles. As this heat builds up, your body temperature rises. During cold-weather training, those nice warm and insulating clothes you wear to keep warm contribute to a rise in body temperature that promotes sweating. Water then acts as a coolant to keep the body from overheating. During exercise, sweating is the body's primary mechanism for getting rid of excess heat.

Sweat losses can easily reach anywhere from 16 to 32 ounces (500 to 960 milliliters) and sometimes even 48 ounces (1.5 liters) or more per hour depending on environmental conditions, exercise intensity, and the sweat rate of the individual athlete. Sweat losses can reach over 64 ounces (approximately 2.0 liters) or more per hour in very cold weather when you wear very warm and insulating clothing.

Even losing as little as 2 percent of your body weight through sweating can impair your ability to exercise. When you sweat, blood volume goes down and stress is placed on your cardiovascular system, which reduces your ability to take in and utilize oxygen. Muscular endurance ability is also impaired with dehydration, and your heart rate may increase at a given level of intensity. When fluid losses through sweat are not replaced, your body temperature rises further and exercise becomes harder. Clearly, not meeting your fluid needs hinders your athletic goals.

Unfortunately, thirst is not a very good indicator of the amount of fluid that your body requires, during exercise or at rest. Some early signs and symptoms of dehydration are light-headedness, headaches, decreased appetite, darkly colored urine, and fatigue. When you are thirsty, you have already lost 1 percent of your body weight through fluid loss. Even fluid losses of 1 to 2 percent of your body weight can adversely affect performance. When fluid losses reach more than 2 to 4 percent of your body weight, increased thirst and symptoms such as irritability and nausea may occur, and can also result in GI upset. Consequently, when you make the effort to drink more after you have become dehydrated, your rehydration efforts can result in stomach discomfort. At losses of 5 to 6 percent of body weight, there will be an increase in heart rate and breathing regulation, and body temperature regulation will be significantly impaired.

Remember, too, that dehydration can affect your mental concentration and ability to perform the skills required for your sport. Clearly dehydration does not support your top performance if it affects movement control, decision making, and concentration.

The longer and harder you train, the greater the risk that your sweat losses can impair your performance. Your sweat losses are also affected by your genetic makeup, fitness level, and acclimatization to the cold, the temperature in which you are training, and, as mentioned, the amount and type of clothing you are wearing. While you will have greater sweat losses in the heat, your hydration can be compromised by exercise in cold weather.

Your hydration can become compromised in cold weather through several physiological mechanisms. One is *cold-induced diuresis*. When you exercise in the cold, the blood vessels that carry blood to your skin, feet, hands, and ears all constrict in order to conserve heat and maintain body temperature. When your blood vessels constrict, your blood pressure increases and the blood pressure specifically in your kidneys rises, which causes you to urinate and lose fluid and sodium.

Water loss in the cold also occurs when you inhale cold air. Your lung passages warm the air and saturate it with water. When you exhale this air saturated with water, there is fluid loss. Fluid losses from your lungs can add up to more than 1 quart (about 1 liter) daily when you are outdoors for a day of training in the cold. These losses increase with intense exercise. Even in the cold air, an increase in your body temperature during exercise can result in sweat losses. Of course sweat losses per hour can vary greatly depending from workout to workout. There are many good reasons for preventing dehydration, including avoiding the following detrimental physiological effects:

• Increased heart rate
• Raised body temperature
• Decreased blood volume
• Heightened perception of effort
• Compromised mental concentration
• Compromised fine-motor skills
• Delayed stomach emptying of fluids
• Greater risk of gastrointestinal upset

Even without the adverse effects of dehydration, training in the cold can adversely affect your coordination, fine-motor skills, strength, power production, and aerobic power. Dehydration levels of over 2 percent body weight can also reduce mental concentration in cold weather. Negative effects from dehydration can be as significant as the effects in warm-weather training when training is hard and insulating clothing does not allow for adequate heat loss.

It is important to gauge your sweat losses during various types of training sessions in a number of environmental conditions. Athletes cannot train themselves to adapt to or tolerate dehydration; it is best prevented or minimized as much as possible.

Just as sweat rates vary greatly among athletes, there is also much variability in efforts to replace fluids during exercise. While your ideal goal is to match your fluid intake to your fluid losses, most athletes fall short and replace only 50 to 80 percent of their fluid losses during practice sessions even in ideal conditions. Even with strong efforts to match your fluid losses, your gastrointestinal system can only absorb a certain volume of fluid per hour. Often, whether or not you can maintain adequate hydration status during exercise is a matter of practicality rather than scientific theory. Consuming the recommended amounts can be challenging due to logistics in obtaining fluid when training and competing, limited opportunities to drink, availability of fluid, taste preferences, and GI tolerances. In cold-weather training, fluids can be even less readily available. You may struggle to keep your fluid from freezing, which it does below 32° Fahrenheit (0° Celsius). Drinking in the cold can also be uncomfortable due to logistics of keeping your hands warm and wanting to avoid pit stops. You are also not as thirsty in cold weather and may not so readily crave fluids.

Clearly, you need to assess drinking opportunities and fluid availability for your own winter sport and specific types of training sessions. Training and preparing for your sport in the gym simply requires that you bring fluids with you for when you train indoors. Matching fluid intake to sweat losses should not prove to be too challenging. Refer to the sidebar for guidelines for estimating both your fluid losses during training and how well your efforts to rehydrate during training are matching these fluid losses. Once you have come up with the best fluid strategies for your various types of training sessions, it is up to you to make the most of your opportunities to drink during training. Regardless of your fluid replacement strategies, you are more likely to consume fluids that taste good and are the proper temperature for your training conditions.

» DETERMINING FLUID LOSSES

This technique for estimating fluid losses is fairly accurate, especially in warmer-weather training. Check your sweat losses for various types of training sessions, whether indoors or outdoors, to better estimate and meet your sweat losses.

1. Check your weight before and after training, and calculate your weight loss.

160–158 pounds (73–72 kilograms)

2-pound weight loss during training (0.9 kilogram)

2. Know the amount of fluid that you consumed during the training session. Fifteen oz. of fluid weighs about 1 lb. (an easier estimate is 1,000-ml fluid equals 1.0 kg body weight). You can also weigh the bottle before and after your training session to determine the actual weight of the fluid you consumed during training.

Let's say you consume 60 oz. (1,800 ml) of fluid during a 2-hour practice.
This fluid weighs 4 lb. (1.8 kg).

3. Add the weight you lost to the weight of the fluid you consumed.

2-lb. weight loss during training, plus 4 lb. of fluid consumed during training equals
6 lb. of fluid lost (0.9 + 1.8 kg = 2.7 kg).

4. 6 lb. equals 90 oz. of fluid divided by 2 hours = 45 oz. per hour for sweat losses (2.7 kilograms equals 2,700 milliliters fluid divided by 2 hours = 1,350 milliliter per hour).

In this example, the athlete sweats about 45 oz., or 5.5 c. (1,350 milliliters), of fluid per hour. Sweat rates can vary from 24 oz., or 3 c. (720 milliliters), of fluid per hour to 80 oz., or 10 c. (2,500 ml or more), per hour.

Not only do you need to focus on how much fluid to consume, you should also be aware of the most optimal and appropriate fluid choice during training in various environments and conditions. Commercial sports drinks often appeal to winter sport athletes and, besides their flavor, also provide fuel and electrolytes in the form of carbohydrate and sodium chloride. Here are some basic hydration strategies designed to maximize your fluid intake during training:

Consume 4 to 8 ounces (120 to 240 milliliters) of fluid during every 15 to 20 minutes of exercise. Practice drinking at regular intervals so that you become highly skilled at consuming enough fluid during training. Try to drink at regular intervals, and take big gulps as larger volumes empty from your stomach more quickly. When training indoors or on the ice, cooler fluids should be more appealing and should assist you in drinking a greater volume.

Start drinking early. This strategy is especially important if the nature of your training session will not allow for frequent drinking breaks and opportunities. Even if you start training adequately hydrated, it does not pay to practice "catch-up" drinking. Once you are dehydrated, fluids empty from your stomach more slowly. In extreme situations, dehydration may lead to GI upset, including a bloated stomach. Because fluids are emptying slowly, you will feel dehydrated and compensate by attempting to drink more, further aggravating stomach upset.

Monitor your sweat rates during training. It is important that you appreciate the rate at which you lose fluid during different types of training sessions and environmental conditions. You can also practice drinking during training sessions that simulate competition conditions. Monitor your weight before and after training to assess how effectively you replace fluids.

Develop a taste for various sports drinks. While you likely have a favorite sports drink brand and flavor that you can consume during training, practice with products and flavors that are also available during competition and get used to their taste and feel during training. This allows for greater flexibility and improved drinking on competition day.

Fluids should be accessible. Ensuring that you have adequate fluid available is fairly simple during an indoor training session. Keeping a squeeze bottle on hand should allow you to drink an ample amount of fluid whether you are training indoors or out.

Monitor your hydration by checking urine volume and color. Athletes should empty several full bladders of urine daily. The lighter the color of your urine, the better your hydration levels. Lemonade-colored urine suggests that you are adequately hydrated, while apple juice–colored urine suggests that you very poorly hydrated.

Prehydrate before training, and rehydrate after training. Despite all your good intentions, behavior strategies, and intent on hydrating adequately, it is best if you start every training session well hydrated. This ensures that you can prevent greater fluid losses during training than is necessary. Rehydrating also allows you to start the next training session with optimal fluid levels.

Fuel Requirements During Exercise

Due to the steady endurance nature of cross-country skiing and snowshoeing, the high-intensity, intermittent nature of hockey play, and the energy needs of a long day of downhill skiing or snowboarding, fuel replacement during winter training is an important consideration. Carbohydrate consumed during training can maintain blood glucose levels and provide fuel to glycogen-depleted muscles. Carbohydrate consumption during training may also provide the opportunity for glucose to be stored in less active muscle fibers during rest periods. For example, when you exercise at low intensity, muscle fibers that fuel higher-intensity efforts can be replenished.

Your brain can also benefit from carbohydrate intake during longer and more intense training sessions, as consuming only water can result in lowered blood glucose levels. Because your brain counts on glucose for fuel, lowered blood glucose can result in some negative central nervous system effects. Having adequate blood glucose to fuel your brain helps to maintain the high level of skill required by many winter sports. Carbohydrate intake can prevent or reverse symptoms of glucose deprivation such as fatigue, perception of increased effort, and poor coordination. Carbohydrate is thought to prevent an increase in brain serotonin levels that can occur during prolonged exercise. Serotonin produces feelings of drowsiness and fatigue in the brain.

Much of the research on carbohydrate intake during exercise has centered on endurance activity. But studies also demonstrate that besides providing performance benefits for exercise lasting 90 minutes or longer, carbohydrate may also improve performance during high-intensity exercise lasting about 60 minutes. Several studies over the past decade measured the performance effects of consuming a sports drink during exercise performed at 80 to 90 percent VO_2max and lasting about 1 hour. Results indicated that the sports drink provided a performance benefit.

Several additional studies measured the performance effects on intermittent, high-intensity exercise lasting about 1 hour, more closely matching the type of training conducted in hockey. Consuming a sports drink at rest intervals allowed the activity to continue longer. Researchers speculated that the carbohydrate drinks provided the fast-twitch muscle fibers, which operate at higher intensities, some fuel to work with at rest intervals between high-intensity efforts. While more research of this type is needed, hockey players can clearly enhance performance by consuming both fluid and carbohydrate during practice as the energy demands of training reduce muscle glycogen and fluid reserves.

Fuel depletion also occurs with the very high-intensity efforts of alpine skiing and snowboarding. While the rest periods between runs are longer than rest periods for hockey, replacing fuel when possible between hard efforts helps to maintain fuel stores and blood glucose levels during a full day on the slopes.

Sports Drinks

Both fluid and carbohydrate can be consumed during specific types of training sessions to maintain hydration and fuel stores. In order for your body to receive both carbohydrate and fluid in a timely and well-tolerated manner, consider several steps in the digestion and absorption of sports drinks. First, when you consume sports drinks, they must empty from your stomach as quickly as possible. Next, they enter your small intestine where they must be absorbed as quickly as possible and then enter the bloodstream. Carbohydrate is then available to maintain your blood glucose levels, supply energy to your exercising muscles, and replenish muscle fuel stores at rest or lower-intensity exercise levels. The fluid from your sports drink maintains blood volume and offsets sweat losses.

In an effort to provide the most scientifically sound formulation, sports drink research has looked at each of the steps in digestion and absorption to see where the flow may actually slow down or speed up. If your sports drink gets bogged down in any one of these steps, it takes the fluid and carbohydrate that much longer to reach your bloodstream and muscles. Consequently, the sports drink is not as performance enhancing. Researchers have determined that the two factors that determine how quickly a drink leaves your stomach are the volume of fluid in your stomach and the concentration of the carbohydrate in the drink.

Concentration

The greater the carbohydrate concentration of the fluid, the longer it takes to empty from your stomach. What research has determined is that carbohydrate solutions of about 4 to 8 percent concentration empty from your stomach very efficiently. Conveniently, most sports drinks fall into this gastrically acceptable range, at about 6 to 8 percent carbohydrate. Solutions in this range deliver an optimal balance of both carbohydrate and fluid. This drink concentration allows fluid to reach your bloodstream pretty much as quickly as water, but it still delivers performance-boosting carbohydrates at a rate that is tolerated when you exercise. Drinks of these concentrations also seem to be well tolerated by most athletes, and tolerance to these products can also improve with practice. In contrast, drinks of 10 to 12 percent concentration, such as soft drinks and fruit juice, are emptied more slowly from the stomach, though they do provide carbohydrates and energy. However, these drinks are not as hydrating and should be diluted if they are consumed during exercise.

Volume

As mentioned previously, volume affects the degree of stomach distention and consequently affects gastric emptying. Increased stomach distention will result in liquids emptying from your stomach more quickly, with about 50 percent of stomach contents being emptied every 10 minutes. To maximize emptying, try to start exercise with a comfortably full stomach and drink at regular intervals of about 10 to 15 minutes if possible. How much fluid an athlete can empty from his stomach is highly variable. However, emptying rates of 24 to 40 ounces, or 3 to 5 cups (720 to 1,200 milliliters), per hour are commonly seen. The most important strategy is to consume fluid whenever the opportunity presents itself. Aim to consume one 20-ounce (600-millilter) squeeze bottle for every hour of practice. Refill your bottle as needed depending on the duration of the practice session.

Intestinal Absorption

Studies measuring intestinal absorption rates have determined that sports drink solutions are as readily absorbed as water. Different forms of carbohydrates are absorbed across the intestinal wall via various transport mechanisms. While the majority of research has demonstrated that the maximum amount of carbohydrate that an athlete can comfortably absorb is about 1 gram per minute, some newer research is currently looking at the effect of two or three sources of carbohydrate on intestinal absorption. Mixing carbohydrate sources could allow for a greater amount of carbohydrate to be absorbed per minute, making more fuel available for training and competition, without sitting in the gut and causing GI problems. This strategy would be especially important during endurance or ultraendurance events in which the athlete needs to maximize fuel absorption in order to keep up with the fuel burned during training or competition.

More research is required to determine just how this improved absorption translates to improved performance. For now, every athlete needs to determine what sports drink and carbohydrate amounts they tolerate best for different types of training sessions.

The sports drink products available does provide a wide variety of carbohydrate sources. These include glucose polymers, glucose, sucrose, and fructose. Many drinks have a mix, allowing various carbohydrate types to be transported simultaneously. These carbohydrate mixes all appear to have a moderate to high glycemic index, handy for quickly raising blood glucose levels and giving you a quick burst of both brain power and energy when consumed.

Glucose polymers do not seem to offer any absorption advantages over glucose, but they are popular because they have a milder rather than overly sweet taste. Fructose is the only beverage not used in high amounts or solely in a sports beverage. Large amounts of fructose are not well absorbed and can lead to GI upset. But drinks that contain some fructose should provide easily tolerated concentrations and additional flavor.

More recently, some sports drinks have been surrounded by claims concerning the drink's effect on blood glucose levels and insulin, in relation to the type of carbohydrate in the drink and the glycemic index of the product. While there is virtually no research comparing the performance effects of sports drinks with various glycemic index levels, the high glycemic effect of most sports drinks would quickly raise blood glucose levels and provide quick fuel for the athlete during training and competition. The number of sports drinks with a lower glycemic index is limited, and the glycemic index of many sports drinks is not available.

Just as has been measured with various food choices, the glycemic index of a carbohydrate source or drink is not necessarily related to whether the carbohydrate source is a "simple" or "complex" carbohydrate. Maltodextrin, which is often promoted as a complex carbohydrate source, has a high glycemic index, whereas the simple sugar fructose has a very low glycemic index. Often, the choice of a sports drink comes down to personal tolerances and preferences, and what drink is available to the athlete or team. Appendix C provides a limited listing of the glycemic index of various sports drinks and various carbohydrate sources that are currently available.

Recently, some sports drinks containing protein have been on the market. Research regarding protein-containing sports drinks and performance in winter sports is limited. More well-designed research studies and data are needed regarding these products.

Amount and Timing of Carbohydrate

Basically the amounts of sports drinks you consume should mimic the water intake guidelines described previously, or about 4 to 8 ounces (120 to 240 milliliters) every 15 to 20 minutes. Drinking at regular intervals can usually take place during training whenever there is adequate opportunity to drink. Performance benefits begin when about 30 grams of carbohydrate per hour is delivered. However, 50 to 60 grams may be optimal to meet fuel needs during higher-intensity exercise and after some muscle glycogen depletion has occurred. Every athlete has his or her own personal tolerances and carbohydrate requirements that maintain optimal energy levels during practice.

Check the labels and instructions of your favorite sports drinks. Then determine what volume you would need to consume in an hour to obtain 30 to 60 grams or more of carbohydrate per hour. Experiment to determine what fluid consumption volume best enhances your performance and maintains adequate hydration levels.

As far as timing is concerned, large single feedings and smaller, regular intakes of a sports drink are both beneficial. Basically, drink whenever possible as the nature of your training session permits. Consuming carbohydrate after depletion has set in can help, but consuming the carbohydrates early on in order to prevent fatigue is smart and prudent. Don't wait until the signs and symptoms of a low fuel tank register before consuming your carbohydrate sports drink.

Form of Carbohydrate

In addition to liquid carbohydrate, semiliquid and solid carbohydrates sports supplements may be consumed before, during, and after exercise, though tolerances to these products can vary depending on the intensity of exercise and timing of the carbohydrate supplement. Obviously, carbohydrate drinks offer the advantage of both hydration and fuel. Although sports drinks are practical, many winter sport athletes may appreciate the more concentrated carbohydrate gels, for situations when energy needs outweigh the desire for fluid, and for a convenient carbohydrate source. These products, however, should be consumed with some fluid. More solid items such as energy bars may take the edge off hunger during training, though most athletes prefer to avoid solid items during high-intensity exercise.

Basically fluid and carbohydrate choices can be somewhat individualized. Often it is possible that fluid needs are of greater significance than energy needs when on the slopes or training indoors. If carbohydrate needs are a greater priority during the end of an intense practice, then a gel taken with water or a more concentrated sports drink may provide the shot of energy required by the athlete.

The Electrolyte Edge

Though your sweat is mainly water, it does contain a number of electrolytes, including sodium, potassium, and calcium. However, the main electrolyte lost in sweat is sodium. Electrolyte losses can also vary greatly among athletes, mostly in regards to salt or sodium content. But, because electrolytes are the major solid component of sweat, research has focused on replacement needs of these nutrients during exercise. Sodium and potassium have been the most frequently studied, though chloride is also a consideration. Sodium has recently become an important consideration for athletes who train in the heat and humidity, which winter sport athletes may do in the warmer months when involved in other sports. Sodium has become an important issue for athletes training in hot and humid conditions who are prone to muscle cramping and developing low blood sodium levels, or hyponatremia. Despite being acclimated to warmer weather, some athletes continue to have high losses of sodium in their sweat. This may be due to genetic or other influences. Sodium losses in athletes are so individual that they can range from 150 to 1,800 milligrams in 1 quart (960 milliliters) of sweat.

Very little information is available on sodium losses when training in colder weather. It is possible that some athletes do have high sodium losses and could develop sodium problems during very long training sessions or ultraendurance competition. This is most likely to occur with excess intake of plain water and inadequate replacement of sodium.

While restricting sodium may be a useful health strategy in sodium-sensitive and sedentary individuals susceptible to high blood pressure, it may not be the best strategy for the winter sport athlete susceptible to muscle cramping or who has moderate to high sodium losses through sweating. Several hours of sweating daily during training can add up to significant sodium losses in some athletes. These sodium losses need to be replaced with a diet adequate in salt. Sports drinks also have varying levels of sodium, and athletes prone to high sodium sweat losses and cramping can choose those higher in sodium. While some physiology laboratories can measure sodium losses in individual athletes, often the only marker to indicate to an athlete that they have high sodium sweat losses are the salt rings and marks on their skin and workout clothing.

» BREAKING THROUGH THE ICE: Winter Hydration Strategies

When training outside for your winter sport, you are often reminded of the cold, hard fact that water solidifies at temperatures of below 32° Fahrenheit (0° Celsius), making optimal hydration a challenge. Winter athletes can practice a few warming strategies to keep the fluids flowing.

Sports drinks can be heated before training and placed inside a thermos or a bottle covered with an insulating warmer. Experiment with drinks and flavors that appeal to you when heated. Warm sports drinks should be easier to down on a cold winter day and can help to maintain your core body temperature. Strategies for having the thermos or bottle readily available depends on your sport and training setting. Hockey players training indoors should do fine with cooler fluids that can be kept available on the sidelines. Cross-country skiers and snowboarders can place bottles in their backpack or fluid belt and keep it as close to their body as possible. Alpine skiers and snowboarders can leave bottles at the bottom of their runs and consume sports drinks during the recovery period.

Newer tube-fed winter hydration systems are also available for training in the cold. Newer models are designed for the cold, but in the coldest temperatures you cannot fight the freeze indefinitely. Hydration systems are handy as they do not require that you reach for your bottle with cold fingers and thick gloves. To prevent the drink tube from freezing, you can now buy products with an insulated hose and bite valves covered with insulating caps. In full-blown winter weather, make sure that you do fill the fluid reservoir with warm or hot fluid. You should also blow back into the drink tube after you have taken a hydrating gulp, to prevent fluid from sitting and freezing in the drink tube. Also, keep the fluid reservoir and hose as close to your body as possible so that your body heat can keep the system warm.

Obtaining adequate fuel and fluid during training sessions, replacing high sodium losses if needed, takes practice, experience, and experimentation. Here are some practical tips for making the most of your fuel and fluid intake during exercise:

Have a plan, and drink on a schedule. Have a squeeze bottle of fluid ready and available for training so that you can consume fluid during breaks or regular intervals during training. Check your intake every hour to determine whether you are keeping up with the required fluid amounts.

Know your sweat losses by monitoring your weight before and after training. It is not necessary to consume more fluid than your body requires, but do try to consume adequate fluid during practice to minimize sweat losses. If you lose more than 2 pounds (approximately 1 kilogram) during an hour or longer practice, you need to drink more. Gaining weight during practice indicates that you are consuming too much fluid relative to your sweat losses.

Start exercise well hydrated. Drink 16 to 20 ounces (480 to 600 milliliters) of fluid in the hour before exercise. Start practice with a comfortably full stomach. This will speed up gastric emptying, as will drinking fluid every 15 to 20 minutes.

Use a sports drink during moderate- to high-intensity practice sessions lasting longer than 60 minutes. Research indicates that this combination of fluid and carbohydrate improves performance by replacing sweat losses and providing carbohydrate fuel for your muscles.

Consume 30 to 60 grams of carbohydrate per hour from a sports drink during moderate- to high-intensity training. This amount will ensure that you do not become dehydrated and provide fuel as glycogen stores become depleted. Most sports drinks provide 14 to 20 grams of carbohydrate per 8-ounce (240-milliliter) serving. One full squeeze bottle would provide 35 to 50 grams and should be consumed over 1 hour of practice.

Start drinking early on during training. Minimizing a fluid deficit makes more sense than reversing dehydration during exercise. Your brain also derives benefits from the carbohydrate consumed, and the carbohydrate spares liver glycogen stores that can be broken down for use later during exercise.

Experiment carefully with other sources of carbohydrate. During intense training sessions or sessions where carbohydrate requirements outweigh fluid considerations, a more solid form of carbohydrate such as a gel may be appealing and provide needed carbohydrate fuel to prevent depletion. Gel servings usually provide up to 50 grams of carbohydrate per gulp. Just remember to consume gels with plenty of water; otherwise they empty from your stomach slowly, as they are a concentrated carbohydrate source.

Know your sweat losses in different environmental conditions and at different times during the season. Monitor your weight before and after practice in various temperatures and types of training sessions and at different times of the year. Train yourself to drink the proper volumes to replace sweat losses in various situations.

Have a squeeze bottle or winter hydration system at each training session, and consume fluids from it regularly. Whenever appropriate, the coaching and training staff should have policies in place that makes fluids readily available to winter sport athletes.

Drink during the warm-up, and have a regular fluid intake when on the bench during hockey practice. Drink a small amount of fluid at each break in play.

Coaches and trainers should remind players to drink regularly, especially those with high fluid losses and low intakes during training or practice.

Experiment with various sports drinks to determine your favorite flavor and best tolerance. Consuming a variety of flavors may minimize the occurrence of taste fatigue during long exercise sessions and competitions. You may find that different products appeal to you in various athletic conditions. Know what works for you under various exercise, temperature, and training conditions.

Pay attention to signs of dehydration. Frequent gastrointestinal problems may indicate that you are not drinking enough. Gastric emptying is delayed when you are dehydrated. It may appear that you do not tolerate a particular product, when what is actually occurring is that the product is unable to empty from your stomach, and further drinking causes bloating.

Note the signs and symptoms of hypoglycemia. Feeling light-headed or experiencing an inability to focus or dizziness can all indicate that blood glucose levels are running low. Be proactive and try to increase your intake of carbohydrate with sports drinks or gels.

Refine your drinking technique. Practice drinking in all types of training situations. Know your limits regarding exercise intensity and the ability to tolerate certain volumes of fluid ingestion. Push your limits and maximize your fluid intake to maintain fluid balance.

Pay attention to your sodium intake if you are susceptible to muscle cramping. Emphasize salty foods and salt foods to taste. Choose higher-sodium sports drinks.

The next sidebar provides some guidelines for using several types of sports nutrition products. Appendix C presents a comparison chart of sports drinks and liquid food supplements. When you consume a wide variety of sports nutrition supplements over the course of a day or even a week, it is important to consider the other nutrients they provide such as vitamins and minerals. Consider your intake in the context of your entire day's food intake and be careful not to oversupplement on vitamins and minerals through use of these products and individual supplements.

» PRACTICAL USES OF SPORTS NUTRITION PRODUCTS

Sports Drinks

Consume 16 to 24 ounces (480 to 720 milliliters) in the hour before exercise.

Consume 4 to 8 ounces (120 to 240 milliliters) every 15 to 20 minutes as your training session allows.

Consume 8 ounces (240 milliliters) during breaks whenever possible.

Consume after exercise with high-carbohydrate food or supplements.

Consume at halftime or play breaks when applicable.

Sports Gel

Consume one packet in the 30 to 60 minutes prior to training or competition.

Consume at breaks during training or practice and during competition.

Consume as part of recovery nutrition snack.

Sports Bar

Include in pretraining and precompetition snack.

Consume as part of daily training diet for a concentrated carbohydrate source.

Consume as part of your immediate postexercise nutritional recovery plan.

Consume during long game days for easy-to-digest source of carbohydrate.

High-Energy Carbohydrate Drink

Consume as part of a pretraining and precompetition meal or snack.

Consume as part of immediate postexercise recovery nutrition.

Consume as part of a high-energy meal plan.

High-Carbohydrate Protein Drink

Consume before and after resistance training for quality protein combined with carbohydrate.

Consume as part of a pretraining and precompetition meal.

Consume as part of a high-energy training plan.

Sports Shake

Use as a pre-exercise meal or snack for a carbohydrate and protein source.

Include in a precompetition menu for easily digested nutrients.

Eat as a recovery snack after practice or weight training.

Include as part of a high-energy training plan.

Use for a quick meal for convenience.

EATING TO COMPETE

Fine-tuning your portions and staying on top of your specific food and fluid tolerances prior to training can set the stage for optimal precompetition nutrition strategies for winter sport athletes who compete in their sport. While the meal(s) and snack(s) you consume on race day are all-important, specific nutrition strategies can benefit your performance in the days and hours leading up to competition. Nutrition strategies during competition can also enhance your race day performance.

Carbohydrate Loading

Depending on your winter sport, training program, and competition schedule, you may or may not have the luxury of tapering training one to several days before competition. At the very least, you may have a rest day or light training day before an important competition. This time period can recharge not only your mental outlook but also your body's fuel stores. Keeping up with your energy needs during hard training cycles and during the competition season can be challenging, and recharging your batteries the day before competition may be necessary for your best competitive performance.

Training sessions and competitions can take place in the early morning after liver glycogen stores become 80 percent depleted when you sleep at night. Because liver glycogen is an important source of blood glucose during exercise, exercising in this fasted state can cause an unwanted drop in blood glucose. Having a high-carbohydrate dinner and perhaps even a light snack high in carbohydrate will fill your liver with glycogen the night before, somewhat diminishing the effect of low morning liver glycogen. Just make sure that any late-night noshes are easy to digest. Research also indicates that muscle glycogen stores return to normal within 24 hours of rest and a high-carbohydrate diet, if there is no significant muscle damage from training earlier in the week.

The day before and especially the night before competition, you do not want to try any new and unusual foods that could result in gastrointestinal upset. Go to bed comfortably full, not stuffed. Avoid consuming large amounts of protein and fat, which take longer to digest and could push out important carbohydrates from your precompetition diet. Be especially careful to eliminate fiber-containing foods and gassy foods, and avoid alcohol. Practice having various high-carbohydrate, low-fiber, easy-to-digest meals the night before an important morning training session. Make simple meals that can be copied when ordering in restaurants when traveling for competition. Pasta dishes low in fat are a common favorite among many athletes, but other carbohydrate choices also work well. Try rice-based dishes, stir-fried noodles, baked potatoes, and low-fiber white breads. You probably want to avoid salads and other raw vegetables and raw fruits the night before an important training session or race.

For your 24-hour rest and glycogen-loading day before an important competition, here are a few guidelines to consider:

- Consume 3 to 5 grams of carbohydrate per pound of body weight (7 to 10 grams per kilogram) in the 24 hours before competition with levels topping off at about 400 to 500 grams daily for female athletes and 600 to 700 grams daily for male athletes. If training prior to this carbohydrate-loading day has been depleting, consume the high end of the recommended amounts.

- Your calorie needs may decrease in this 24-hour period due to light or no training, but the proportion of carbohydrate from your diet should increase.

- If training is not tapered before competition, be especially diligent with consuming the optimal amount of carbohydrate and calories the day before an important competition.

- Be aware that for every gram of glycogen stored in your muscles, you also store up to 3 grams of water. This can result in weight gain and helps to delay dehydration during the event.

- Light exercise the day before competition keeps your muscles light and can reduce the stiffness that comes with fluid stored in your muscles from a high level of glycogen storage.

» HIGH-CARBOHYDRATE, LOW-FIBER FOOD CHOICES

The following precompetition foods provide 30 grams of carbohydrate per serving:

Bagel, 2 ounces (60 grams)

Bread, white, 2 slices (60 grams)

Pita pocket, 1.5 rounds

Dinner rolls, 2

English muffin, 1

Muffin, low-fat, low-fiber, 3 ounces (90 grams)

Tortillas, 2 small

Cooked cereal, 1 cup (240 milliliters)

Apple, 1.5 medium

Applesauce, sweetened, ½ cup (120 milliliters)

Grapefruit, peeled, 1 large

Canned fruit, 1 cup (240 milliliters)

Cold cereal, low-fiber, 1.5 ounces (45 grams)

Graham crackers, 6

Saltines, 8

Rice, cooked, white, ⅔ cup (200 milliliters)

Pasta, cooked, 1 cup (240 milliliters)

Pretzels, white flour, 1.5 ounces (45 grams)

Potato, baked, no skin, 1 medium

Sweet potato, no skin, 4 ounces (120 grams)

Apple juice, 8 ounces (240 milliliters)

Carrot juice, 10 ounces (300 milliliters)

Grape juice, 6 ounces (200 milliliters)

Cranberry juice cocktail, 8 ounces (240 milliliters)

Milk, skim, 20 ounces (500 milliliters)

Yogurt with fruit, 1 cup (240 milliliters)

• If needed according to your tolerances, emphasize low-fiber and compact carbohydrate sources to minimize gastrointestinal upset and to ensure that you consume the prescribed amounts.

The sidebar emphasizes some good high-carbohydrate (30 grams) food choices that are also low in fiber. Starches, cereals, and breads are fairly concentrated carbohydrate sources, and fruits and fruit juices are also good sources of carbohydrate. Sports nutrition supplements such as sports bars, gels, concentrated carbohydrate drinks, and liquid meal replacements can also fit nicely into your plan.

Having a sound menu plan in mind can lessen any stress associated with making food choices the day before an important competition. You may want to consider having moderate portions of proteins and fats when replenishing carbohydrates on a rest day or a light training day. This prevents unneeded calories from being consumed and leaves room for important carbohydrates. Consuming between-meal snacks can help in reaching the

TABLE 4.3 » HIGH-CARBOHYDRATE, PRECOMPETITION MENU

Breakfast	Orange juice, 1 c. (240 ml) Cornflakes, 1 c. (240 ml) Banana, 1 large Skim milk, 1 c. (240 ml) Toast, 2 slices (60 g) Margarine, 1 t. (7 ml) Jelly, 2 tbsp. (40 ml)	147 g carbohydrate, 750 calories	›
Snack	Yogurt with fruit, 6 oz. (200 ml)	20 g carbohydrate, 150 calories	›
Lunch	Lean turkey, 3 oz. (100 g) White bread, 2 slices (60 g) Pretzels, ¾ oz. (20 g) Pear, 1 large Apple juice, 8 oz. (240 ml)	105 g carbohydrate, 585 calories	›
Snack	Energy bar, 1 medium	40 g carbohydrate, 200 calories	›
Dinner	Rice, cooked, 2 c. (480 ml) Ground turkey, 3 oz. (100 g) Cooked peas, 1 c. (240 ml) Bread, 2 slices (60 g)	160 g carbohydrate, 961 calories	›
Snack	Frozen yogurt, 12 oz. (360 ml) Fig Newtons, 2	102 g carbohydrate, 460 calories	›

TOTAL:
574 g carbohydrate,
3,100 calories

required carbohydrate amounts. Table 4.3 provides a sample precompetition menu ranging from 400 to 600 grams of carbohydrate daily. For the lower carbohydrate level, trim or eliminate the snacks on the menu.

Eating the Day of Competition

Meal timing and portioning is especially important the day of competition. It is important that you have a game plan for eating times and portions on the day of competition. Experiment with meal and snack timing in training, and try to mimic the schedule of an upcoming competition. For earlier start times, you may want to consider one moderate-sized meal several hours before the start time. If you do not want to rise as early as this strategy requires, a smaller meal can be consumed closer to the start time.

Later start times could necessitate eating one larger meal earlier in the day and then consuming a series of snacks as the competition start approaches. On competition day, you can enjoy many sports nutrition supplements that are easily digested and well tolerated. Liquid meal replacements, high-carbohydrate energy drinks, and sports drinks and gels can be consumed leading up to the start time. Table 4.4 offers some meal- and snack-timing suggestions.

Replacing Fluid and Fuel During Competition

How you intake fuel and fluid during competition depends on the nature of your competitive event. Endurance athletes such as cross-country skiers and snowshoers may find that fluids and fuel are accessible during competition lasting longer than 60 minutes and want to consume a sports drink whenever possible during a race. Hydration and fuel intake during longer races can significantly improve performance. Alpine skiers and snowboarders should rehydrate and refuel between runs as much as necessary so that each run is completed when well hydrated and optimally fueled.

It is important to maintain blood glucose levels for concentration and focus, and to maintain the high skill level required of these sports. Proper precompetition eating should be combined with strategies to time fluid and fuel intake properly during competition. Hockey players can rehydrate and refuel on the bench and during periods of rest when off the ice. They can consume 8 to 16 ounces (240 to 480 milliliters) of fluid during breaks between periods. Carbohydrate gels can also replenish fuel stores between periods.

More specific competition day fuel strategies for individual sports are covered in Part II. Most important, each athlete needs to practice nutritional strategies for fueling and rehydrating when training. Rehearse your competition strategies as closely as possible so that you can develop an optimal personalized plan.

TABLE 4.4 » MEAL TIMING BEFORE TRAINING AND COMPETITION

Timing	Food Recommendations	Sample Foods	Start Time
Night before	High-carbohydrate meal 300 g carbohydrate Low in fiber Plenty of fluid	Pasta dishes Rice dishes Lean protein Easy on fat Cooked vegetables	Essential for early starts Helpful for any start time
3–4 hours prior	Carbohydrates: 1.5-2 g/lb. weight (3-4 g/kg) Low-fat proteins Low-fat Low-fiber Plenty of fluids	150-pound athlete: 225-300 g carbohydrate Cereals, bread, crackers, milk, yogurt, fruit, juices, jelly, muffins, bagels	**For midmorning starts:** Eat at 7:00 a.m. for 10:00 a.m. start **Midafternoon starts:** Eat at 10:00 a.m. for 2:00 p.m. start **For evening starts;** Eat at 4:00 p.m. for a 7:00 p.m. start after adequate carbohydrate meals
2 hours prior	Carbohydrates: Up to 1.0 g/lb. weight (2 g/kg) Minimal low-fat protein Low-fat and low-fiber Plenty of fluids	150-pound athlete: 130-150 g carbohydrate Cereals, bread, milk, yogurt, fruit, juices, jelly, crackers	**For midmorning starts:** Eat at 8:00 a.m. for 10:00 a.m. start **For midafternoon start:** Eat at 12:00 noon for 2:00 p.m. start after a large morning breakfast **For late starts:** Eat at 6:00 p.m. for 8:00 p.m. start after adequate carbohydrate meals throughout the day
1 hour prior	Carbohydrates: 0.5 g/lb. weight (1.0 g/kg) Emphasize liquids Easy-to-digest carbohydrates Avoid protein, fat, and fiber	Sports drinks, concentrated carbohydrate drinks and gels, sports bars, tolerated fruits	**For early starts:** Eat at 6:00 a.m. for 8:00 a.m. start **For midmorning starts:** For 10:00 a.m. start, have snack/liquid at 9:00 a.m. in addition to 6:30-7:00 a.m. meal
Immediately prior	Carbohydrates	Sports drinks Energy bars if exercise starts at moderate intensity for at least 30 minutes	For any start time

Timing Matters

Nutritional recovery does take 24 hours and is impacted by what foods and fluids you consume in the hours after exercise and in your daily diet. But, clearly, specific sports nutrition strategies in the hours leading to the training session and during training and competition can benefit winter sport athletes. Consuming properly timed meal(s) or snack(s) at various intervals in the 4-hour time period before practice or competition boosts fuel stores for exercise and supports optimal performance. Replacing fuel and fluid that become depleted during practice and competition is also crucial for top performance and effective strategies, and fluid and fuel choices vary from team sport to team sport athlete and are specific to each sport.

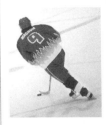

5 Weight, Muscle Building, and Changing Body Composition

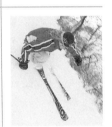

Winter sport athletes, like all of us, come in a variety of shapes and sizes, and many may begin participating in their sport in grade school or high school when body composition is still in flux. As one of these athletes, you may participate in your winter sport well into your years as a masters athlete. You may find that focusing on body composition changes can improve your strength, fitness, and performance. Many winter sport athletes may emphasize building muscle and decreasing body fat to improve athletic performance, particularly alpine skiers and snowboarders who need to develop strength and hockey players who routinely weight train in the preseason. Some winter sport athletes may arrive easily toward the body composition physique that is appropriate for their sport, while others need to work hard and be focused on building muscle and strength and decreasing body fat.

There are smart and sensible ways to attain a lean and strong body. However, many destructive ways can also be used to attempt to attain an overly idealized body composition that may not be realistic for your age, growth and development, level of training, and genetics. It is easy to assume that dropping a few "extra" pounds will improve your performance and that intense training builds muscle strength, but athletic success is not always that simple. Examples abound of athletes at all levels who have restricted their diet or increased their training in an attempt to improve body composition, with the end result being a decrease in energy levels and performance. It is important that you keep an open mind regarding your "best weight." Don't compromise your recovery and energy to build a few pounds of muscle or lose a few pounds of fat.

BODY COMPOSITION, WEIGHT, AND PERFORMANCE

Athletic performance in winter sports does depend on a number of interrelated factors, including your ability to sustain power and move your body weight at high speeds, strength, skill, speed, and cardiovascular development. While some sports place a greater emphasis on specific training components more than others, several of these factors, including power, speed, and strength (which are emphasized in downhill skiing, snowboarding, and ice hockey), can be affected by your muscle development. Endurance athletes also benefit from muscular endurance and lean bodies or optimal body composition. An athlete carrying excess weight or lacking in muscle strength can be at greater risk for injury when performing the skills required for winter sports, as well as the adverse performance effects.

When striving to make body composition changes, you should appreciate that you will perform your best at your own optimal body composition, and not at some idealized body composition that would require excessive training efforts and restrictive food strategies. Severe food restriction and excessive training can result in low energy levels and poor-quality training sessions, increase the risk of injury, and pose both short-term and long-term health risks.

While athletes may desire to achieve a certain level of body fat for optimal performance, strength training or resistance training is a common element of a training program for many winter sport athletes. The high level of muscle mass and strength that can be achieved with resistance training are important factors in athletic performance whether on the slopes, snow, or ice. Optimal and effective methods for gaining muscle mass have long intrigued sports nutritionists and the muscle and supplement industries that pay for heavy marketing and promotion of muscle-building products. However, the key ingredients for maximizing muscle building and strength include your genetic potential, an appropriate resistance-training program, and specific muscle-building nutritional strategies supported by solid scientific research.

Clearly there are advantages for many winter sport athletes in building muscle and maintaining optimal levels of body fat. Let's take a look at some strategies for building muscle and assessing body composition, along with the science, hype, and possible health risks behind some of the supplements marketed to athletes interested in changing body composition and improving performance.

Building Muscle

Hormones—specifically, growth hormone, testosterone, insulin, and insulin-like growth factor—largely control muscle growth. Nutrition can very effectively support your efforts to increase lean body mass by affecting these hormone levels and providing your body with the nutritional tools required for optimal muscle building. Much of the nutritional strategies for muscle building center not only on your daily training diet but also on the intake of certain nutrients timed specifically around your weight-training sessions to optimize your muscle-building efforts.

Some of the keys to optimizing muscle-building efforts include the following:
- Attaining enough calories so that your body has the energy required to build muscle
- Consuming enough carbohydrates so that you meet the fuel demand for both resistance training and training for your sport
- Having enough protein in your daily diet
- Timing your nutrient intake before and after resistance training, particularly for protein
- Consuming fluids and carbohydrate during your workout

Nutritional Requirements for Building Muscle

Calories and carbohydrates. When you strength train, you likely are also participating in regular training for your sport and could be burning significant amounts of stored body fuel from various types of exercise sessions. During weight training, the stored fuels of creatine phosphate and muscle glycogen serve as important energy sources. When combined with other components of your training program, resistance training can provide a further drain on your body's carbohydrate fuel stores. Although you may typically think of increased protein intake in relation to strength training, your first focus should be on consuming adequate energy to build muscle tissue.

One of the most important nutrition guidelines for effectively building muscle is to consume enough calories. Because of the increased energy it takes to build body tissue, falling short on your calorie requirements will impair your rate of muscle building. An additional 350 to 500 calories daily are needed to gain 1 pound of muscle mass per week. Further increases in muscle building require additional calories. Once you gain the muscle and strength that you desire for your sport and performance, it also takes an adequate amount of energy to maintain this increased weight. Keep in mind that these additional calories are the calories required above your energy needs for training and recovery in your sport. The combination of both your winter sport training program and weight training can have a significant impact on your energy needs.

Often the perception is that extra calories consumed to build muscle should be protein calories. Although protein *is* required to build muscle tissue, it is only one of the required tools for the tissue-building process. The amounts of protein that you require as a winter sport athlete should be adequate to cover your daily needs for muscle building, and your protein needs may increase only slightly, if at all. In fact, many of the extra calories needed for muscle building should come from carbohydrates in your diet. The most important factor in your protein intake is timing.

Muscle glycogen is an important fuel source during weight training, and an intense session may deplete 30 percent of your muscle glycogen stores. Clearly when this type of training is combined with your winter sport training, muscle glycogen stores can become significantly depleted in a day or over several days. Regardless of how quickly you deplete these stores, it is important that you replenish glycogen stores adequately after training, whether in the weight room or gym or on the slopes, snow, or ice, so that you continue high-quality training sessions.

Protein. Strength training calls for increased carbohydrate intake, but protein is also an important construction material for the repair and growth of your muscle fibers. Strength training causes the breakdown of muscle fibers, which respond by making bigger and stronger muscle fibers to protect against further stress. Protein is one of the major construction materials for this repair process. While this means that athletes who strength train have higher protein requirements than sedentary individuals, the amount of protein that you consume for your regular winter sport training is likely more than adequate to put you in positive protein balance. Positive protein balance means that you consume enough protein to meet all the protein requiring processes and functions in your body, including synthesizing new muscle tissue.

Your protein needs may increase slightly, if at all, when weight training becomes part of your program. If you do consume protein in excess of what is required for both your strength training and winter sport training, this extra protein is burned for energy, which is not a very efficient process, or simply stored as fat. More is not better, and eating twice as much protein as your body requires won't make your muscles twice as big. Strength training also makes your body more efficient at utilizing protein.

Real foods can easily be part of a well-balanced diet that meets your protein requirements for both weight training and team sport training. Stick with the good high-quality sources of protein mentioned in Chapter 1, such as lean red meat, poultry, fish, and skim milk dairy products. You will also obtain protein from some plant foods, all of which contribute to your total protein intake. Fat in your diet should continue to round out your calorie choices just as it would for your regular training diet.

Timing Your Nutritional Intake

After weight training, your body synthesizes new muscle protein and replenishes muscle glycogen. Several research studies indicate that your nutritional intake in the hours before and after weight training can have a significant impact on supporting your muscle-building efforts. Consuming a combination of carbohydrate and protein both before and after weight training may be more effective in improving protein building than just increasing your overall daily protein intake to build muscle.

Consuming some protein prior to and after your resistance training efforts is probably the most important nutrition strategy to facilitate improved protein synthesis. Aim for about 15 to 20 grams of protein, emphasizing high-quality sources such as skim milk dairy products, whey protein, and protein from animal foods, as essential amino acids are the most potent stimulators of muscle protein synthesis. Combine this protein with at least 35 to 50 grams of carbohydrate.

You can also include both carbohydrate and protein in the next snack or meal that you consume after weight training to continue to facilitate the recovery and muscle building process. Aim for some recovery nutrition foods and fluids within the 1 to 2 hours after weight training. Carbohydrate and protein consumed after resistance training should also work to stimulate both muscle glycogen synthesis and protein synthesis. This form of supplementation increases blood levels of insulin and growth hormone, both of which are tissue-building agents. High-glycemic carbohydrates can be emphasized after resistance training, just as they can after your regular training sessions. Aim for 15 to 20 grams of protein and 50 grams or more of carbohydrates in your recovery snack or meal.

Often your nutritional choices before and after weight training may be related to the practicality of your food and fluid choices and availability. Keep snacks on hand to consume both before and after resistance training. Aim for convenience choices like a low-fat shake or smoothie. Pack protein-containing snacks such as yogurt with fruit, a peanut butter and honey sandwich, or low-fat cheese and crackers. A commercial sports supplement containing a mix of carbohydrate and protein is convenient and meets your nutrition requirements in the hour before and after weight training.

What you consume during resistance training may also be beneficial to your recovery and the quality of your training sessions. While ATP and creatine phosphate in the muscle are your primary fuel sources during weight training sessions, muscle glycogen can become somewhat to significantly depleted between training sets, depending on the intensity and duration of your training. Between sets, your muscle will use the glycolysis energy pathway to regenerate ATP stores. Consuming a sports drink for the carbohydrate it provides can help you maintain muscle glycogen stores and provide energy during your workout. These drinks also provide fluid and assist you in maintaining adequate hydration levels. Of course, consuming plain water during resistance training is also rec-ommended. As with any training session, try to start your workout well hydrated.

Protein Supplements and Weight Training

Protein supplements, currently available in a variety of forms, are a convenient way to con-sume protein before and after resistance-training workouts. As discussed previously, this nutritional strategy can optimize muscle building because the timing of protein intake is key. This protein can be consumed with moderate amounts of carbohydrate in conjunc-tion with both strength training and a hard training session or competition for your sport.

Whey protein is an increasingly popular protein supplement. Whey is the component of milk that is separated when making cheese and other dairy products. It is a high-quality protein and easy to digest. Whey protein can also be lactose-free in the form of whey pro-tein isolate. Soy protein is also an excellent source of protein, especially soy protein iso-late. It is also a high-quality protein choice for vegetarians and is lactose-free. Casein is another protein obtained through cheese production. It does not have as strong of an amino acid profile as whey protein but is still a good protein source. Egg protein is obtained from egg whites and considered the reference standard against which to compare other proteins. Eggs may not be as convenient a protein source as other supplements depending on the timing and location of your training. Other high-quality protein can be obtained from real food sources, such as milk and yogurt, tofu and other soy products, and poultry and lean meats.

Like many other sports nutrition strategies and choices, use of protein supplements before and after resistance training may be a matter of convenience. These products should be taken with a carbohydrate source such as juice. Often, only a small scoop of the pro-tein supplement is needed to provide the required 15 to 20 grams, though higher doses may be encouraged on the label.

Some practical protein and carbohydrate combinations to be consumed before and after weight training include homemade smoothies that use a variety of quality protein ingre-dients such as soy milk, yogurt, and dairy milk. Fruit juice or fruit can be added for car-bohydrate. A generous serving of yogurt with fruit can make a good protein and carbohydrate combination. Low-fat cheese is also a high-quality protein source that can be consumed with fruit or a granola bar.

Your Weight-Training Diet

Clearly your nutritional strategies for optimizing muscle building and increasing strength are complex and interrelated. Consuming adequate calories is key to providing your body with the energy to build muscle. However, your daily protein needs must be met, and the

timing of your protein intake is also important, particularly before a
Weight training is also a fuel-depleting exercise. Consuming carbohydrate
training with protein can facilitate energy and recovery, while consuming ca
ing training also fuels your efforts.

To gain muscle mass while following a strength-training program, you require an additional 350 to 500 calories daily for a muscle gain of one pound per week. These additional calories can come mainly from carbohydrate and some protein. Here are some strategies for obtaining additional calories:

- Adding a bit more protein to sandwiches and dinners
- Topping carbohydrate foods such as bagels with jams and honeys
- Adding another snack to your meal plan
- Adding a fruited yogurt, fruit smoothie, low-fat shake, or instant breakfast drink to your meal plan
- Adding a pasta or rice salad side to your lunch
- Considering a high-calorie shake or meal replacement
- Making oatmeal and soups with milk
- Adding wheat germ, sunflower seeds, and dried fruit to cereals
- Choosing higher-calorie juices such as apple, cranberry, and nectars, and blends
- Choosing calorie-dense cereals such as muesli, granola, and Grape-Nuts
- Having the higher-calorie starchy vegetables such as peas, corn, and winter squash

Table 5.1 summarizes the nutritional strategies for building muscle mass.

Stepping on the Scale

Just as you may be focused on muscle building for your winter sport, you may also monitor your weight and attempt to become leaner in hopes of improving your performance. Often, your efforts at body composition change result in frequent weight checks on the scale. It is important that you keep the scale in perspective as it provides only a rudimentary measure of your body weight and some of the body markers that you monitor during the training season.

The scale obviously weighs all of you—muscle, fat, bone, water and fluid fluctuations, and body organs—and does not differentiate among these body tissues. For this reason, highly muscular athletes may weigh at the high end of their "ideal" weight. Conversely, thin, small-boned people weigh less and are favored by the scale. Your body weight is influenced by much more than what you eat and how much you train. Many of the factors that affect your weight are determined by genetics and are often out of your control.

The best use of a weight scale is to monitor long-term changes over time as they coincide with monitored body composition changes and to measure short-term changes

TABLE 5.1 » NUTRITIONAL FACTORS IN MUSCLE BUILDING

Daily Diet

Nutrient	Role
Calories	Provide additional 350-500 calories in daily diet to build 1 pound muscle per week
Carbohydrates	Fuel source during weight training; require adequate carbohydrates in diet to replenish glycogen stores for comprehensive training program that includes aerobic and anaerobic conditioning.
Proteins	Increased requirements for muscle building; protein needs easily met on well-planned diet for comprehensive training program that includes weight training and aerobic and anaerobic training
Fat	Adequate fat to maintain hormone levels, including testosterone; healthy fats for cardiovascular health

One Hour Before Weight Training
Consume 10-15 g high-quality protein from whey, dairy, or soy source
Consume 25-50 g carbohydrate
Prehydrate with 16-24 oz. (600-720 ml) fluid

During Heavy Training
Consume 16 oz. (600 ml) carbohydrate-electrolyte beverage per hour if desired
Can consume gel and water for carbohydrate and fluid sources

After Training
Consume 15-20 g high-quality protein from whey, dairy, or soy sources
Consume 25-50 g carbohydrate
Rehydrate with 20 oz. (600 ml) fluid for every pound (0.5 kg) of weight loss

related to your hydration status. As mentioned previously, weight loss after a hard training session provides feedback regarding your level of hydration. It is recommended that for every pound (0.5 kilogram) of weight lost during exercise, you rehydrate with 24 ounces (720 milliliters) of noncaffeinated fluid.

Long-term weight changes as measured by a scale can provide you with a crude indicator regarding changes in body composition over time or even help you determine whether you are keeping up with your energy needs or possibly exceeding your energy needs. Chronic unwanted weight loss can indicate that you are not meeting your caloric requirements, and perhaps pushing yourself to an overtrained state. It is also important not to get overly focused on an idealized weight obtained from a height and weight chart, or on the weight and body fat levels of the top athletes in your winter sport. While certain body fat level averages have been measured for specific sports, a number of individual and interconnected factors other than body fat affect an athlete's performance. Averages also indicate that athletes can be successful at varying degrees of reasonable body fat levels, with some competitors at the low end of the body fat range and others at the high end. Top athletes do not always fit the lean and muscular ideal for their sport, and a low body fat level does not guarantee success.

Techniques for Measuring Body Fat Levels

Regardless of the body fat measurement technique that you employ, you should keep in mind that they all measure your body fat indirectly. When choosing a body fat measurement technique, you should consider the following guidelines:

- The technique and formula used to estimate your body fat should be valid for athletes in your sport, your gender, and for your age.
- A reliable technician should perform the technique.
- The same technique should be repeated over time to obtain long-term data and to measure progressive changes.
- The results should be interpreted by a knowledgeable expert who is aware of the limitations of the technique and can advise you appropriately.

Clearly, the measurement of body composition is far from being an exact science. For example, a commonly utilized technique is skinfold testing, which has a standard error of 3 percent. If an athlete were to test at 15 percent body fat, actual body fat levels could range from 12 to 18 percent body fat. Body fat assessments provide a possible range of body fat, rather than an absolute number. When monitoring your body composition over time, it is very important that you do not try to compare various body fat levels measured using different techniques and technicians. Table 5.2 provides the measured body fat levels of athletes from various winter sports. Each athlete has his or her own individual body fat level at which that athlete performs best.

The following body fat measurement techniques are the most commonly used. They all contain some inherent error in their technique and provide only an *estimate* of body composition. Accuracy also can vary among techniques.

Hydrostatic Weighing

Hydrostatic or underwater weighing is a water displacement technique often cited as the "gold standard" of body fat assessment, despite having a standard error of at least 2 percent.

Hydrostatic weighing involves being weighed underwater after expelling all the air from your lungs. Your body density is estimated from the difference between your weight on land and your weight underwater. Your body fat is then extrapolated from this information.

Like all methods, hydrostatic weighing is not error-free. This method assumes a constant fat-free body density and may not be appropriate for all population groups. There is some potential error related to your hydration status, and how much air is actually left

TABLE 5.2 » BODY FAT LEVELS FOR HEALTH AND WINTER SPORTS

Rating	Body Fat
At risk (low levels)	Males: <5% Females: <9%
Below average	Males: 6%-10% Females: 10%-15%
Good	Males: 11%-14% Females: 16%-19%
Average	Males: 15%-18% Females: 20%-25%
Above average	Males: 19%-24% Females: 26%-29%
At risk (high levels)	Males: 25% or more Females: 30% or more

Sport	Body Fat
Alpine skiing	Males: 7%-14% Females: 21%
Snowboarding	Alpine: Males: 11%-13% Females: 21%-25% Freestyle: Males: 6%-9% Females: 15%-18%
Cross-country skiing	Males: 7%-12% Females: 16%-22%
Snowshoeing	Recreational snowshoers: Masters males: 19% Masters females: 23% Competitive or physically active, similar to warm-season
Endurance sports	Cycling: males: 8%-10%; females: 15% Running: males: 6%-13%; females: 10%-19% Triathletes: males: 5%-11%; females: 7%-17%
Hockey	Males: 8%-15% Females: 15%-20%

in your lungs when being weighed underwater, when assuming a standard body density.

Underwater weighing can be a bit uncomfortable, but is offered at some sports medicine centers and universities. Your health club may have someone perform this technique several times throughout the year. This can be a useful body composition technique as measured over time by a skilled technician.

Air Displacement

Also known as body plethysmography, this technique measures body density, too, but by air displacement rather than water displacement. Your body fat percentage is calculated based on equations. This technique provides body fat estimations similar to underwater weighing, though more data are needed on competitive athletes. You sit in an enclosed capsule (a Bod Pod) while a computer measures the amount of air displaced.

This is an expensive system, but is less inconvenient than underwater weighing. However, this technique may not be widely available, but may be at some universities and health clubs.

Bioelectrical Impedance Analysis (BIA)

Use of bioelectrical impedance has markedly increased over the past 10 years because it is relatively inexpensive, portable, and convenient. BIA is based on the conductive property of different tissues within the body. Because muscles contain a high percentage of water, they conduct current more quickly than fat stores. The BIA machine passes a small and undetectable current through the body and analyzes the resistance to the flow of the current. The slower the signal, the more body fat you have.

While BIA is relatively quick and simple, it may overestimate body fat in lean individuals, and the results are affected by hydration levels. If you are not well hydrated, you will appear to have a higher level of body fat than you actually have. You should be well hydrated for the test, but also not drink fluids 4 hours before the test to empty your bladder. It is best if you do not exercise within 12 hours of the test. Alcohol, diuretics, and caffeine should also be avoided prior to this measurement.

Many individuals are now purchasing a home scale (Tanita brand) that measures body fat with this technique. You should take the readings at the same time of day, be well hydrated, and have an empty bladder. Avoid early-morning readings when you are most likely to be dehydrated.

Skinfold Calipers

The skinfold caliper method is the most widely used technique and the most inexpensive and convenient method for measuring body fat. A skilled technician uses calipers to indirectly measure the double thickness of subcutaneous fat underneath the skin. Several standard skinfold sites have been identified on the body: abdomen, arm, thigh, hip area, and back of shoulder. They must be accurately marked, and the skinfold is then pinched and gently pulled away from the body. The sum of several skinfolds (anywhere from three to seven sites) is plugged into a formula that is then used to estimate total body fat.

This technique has several disadvantages. It requires a skilled technician. It assumes that subcutaneous fat is proportional to total body fat. The formulas for skinfold measurements are also based on body composition measurements from the indirect measurement of underwater weighing. Formulas used for skinfold measurements should be appropriate for athletes and their sport. When formulas for the general population are used, body fat is often underestimated in athletes. Skinfold measurements may also underestimate body fat in very lean athletes.

However, when kept in perspective, this technique can be reliable and accurate. When this technique is utilized, you cannot only calculate the body fat percentage but also obtain a number that is the sum of all the skinfolds measured. This absolute number is not formula-dependent and can be monitored over time. For example, a 20-year-old male hockey player may have a three-site skinfold sum of 40 and estimated body fat of 11 percent. A follow-up measurement at several months may show an increase in body weight, while total skinfolds decreased to 36 millimeters. These results would indicate a probable loss in body fat and increase in muscle mass. This trend can be monitored every several months and over a year's time, providing useful feedback regarding training and diet.

Tape measure readings can also be combined with skinfold assessment. Measurements are taken at thigh, arm, and abdominal sites. The more skinfold measurement sites required by the formula, the better. You should never compare body fat estimations made over time using different formulas.

Changing Body Composition

Because your body composition is the result of genetics, as well as training and diet, some athletes may fall naturally at an optimal body composition, while others may struggle due to hereditary factors. Extreme efforts to maintain a set body composition may not be worth the energy as intense weight loss approaches and may compromise the quality of your diet and training. It is also important to keep a perspective on body fat. Aim for a healthy and appropriate range rather than a specific number. Body fat levels may also change over the course of a season and during your years participating in your winter sport depending on the phase of your training, your age, and, if applicable, the stage of your competitive career.

If you are considering improving your body fat composition, have it assessed by a skilled technician. An optimal goal weight can be determined, but it is important to be realistic regarding how much body fat you want to lose, and how quickly you should reach your goal. This may require some professional advice and some realism on the athlete's part.

First, consider your genetics. Experts suggest that 25 to 40 percent of how much fat our body stores is related to our genetics. If you have a history of struggling with body fat loss and maintenance or can say the same of your family members, you should consider a moderate and gentle weight loss goal. Next look at your lifestyle. Food choices are heavily influenced by your schedule, commitments, environment, and stress levels. It is important for your weight loss and body fat goals to be reasonable, as you have to meet the energy demands of not only training but life in general—and work or school—as well.

Dieting Pitfalls

Dieting certainly presents several pitfalls for the winter sport athlete. An athlete who is glycogen depleted, electrolyte depleted, low on protein, and dehydrated from dieting will not perform at his or her best and likely will perform poorly. Rigid dieting and too much calorie restriction can deplete body fuel stores. Intense weight loss efforts can also result in hormonal imbalances, iron deficiency anemia, compromised bone health, and loss of muscular strength and power. Severe dieting can also make you crabby and tired. Dieting just isn't fun.

Food is fuel for your hardworking body, and your body does not respond positively when fuel runs low. A low fuel gauge sends out a slew of appetite-triggering brain chemicals that drive you to eat. What many dieters perceive as a lack of willpower is really the body's drive for self-preservation. Restricting foods can lead to overeating and even binge eating, thwarting weight loss efforts. Besides playing games with the body, dieting wreaks havoc with the mind. Restrictive eating can lead to feelings of deprivation and a preoccupation with food.

Besides triggering overeating, drastic calorie reduction can break down body protein stores for energy. This muscle loss not only hinders your strength and power, but also negatively impacts your metabolism. Muscle is what keeps your furnace burning. Your body also responds to calorie restriction by lowering its resting metabolic rate. Eating normally can restore your metabolism, though this may be difficult if you have a history of repeated dieting. Over time your body may become more efficient at utilizing calories and storing body fat.

Healthy Weight Loss Guidelines

A healthy weight for an athlete is about how you feel and perform, not just about how you perceive how you look or the weight reading on the scale. Keeping a healthy perspective on weight can be confusing these days. The ideal in our society has become more muscular and leaner than ever, while as a whole the population has increased in body weight. Often the ideal portrayed in the media is unhealthy and unrealistic, and this so-called ideal can only be attained through excessive exercise and overly restrictive eating.

Healthy weight loss starts with setting a realistic goal and avoiding quick, unbalanced, and extreme weight loss approaches. Try to accomplish a realistic weight loss in a reasonable amount of time and at an off-season time of year. Let's take a look at some sensible weight loss guidelines.

Set a realistic body composition and weight goal. It is very likely that your training program emphasizes both muscle building and maintaining a low level of body fat. Often, real body composition changes do not result in drastic body weight changes, as the scale measures all body tissue, not just body fat. Elicit the advice of a qualified professional who can assess your body composition results and provide recommended changes in body composition that are appropriate for your age; growth and development, if appropriate; current training program; and sport.

Set a realistic calorie deficit. Keep in mind that when you attempt to lose body fat, you have to restrict calories; however, when you desire to build muscle, you need to consume adequate calories, so it is important to find a balance between your body composition goals. Females should not exceed a weight loss of 1 pound weekly and males, 2 pounds weekly, especially during heavy training periods. Losing 1 pound weekly requires a deficit of 500 calories daily. Greater weight loss requires even more restriction. Losing 2 pounds weekly requires a daily 1,000-calorie deficit, clearly calling for some intense calorie-cutting and calorie-burning efforts that are not always appropriate during periods of growth and/or heavy training cycles.

Trimming no more than 200 to 300 calories daily may be the safest and most effective long-term weight loss approach. This mild reduction should have no metabolism-lowering effects and will not precipitate feelings of hunger and deprivation. However, if you are stepping up your muscle-building efforts, your best results may be obtained by following the proper training program and the nutrition program that is optimal for building muscle mass.

Keep a food journal to assess your current eating habits. Write down your food intake, times eaten, and portions for 1 week. Record your training sessions, noting the duration and intensity of training in conjunction with your food intake. You can also record your moods, thoughts, and feelings that correlate with your food intake to determine some of your eating triggers such as stress or fatigue. It may also be helpful to make a note of your energy levels and recovery during and after various types of training sessions.

Assess your intake. Make sure that you are following the principles of postexercise recovery nutrition. Monitor your hunger and fullness patterns. Do you often wait until you are ravenous before eating? Do you get overfull at meals? Do you eat for comfort or in reaction to stress fairly often? Do you have significant drops in your energy levels during the day?

You may be surprised at how much you actually consume during the day. Writing your food down can also be very helpful in keeping you on track while you are trying to lose weight and, more important, improve the quality of your diet and nutritional strategies, as it makes you accountable and conscious of your food choices.

Have a healthy strategy or plan for reducing your caloric intake and improving your diet. There are a number of effective ways to reduce your caloric intake and improve your diet. It is important that you do eat well postexercise and practice the recovery nutrition guidelines reviewed, as well as time your meals and snacks appropriately before training. If you eat out frequently or consume too much fast food, you may be consuming a large amount of hidden fat in your diet.

Other techniques for reducing fat intake include choosing leaner meats, switching to low-fat dairy products, minimizing added fats and those used in cooking, and decreasing the frequency of sweets. You can also cut back on high-calorie fluids. Alcohol is an obvious choice, as are sodas and perhaps juices.

Pay attention to portions when you eat out or grab items on the run. A bagel or muffin can easily provide over 300 calories.

Plan ahead. Preparing meals ahead of time can help you avoid fatty restaurant foods. Learning how to shop for quick, low-fat, and nutritious foods is also extremely helpful in improving your diet and changing your body composition. You can also pack healthy snacks such as fresh fruits and vegetables. Programming your food environment for success or learning how to manage the environment in which you make your food choices will go a long way to supporting you in reaching your weight loss goals.

Eat balanced meals at the right times. Having real meals will leave you feeling satisfied. Make sure that you consume meals throughout the day, and don't set yourself up for periods of intense hunger. Have a full breakfast and lunch, and don't consume all your calories in the evening. Your body works best on a steady supply of fuel throughout the day. As you can see from the nutrition guidelines outlined for pretraining eating, recovery nutrition, and nutrition strategies designed to optimize muscle building, eating small, frequent meals is ideal and effective.

Have some protein and fat with your meals and snacks. These foods will keep you feeling full longer and help prevent the hunger that leads to an unplanned trip to the vending machine. Choose lean proteins and small amounts of healthy fats. Look at your food journal to determine what times of day you get too hungry. Add a bit more protein or fat to the preceding meal or snack if hunger sets in quickly at specific times.

Pay attention to hunger and fullness. Your body's inner physiological signals are one of the best ways to gauge when it is best to start eating and when your body has had enough food at that particular meal. Of course, you must also plan when you eat around your training and schedule, but paying attention to your hunger and fullness can also provide some valuable direction regarding your food intake and portions. You can also use the 20-minute rule to wait and see whether your meal has been filling and satisfying.

Enjoy the meal, and have some treats. Food is not only fuel but also a source of enjoyment. This means sitting down and enjoying your meals whenever possible, eating slowly and savoring the food, and making sure that favorites are regularly included in your diet.

The Spectrum of Disordered Eating

When you train and compete, being able to move your body quickly over a given distance for a set amount of time offers a performance advantage. So having a lower level of body fat is considered to be a mechanical advantage. However, athletes can become overly focused on their weight and body fat levels. Because athletes may be driven, goal oriented, perfectionistic, and highly competitive, some of the qualities that promote athletic success may manifest in unrealistic weight and body fat goals, and placing a high degree of importance on losing a few pounds. Pressure to lose this weight may come from a number of outside sources, including trainers, coaches, athletic peers, and ideals promoted in the media. Female athletes seem especially at risk of being dissatisfied with their body image, though males are also susceptible.

The estimated prevalence of eating disorders in athletes ranges greatly depending on the screening technique used, the athletes studied, and how an eating disorder was defined. Estimates in female athletes range from a low of 1 percent to a high of 62 percent, and from 0 percent to 57 percent in male athletes. Despite these wide-scale ranges, most experts agree that eating disorders pose a significant health risk to too many athletes. It is also important to appreciate that there is a full spectrum of disordered eating that differs from the full-blown eating disorders of anorexia nervosa, bulimia nervosa, and eating disorders not otherwise specified (EDNOS). *Disordered eating* is a broader term that describes misguided and unhealthy strategies for weight loss, or even occasional bingeing and purging.

There are many gray areas in the area of disordered eating, and it can often be difficult to differentiate when a true eating disorder begins. Often behavior that begins as an attempt to lose weight takes on a life of its own and develops into unhealthy groups of behaviors known as *disordered eating*. Disordered eating represents a full spectrum of eating behaviors, with poor eating habits at one end, and full-blown anorexia nervosa and bulimia nervosa at the other end.

Although full-blown eating disorders are not exceptionally high in most sports, studies indicate a high prevalence of disordered eating behavior and distorted concerns regarding body weight, body fat, and body shape among athletes. Some common disordered eating behaviors may include skipping meals, constant weighing, eating very little fat, and fearing that specific foods may promote unwanted weight gain. Binge eating, as characterized by consuming large amounts of food while feeling out of control, can be part of disordered eating.

Another term, *anorexia athletica*, describes a syndrome characterized by disordered eating and compulsive exercising. It is associated with an intense fear of gaining weight, despite being at normal or below normal weight, and is characterized by food restriction, often fewer than 1,200 calories per day, and excessive exercise. Bingeing, self-induced vomiting, and use of laxative and diuretics may also occur. Some athletes are able to stop these behaviors when participation in a sport stops. But for other athletes, this behavior continues to develop into a full-blown clinical eating disorder.

Eating disorders are complicated and multifactorial. Psychological and emotional issues such as anxiety and depression, an inability to cope with family and personal problems, life stresses, biochemical imbalances, and the pressure to be thin or lean from both sport and society may be involved. Some triggers associated with eating disorders in athletes include traumatic life events such as relationship and family problems, recommendations to lose weight, prolonged periods of dieting, and a large discrepancy between actual weight and a self-defined ideal weight. It is possible that individuals at high risk for eating disorders may gravitate toward certain sports, but being involved in a sport may also trigger the eating disorder in a susceptible athlete. Some risk factors that are more specific to athletes than the general population include prolonged periods of dieting or weight cycling; an increase in training volume; stress related to their sport and training, such as the loss of a coach; weight loss pressures from coaches and trainers; and lack of guidance on appropriate weight and body composition goals and healthy weight management strategies.

While eating disorders in men and male athletes are not as high as in females, it is still a concern, and the figures available may underestimate the true prevalence of eating disorders in men. Males who develop disordered eating are more likely to previously have been overweight or even obese, and the fear of gaining weight may relate to this past experience. Male athletes may also diet in an attempt to improve performance or in response to an injury that limits training.

A recently identified body image disorder in male athletes is *muscle dysmorphia*. Muscle dysmorphia is characterized by an intense preoccupation with body size and degree of muscularity. Individuals with this disorder attempt to increase body size and may abuse performance-enhancing drugs or dietary supplements that promise to increase muscle mass or decrease body fat. This disorder is more common in male weightlifters and bodybuilders.

Several common warning signs may signal the start of an eating disorder. They include repeatedly expressing concerns about body weight, refusal to maintain even a minimal weight, periods of severe calorie restriction, and excessive physical activity that is not part of a balanced training program. Other warning signs may include food rituals, self-induced vomiting, and abuse of laxatives and diet pills. Many of these behaviors by themselves do not prove the presence of an eating disorder, but they justify further attention to the

» EATING DISORDERS

Anorexia Nervosa
– Resistance to maintaining body weight at or above a minimally normal weight
– Intense fear of gaining weight or becoming fat even though underweight
– Distortion in the way in which one's body weight or shape is experienced; denial of the seriousness of current low body weight
– Infrequent or absent menstrual periods in females who have reached puberty

Physical Characteristics of Anorexia Nervosa
Hair loss and growth of fine body hair | Low pulse rate | Sensitivity to cold | Stress fractures, osteopenia, or osteoporosis | Overuse injuries | Abnormal fatigue | Gastrointestinal problems

Bulimia Nervosa
– Recurrent episodes of binge eating, characterized by a sense of lack of control and an excessive amount of food within a short period of time
– Purging behavior such as self-induced vomiting, misuse of laxatives, diuretics, enemas, or other medications
– Binge eating and purging behavior occurring

on average at least twice weekly for 3 months
– Self-esteem being inappropriately influenced by body shape and weight

Physical Characteristics of Bulimia Nervosa
Frequent weight fluctuations | Difficulty swallowing and throat damage | Swollen glands | Damaged tooth enamel from gastric acid | Electrolyte imbalances and dehydration | Menstrual irregularities | Diarrhea or constipation

Eating Disorder Not Otherwise Specified (EDNOS)
This category includes disorders of eating that do not meet the criteria for a specific eating disorder.
– Binge eating disorder and episodes of binge eating without the use of compensatory behavior as seen in bulimia nervosa
– Repeatedly chewing and spitting out, but not swallowing, large amounts of food
– The criteria for anorexia nervosa are met except that the individual has regular menstrual periods.
– All the criteria for bulimia nervosa are met except that the frequency of binge eating and

possible presence of a problem. The sidebar describes some of the characteristics of full-blown eating disorders.

Disordered eating and eating disorders can lead to poor performance related to glycogen and electrolyte depletion, dehydration, and loss of lean body mass. Nutrient deficiencies can result, as can increased risk of infection, illness, and injuries. Other health-related effects are decreased metabolism, gastrointestinal complication, menstrual dysfunction in females, and decreased bone mineral density. To avoid these harmful effects, an athlete with an eating disorder requires the help of a team of skilled professionals trained in treating this condition, including a physician, dietitian, and psychologist or therapist.

purging behavior occur less than twice weekly and for less than 3 months.
– Regular purging behaviors occur after consuming small amounts of foods.

Muscle Dysmorphia
This term describes a form of body image disturbance described in male bodybuilders and weightlifters.
– Preoccupation with not being sufficiently lean and muscular
– Preoccupation with muscularity causes significant social impairment
– Characterized by excessive exercise, preoccupation with food, abuse of steroids, and abuse of dietary supplements aimed at increasing body size or decreasing body fat

Anorexia Athletica
This term has been used to describe a condition that is not a full-blown eating disorder.
– Characterized by disordered eating and compulsive exercise
– Intense fear of weight gain despite weighing below the expected weight for age and height

– Weight loss achieved by food restriction and extensive compulsive exercise
– May involve self-induced vomiting and use of laxatives and diuretics

Binge Eating Disorder
This disorder is currently a subset of EDNOS, but it is expected to be classified as a separate diagnostic entity.
– Recurrent episodes of binge eating during a discrete period of time and characterized by a large amount of food and a sense of lack of control
Binge episodes characterized by the following behaviors:
   – Eating more rapidly than normal
   – Eating until uncomfortably full
   – Eating large amounts when not physically hungry
   – Eating alone because of embarrassment of the volume of food
   – Feeling disgusted, depressed, or guilty after eating
   – Marked distress regarding binge eating
   – Bingeing occurs 2 days weekly for 6 months

EVALUATING NUTRITIONAL SUPPLEMENTS
Sales and Marketing of Ergogenic Aids

The term *ergogenic* means "to produce work." Nutritional ergogenic aids are promoted as increasing muscle size, increasing strength, promoting fat burning, and improving speed. For example, it is claimed that several ergogenic aids such as carnitine "enhance fat burning." Creatine is reported to enhance muscle building when taken during a strength-training program.

Apparently many consumers have believed the promise that nutritional ergogenic aids promote, as nutritional ergogenic aid sales have become a serious and lucrative business. U.S. sales from one such product, creatine, increased from $30 million in 1995, to $180 million in 1998, to a high of $400 million in 2001. In fact, sales for the entire dietary supplement industry, which include these ergogenic aid products, grew to nearly $18 billion in 2002, of which sports nutrition sales exceeded $6 billion for that same year. With all sports nutrition product sales, not just ergogenic aids, expected to have surpassed $7.2 billion in 2004, athletes have clearly embraced a wide selection of these products as an important component of their training programs.

One study of female collegiate varsity athletes determined that more than 60 percent of them used some type of nutritional supplement at least once a month. Good health was the reason most frequently cited for supplement use. Over one-third of the female athletes took a multivitamin mineral supplement with iron, but there was also use of amino acid and protein supplements, and herbal products.

Chapters 3 and 4 outline practical uses for a wide variety of sports nutrition products such as sports drinks, gels, and bars, and high-carbohydrate and meal replacement supplements that are backed by both research and the practical experience of athletes. Using these products knowledgeably and appropriately carries minimal risk and some clear performance benefits that support your training and competition goals (see the sidebar in Chapter 4). However, some sports drinks and recovery drinks may also contain ingredients that are not necessary or even safe for some athletes to consume, especially young and developing athletes.

Ergogenic aid sales are a serious business for both male and female athletes. It is important that when you ingest a product in the quest for top performance, you have verified that it is legal, effective, and safe. Unfortunately, many of these products are backed solely by strong and enticing claims, anecdotal hearsay, high-profile athlete and coach testimonials, and referenced "research" that has not been published in full in a reputable scientific journal. In reality, the majority of these supplements have *not* been thoroughly and appropriately tested. Moreover, many of the supplements that are tested independently of the manufacturers who supply them don't live up to their performance claims.

But despite this lack of plausibility, it can be tempting to top off all your hard work with an easily ingested supplement that promises a quick and effective performance boost.

With new products coming out monthly, athletes need to be discerning when evaluating nutritional ergogenic aids or performance enhancers. It is important that you can make knowledgeable choices about these products. Keep these tips in mind before you use them:

- Understand how the ergogenic aid purportedly functions.
- Know the summary of the current research support on the supplement.
- Be aware of any safety concerns surrounding the product.
- Know whether the product is a legal supplement for athletes.

Chances are you may try a supplement because it is widely talked about among other athletes that you train with or compete against, or because it is surrounded by enticing marketing claims for building muscle, burning fat, and increasing energy output. But these supplements are never going to be an effective substitution for a solid training program and an optimal performance diet.

Another important consideration when evaluating the safety of these supplements is the age of an athlete. The American Academy of Pediatrics does not recommend high-performance supplements in the diet of child athletes. These supplements are also routinely tested on adults (if at all) and not on young and growing bodies, or athletes of high school age. Studies of collegiate athletes are limited, as are long-term safety data. What safety information is available would not address safety issues in high school athletes. Some supplements are also banned by the National Collegiate Athletic Association (NCAA) and can be varified on their Web site (www.ncaa.org).

Regulation of Dietary Supplements and Nutritional Ergogenic Aids

Athletes are bombarded with claims of the magical effects of nutritional ergogenic aids on performance. Advertising and claims surrounding these products have increased exponentially since the Dietary Supplement Health and Education Act (DSHEA) was passed in 1994. DSHEA significantly changed how all dietary supplements such as vitamins, minerals, herbs, amino acids, metabolites, and even hormones were tested, marketed, labeled, and manufactured.

Unlike regulation of makers of a drug or food additive, supplement manufacturers are not required to prove that a dietary supplement works. Under DSHEA, manufacturers are responsible for making sure that products are safe. The government does not review these products before they are put on the market, but the Food and Drug Administration (FDA) can take action against any unsafe dietary supplement products. However, the FDA cannot evaluate the thousands of products on the market, and it makes selective use of time and resources. It is more likely that it will respond only to products that have resulted in significant adverse health effects that occur on a large scale.

You may also notice on the label a somewhat loosely defined "nutrition support claim." These claims may relate to the "structure and function" of the body and "general well-being." While a certain set of conditions must be met to make these claims, they do not require prior FDA approval. Manufacturers must be able to substantiate that the claim is "truthful and not misleading," but they cannot promise to prevent or cure a disease. Some nutrition support claims may include "maintains a healthy circulatory system," or "helps maintain a healthy intestinal flora." Note that supplements providing these types of claims must also state: "This product is not intended to diagnose, treat, cure, or prevent any disease."

The FDA also recommends that the discerning consumer realizes that it is up to each company to decide how their manufacturing practices will prepare and package supplements, thereby affecting their purity, safety, potency, and therefore overall quality. According to the FDA, consumers can contact the manufacturer and request product safety information and research support, which would preferably not be only in-house published data. They can also question whether the firm has a quality control system in place and whether any adverse event reports have resulted from use of their product.

Starting in 2003, the FDA is in the process of developing Good Manufacturing Processes (GMPs) in coordination with the supplement industry. Two Web sites, www.nsf.org and www.consumerlab.com, currently list products that have been evaluated for appropriate quality control. Both of these sites also test products for banned supplements and can certify products do not contain banned supplement for athletes. Some supplement companies have their own GMPs in place and may be regulated under the National Nutrition Foods Association (see www.nnfa.org).

You should also review the "Supplement Facts" labels on the package of dietary supplements. Unlike conventional foods, the dosage on labels is not standardized. So remember that higher amounts than needed or are safe may be recommended. The label will provide the following information:

- Statement of identity
- Net quantity of ingredients
- A structure and function claim statement
- Directions for use
- Supplement Facts Label
- Other ingredients listed in descending order of predominance
  by common name or proprietary blend
- Name and address of packer, manufacturer, or distributor

Unfortunately, even if companies are accused and fined regarding false claims on dietary supplements, they may not be deterred from promoting new products. Often fines may be rendered insignificant by a large volume of sales generated while claims are investigated.

Is It Effective?

Valid scientific testing of a nutritional ergogenic aid costs time, money, and resources. Tests of a supplement's effect on performance should be conducted with well-trained athletes and can be specific to the type of sport. For these and other reasons, much of the supplement industry forgoes testing and relies heavily on testimonials, anecdotes, and untested scientific theories, rather than research studies to promote their product. But, a theory is not proof. A theory is a hypothesis or intriguing idea that requires testing. "Scientific breakthroughs" may be new and interesting ideas with little or no basis in fact.

A scientific trial remains the best way in which to examine the effectiveness of ergogenic aids on performance. Here, athletes' experiences can be helpful to researchers who desire to focus on potentially effective substances. Scientists can use them to determine what products are worth testing and what dosages are appropriate for test protocols. Testing should closely mimic real athletic performance conditions as much as possible. Researchers should control for age, level of training, and nutritional status. Various dosages, supplementation periods, types of exercise, and performance testing may need to be incorporated.

Studies should control for the placebo effect as much as possible by incorporating a double-blind design. In this approach, subjects receive both the substance being tested and a placebo. To minimize bias, subjects and researchers don't know which product is being administered when. In addition to a placebo trial, there may be a control (no treatment) group. These are only some of the needed features of well-designed testing that satisfy the scientist, but not always the athlete. A large change in performance is required for outcomes to be considered statistically significant. In many cases, however, changes produced by nutritional supplementation are likely to be smaller. Although a 1 to 3 percent change may not be statistically adequate, it may be useful in elite competition. Researchers also report the overall performance effect within a group. Positive results of individuals within a group may be diluted by the negative or neutral responses of other subjects. Not all subjects respond in the same way to a particular substance.

Unfortunately, even well-designed studies can be quoted out of context. Research findings are extrapolated to inappropriate conclusions. Companies often state that they are in the process of conducting research. Other times they say that research is "in-house" or has simply never been published in reputable peer-reviewed journals. And even well-designed preliminary studies require verification through additional sound research.

Unfortunately, even studies published in reputable journals can provoke criticism when placed under close scrutiny. Additionally, patented nutritional ergogenic aids may also look impressive. Yet patents are not granted based on the effectiveness of the product, but rather on its distinguishable differences. Patents can be obtained with a theoretical model rather than objective double-blind research.

Is It Safe?

False claims aside, the next step in determining whether you should use an ergogenic aid is safety concerns. As previously mentioned, supplement manufacturers are not required to prove a product's safety. Negative effects from products may be acute, mild, or temporary, but they can also be serious and chronic. Some dietary supplements may be toxic or decrease the absorption of other nutrients, especially in high doses, where the "more is better" belief prevails. Ironically, independent testing has also found that many supplements do not contain the ingredients marked on the label. Often products are watered down or contain other unlisted ingredients that may be harmful or illegal. Hopefully this concern will be resolved when all companies comply with adopted GMPs.

Is It Legal?

As a competitive athlete, particularly if you may be drug tested, you do not want to inadvertently take a dietary supplement that contains a banned substance. The past several years have seen a significant increase in the number of positive tests at the elite and professional levels, claimed to be the result of contaminated or mislabeled dietary supplements. All athletic governing bodies have some regulation regarding the use of ergogenic aids. (Products banned by the NCAA, for example, are listed at www.ncaa.org.) Even if you avoid illegal products such as ephedra or androstenodione, reading labels is not a 100-percent guarantee of avoiding banned products. Cross contamination can occur in the manufacturing process, and the purity of these supplements is often questioned.

Specific nutritional ergogenic aids can benefit athletes under certain conditions. However, the supplement industry is an extremely profitable business that relies on theories and testimonials to market products. Ergogenic aid theories may even be extrapolated from clinical research on disease states or nutrient deficiencies. To say that this product will then produce a performance improvement is not a scientific breakthrough but a leap in logic. Even with proven ergogenic aids, it is important to keep their role in perspective. While they may produce small performance improvements, ergogenic aids are no substitute for proper training, nutrition, and psychological preparation.

Supplement Research Support, Safety, and Practical Issues

This section will review several popular nutritional ergogenic aids for scientific validity as determined by quality research. Any safety concerns and any practical issues regarding the use of these supplements will also be reviewed in this section. Not surprisingly, many sports physiologists and sports nutritionists do not provide overwhelming support for the majority of these supplements. They would rather that you trained and ate properly as this very effectively improves performance! Many professionals also have concerns about younger and developing athletes taking supplements that have not been proven safe, as supplement testing is usually done in adults.

Many ergogenic aids marketed to team sport athletes are designed to increase muscle mass and strength and decrease body fat. Some ergogenic aids are also reported to improve performance by increasing power output during exercise. Table 5.3 summarizes several ergogenic aids that are discussed in more detail here.

Ergogenic Aids that Affect Body Composition
Creatine

With sales in the United States at $400 million in 2001, creatine is clearly a supplement that came out of the starting blocks and shifted into high gear. Fortunately, creatine is one of the best-researched ergogenic aids, making it possible for sports nutritionists to provide clear and confident recommendations regarding this sports nutrition supplement.

TABLE 5.3 >> SUMMARY OF ERGOGENIC AIDS

Supplement	Claims	Scientific Data	Safety
Creatine	Supports training for increased muscle mass	Well supported by scientific data	Can be used safely by adults when following scientific protocols
HMB	Builds muscle strength; inhibits breakdown of muscle and protein	Limited human data supporting claims; several studies found no benefits	Doses at 3 g daily taken for 6-8 weeks appear safe
Protein supplements	Facilitates muscle building	Can consume 10-20 g high-quality protein in conjunction with carbohydrate before and after weight training	Can consume protein from real foods, supplements not required; exceeding recommended dose provides no additional benefits

CONTINUED

TABLE 5.3 continued

Amino acids	Facilitate muscle building and exercise recovery	Not supported by well-designed research	Can upset balance of amino acid metabolism when taken in large doses
Ribose	Improved muscle recovery, energy and endurance enhancer; rebuilds ATP	Published research is limited; current data far from conclusive	Not enough safety data
Glutamine	Supports the immune system; promotes protein synthesis	May benefit athletes with a true glutamine deficiency; more data required	Often incorporated in many sports nutrition supplements; too much could upset amino acid balance
Carnitine	Metabolic fat burner	Not supported by well-designed research	L-carnitine form only; can be consumed at 1-2 g daily for 6 months
Chromium	Builds muscle and burns fat	Not supported by well-designed research	Not to exceed 200 mcg daily
Pyruvate	Improves endurance; promotes muscle building and fat loss	Not tested on athletes; not supported by research	Not much safety data
Prohormones	Promotes muscle building	Illegal products	Banned by the USADA and IOC; long-term safety concerns and possible adverse health effects
Weight loss supplements	Promotes body fat loss and weight loss	Many ingredients not supported by well-designed research; risks may outweigh benefits	Risks of supplements may be serious; some ingredients may be banned
Caffeine	Promotes endurance; may improve power output for shorter distances	Good data on endurance exercise; limited data on power sports indicate need for more research	Can be used safely in moderate doses; high doses are not required for ergogenic effect
MCT oil	Provides fuel during training and spares muscle glycogen; enhances fat burning	Tested mainly for endurance exercise; not supported by well-designed research	May cause mild gastrointestinal symptoms

Creatine is often advertised as a steroid alternative, but it is really more comparable to glycogen loading. Just as carbohydrate ingestion maximizes glycogen content of the muscle, "creatine loading" can increase muscle creatine stores. Your normal intake of creatine is about 2 grams daily (perhaps less for vegetarians), and it is also synthesized in the liver and kidney. Creatine is an essential fuel of the ATP creatine phosphate system. Loading the muscle with creatine is designed to increase ATP resynthesis. This power system typically stores enough fuel to last 6 to 8 seconds. Creatine can also buffer lactic acid and transport ATP to be utilized for muscle contraction.

Muscle biopsies have confirmed that rapid loading can be achieved with 25 to 30 grams of creatine daily divided into five to six doses. A more gentle loading protocol is 3 grams daily over 28 days. Unlike carbohydrate, creatine appears to remain trapped in the muscle without supplementation for 4 to 5 weeks. About 30 percent of individuals who creatine load appear to be "nonresponders." Ingesting about 75 to 100 grams of carbohydrate has been demonstrated to enhance creatine accumulation in the muscle. You should also be aware that a 2- to 5-pound (1- to 2-kilogram) weight gain is associated with creatine loading. Scientists believe this to be water gain, as urine output decreases during the loading phase.

Though not documented in the scientific literature, anecdotal reports abound that creatine loading is associated with muscle cramping and GI upset. When loading with creatine, make sure that you consume plenty of water to help prevent any side effects. Taking more than 30 grams of creatine daily over 5 days offers no additional benefits for loading. As is often the case with many nutritional supplements, more is not better. In fact, there are some concerns that chronic and high doses of creatine can lead to liver and kidney damage. People with existing kidney disease should not take creatine.

We know that creatine ingestion can load the muscle, but how does it affect performance? Creatine loading appears to increase the rate of creatine resynthesis during recovery (20 seconds to 5 minutes) from bouts of high-intensity exercise (6 to 30 seconds). Creatine loading delays fatigue during activity that includes repeated, all-out surges of energy interspersed with rest periods.

Creatine could potentially assist team sport players, such as hockey players. Creatine loading appears to benefit resistance training, allowing more repetitions to be performed and consequently increases in strength. Of course, resistance training is commonly part of a winter sport athlete's training program.

It is not recommended that you supplement for more than 60 days, and it should be at a low dose of 3 grams during this time period. Creatine loading may also only be necessary once or twice yearly due to the cyclical nature of your training and the muscle's ability to hold creatine for several weeks.

Creatine is currently legal. However, there have been some concerns of cross con-tamination of creatine products in recent years, as athletes ingesting this supplement have tested positive for banned prohormone products. No creatine studies have been done with high school athletes or athletes who are still growing and developing. Many high schools and colleges likely have their own policy regarding creatine supplementation in their ath-letes. The NCAA does not allow use of creatine (see the sidebar later in this chapter).

Beta-Hydroxy-Beta-Methylbutarate (HMB)

HMB is primarily marketed to strength and power athletes and is one of the fastest-selling supplements on the market. Winter sport athletes who weight train and want to facilitate muscle recovery may be interested in this supplement.

HMB is not actually a nutrient but a metabolic by-product produced in small amounts when the amino acid leucine is metabolized. You produce only about 0.2 to 0.4 gram of HMB daily. HMB was first developed by scientists and then patented by the company that produces HMB, which has sponsored much of the research on HMB.

Much of the initial HMB research was done on animals, but there are also human data. Some research has found greater increases in muscle mass and fewer markers of muscle damage; however, these studies did not always control for diet, which can have a signifi-cant impact on muscle gain in conjunction with weight training. Several studies found no ergogenic benefit from HMB supplementation. In one study on collegiate football play-ers, for example, no improvements in muscle strength and body composition were seen with HMB supplementation. Another study in elite male rugby players found that both aerobic and anaerobic capacity was unaffected by HMB supplementation, as well as a com-bination of HMB and creatine supplementation.

Further published data on this supplement are needed. A daily dose of 3 grams ap-pears to be safe when taken for a 6- to 8-week period.

Amino Acids

Marketing of amino acid supplements is heavily targeted to strength athletes and other athletes who benefit from building muscle mass. Supporters of amino acid supplemen-tation claim that these products are more readily digested and absorbed than the protein found in foods. This statement simply is *false*, because your body is well equipped to han-dle protein from whole foods by secreting a number of enzymes that renders amino acid absorption at a high level of effectiveness. It is true that the timing of your protein in-take before and after weight training can facilitate muscle building and recovery. However, full muscle recovery entails following specific nutrition guidelines to obtain enough calories and protein in your daily training diet. Purchasing expensive amino acid supple-ments simply isn't necessary.

It is also important for you to appreciate that amino acid or protein metabolism is very complex. It is affected by a variety of factors including amino acid concentration in the blood, competition with other available amino acids, and the presence of other nutrients. Amino acid mixtures could potentially lead to nutritional imbalances, as an excess of one amino acid may negatively affect the absorption of another.

Amino acid supplement dosing may also be misleading. A bottle listing up to 500 milligrams in a capsule actually contains less than 1 gram of amino acids, whereas only 1 ounce of chicken contains 7,000 milligrams, or 7 grams of amino acids in the form of whole protein. Clearly, amino acid supplements cannot meet the dosing found in a compact source of natural protein.

The amino acids arginine, lysine, and ornithine are often sold individually or in combination as "legal anabolic compounds" and "recovery agents." Claims surrounding these products include promoting release of growth hormone and a subsequent increase in lean body mass and decrease in body fat. These claims surfaced after two studies found that infusing these amino acids directly into the bloodstream stimulated the release of human growth hormone, which is involved in building muscle tissue.

The effects of oral supplementation on human growth hormone are very questionable. Several well-controlled studies have verified that oral supplementation is not comparable to intravenous infusion. Other studies using oral supplementation have been criticized for their design. One study that provided a large oral dose of arginine and ornithine found a slight increase in growth hormone release. However, this was most likely stimulated by the resistance training rather than the amino acid intake. High oral dosages of these amino acids are also associated with gastrointestinal problems.

Arginine, lysine, and ornithine are available individually or in mixtures in powder or tablet form. Dosages used in several research studies were 2 to 3 grams, and 6 grams may cause gastrointestinal distress. High doses of amino acids may also inhibit absorption of other amino acids. Doses used in several studies are also easily obtained by consuming high-protein foods. Use of these supplements or any other amino acid supplement combination is unlikely to be beneficial, and they are not recommended.

Ribose

Ribose is hyped as a supplement that can improve muscle recovery, boost energy, enhance endurance, support cardiovascular fitness, and rebuild ATP. A sugar formed from the conversion of glucose, it is considered the starting substance for ATP production and is part of the metabolic pathway that results in ATP resynthesis.

However, published research on the effect of ribose in athletic performance is relatively limited. Ribose did benefit one group of men who suffered from cardiac ischemia, which is not applicable to athletes. Three published studies measured sprint or repeated high-intensity exercise in trained male athletes. Ribose supplementation did not affect power output. Another study that combined the ribose supplements with creatine and glutamine found no improvement in muscular strength and endurance or in body composition.

Ribose is for sale, so safety must be considered. Ribose has not been used for long periods of time, though doses of up to 20 grams appear to be tolerated. Higher doses may result in gastrointestinal side effects. Manufacturer recommendations are often 3 grams prior to and 3 grams after exercise. The patent holder recommends that it be consumed with carbohydrate on an empty stomach. Current data are far too limited to safely recommend a cycling or maintenance dose. In fact, much more data and solid proof are required before this supplement can be recommended.

Glutamine

Glutamine is an amino acid synthesized in the muscle tissue. It is the most abundant amino acid in the body and used as a fuel source by the cells of the immune system. Impaired glutamine status has been associated with the overtrained state in athletes. Overtrained athletes are thought to be more susceptible to upper respiratory tract infections and other infections.

Blood glutamine levels fall during endurance exercise and remain lowered during the recovery phase several hours after exercise. Glutamine depletion is thought to become cumulative if recovery between sessions is inadequate, because overtrained athletes have lower blood glutamine levels. However, adequate daily carbohydrate consumption is thought to possibly be the most effective means for preventing glutamine depletion.

The theory maintains that glutamine supplementation could help prevent the immune problems suffered by overtrained athletes. Research data, however, are not consistent in proving this true. Only one study has reported that supplementation reduced the incidence of infection the week following a heavy exercise session. What is likely is that glutamine supplementation benefits those athletes with a true deficiency and that it is not a general cure for immune system problems.

Another theory regarding glutamine supplementation is that it promotes protein synthesis and helps maintain positive protein balance in the muscle by preventing protein breakdown. Glutamine may also stimulate the synthesis of muscle glycogen. Obviously glutamine performs some very important functions in the body. However, more research on glutamine supplementation in athletes is needed.

Carnitine

Often promoted as a "metabolic fat burner," carnitine is a nonessential nutrient formed in the liver from two amino acids. Your skeletal muscles contain at least 90 percent of the carnitine in your body. Carnitine is of interest to athletes because it carries fat into the cells to be burned for energy during exercise. If carnitine supplementation did increase fat burning, and decrease your body's reliance on glycogen and blood glucose, it could enhance performance.

Carnitine is unlikely to be an effective ergogenic aid, as carnitine supplementation does not appear to increase muscle carnitine levels (as measured by muscle biopsies). Glycogen sparing with carnitine supplementation was also not found in the studies conducted on its use. Only one study found a slight increase in muscle carnitine content after supplementation with 2 grams daily. Other studies found no improvements in exercise performance with carnitine supplementation. Two studies that did find a positive performance effect have been criticized for their methodology and design.

Carnitine supplementation appears to be safe if you consume the L-carnitine form of the nutrient only. DL-carnitine can be toxic as it depletes L-carnitine and may lead to a deficiency. Two to 4 grams daily can be consumed for one month, though 1- to 2-gram doses have been taken for 6 months.

Chromium

Chromium is a trace mineral, often marketed as a legal alternative to anabolic steroids and human growth hormone. Scientists have long known that chromium enhances the effects of insulin, which regulates glucose metabolism. Adults with impaired glucose regulation have been measured to have positive responses with chromium supplementation. Insulin also promotes the uptake of amino acids into muscle cells and regulates protein metabolism. This protein-building function has linked chromium to an increase in muscle mass.

Proponents of chromium supplementation for athletes maintain that many are chromium-deficient and that a supplement would improve protein building. Other proponents believe that high chromium doses could stimulate greater than normal muscle building. It has not been firmly established that athletes are chromium-deficient; however, the North American diet is high in refined grains, which may trigger a higher release of insulin and require more chromium in the diet than is normally consumed.

Studies on chromium supplementation have produced mixed, but mostly negative results. The more recent and better-designed studies monitored and controlled for exercise training and carefully measured body composition. These studies found no significant gains in muscle mass with chromium supplementation. Earlier studies, which showed some positive results, were not as carefully controlled. Higher doses of chromium in several studies have also not shown significant gains in muscle mass.

With high sales of chromium picolinate and large doses recommended by manufacturers, safety concerns regarding chromium supplementation have been raised. We do not have much long-term data on chromium doses beyond 200 micrograms. Because chromium is a mineral, concern has been raised about large chronic doses. Minerals often compete with one another for absorption, and one study did find that iron status was compromised with chromium supplementation.

Clearly, adequate chromium intake is important. Especially good sources are wholegrain breads and cereals, mushrooms, asparagus, apples, raisins, cocoa, peanuts, peanut butter, and prunes. Various sports nutrition supplements such as recovery drinks and bars are often supplemented with chromium, and many regular multivitamin mineral supplements also contain it. Try not to exceed 200 micrograms daily from supplemental sources. Most diets likely do not exceed 50 micrograms of chromium daily.

Overall, chromium's ability to build muscle mass in athletes appears highly doubtful. Supplementation in safe doses is only appropriate to correct a deficiency and compensate for an inadequate diet.

Pyruvate

Pyruvate is commonly sold as DHAP, which is a combination of pyruvate and dihydroxyacetone. This supplement is promoted to improve endurance exercise, promote fat loss, and increase muscle mass.

Studies that have tested pyruvate on endurance performance need to be put in perspective. These studies, using a small number of untrained subjects exercising at moderate intensity, may not have much relevance to endurance athletes. In addition, several of the study protocols used 25 grams of pyruvate combined with 75 grams of dihydroxyacetone. Many commercial preparations contain much smaller doses. However, these studies did measure an increase in endurance with the supplement.

Pyruvate does not appear to have much validity as a fat burner, either. One oftenquoted study restricted participants to a 1,000-calorie diet daily and no activity—a result not applicable to an athlete participating in winter sports.

Prohormones

Prohormones are widely sold in dietary supplements and are currently banned by the International Olympic Committee (IOC), U.S. Antidoping, and other sport governing bodies. These products include the "andro" and the "nor" prohormones. Andro products, namely androstenedione, are testosterone precursors, and they transform to this hormone in the body. Other androgenic products include androstenediol and dehydroepiandrosterone (DHEA). Nor products are precursors to the steroid nortestosterone (nandrolone), which is similar in structure to testosterone. Available nor-prohormones are 19-norandrostenediol and 19-norandrostenedione. These nor products break down to the same metabolites used to detect nandrolone usage. Andro prohormones may lead to an elevated testosterone-to-epitestosterone ratio. All of these substances carry the risk of a positive drug test and potential negative side effects.

Prohormones are easily purchased in the United States and over the Internet because they are classified as dietary supplements. Often these supplements are geared toward building muscle, enhancing recovery, and "maintaining hormone levels."

Since the late 1990s, a rash of elite athletes have tested positive for the steroid nandrolone. Many of these athletes have claimed that it occurred through the inadvertent ingestion of the dietary supplements that contained nor hormones. Although athletes can read labels carefully to avoid these banned products, it is becoming clear that this may not be enough. A study conducted at the UCLA Olympic Laboratory checked urine tests after supplementation with androstenedione and 19-norandrostenedione. As expected, the 19-nor produced nandrolone metabolites exceeding IOC limits. But the results of the andro supplementation were especially concerning. This test actually produced nandrolone metabolites in the urine! Twenty of 24 positive urine samples exceeded IOC limits. Based on these findings, researchers tested several andro supplements. Seven of eight tested capsules contained varying amounts of 19-nor. Researchers speculated that the supplements had been contaminated with 19-nor in the manufacturing process. Many supplement companies use the same equipment to blend, encapsulate, and bottle both prohormone and nonprohormone products. Quality control is entrusted to supplement companies.

Other than inadvertently testing positive, some of these prohormones may carry some unwanted side effects. One study that supplemented with andro did not find higher testosterone levels or increased muscle strength, but actually a rise in blood estrogen and reduction in the good HDL cholesterol in male subjects. These side effects could result in potentially serious health effects. A second study tested andro combined with an herbal product designed to decrease estrogen production. The estrogenic profile was not reduced from the herbal supplements despite claims from the manufacturer.

Of course, you should not take prohormones because they are illegal. But read labels carefully to ensure that they are not inadvertently consumed in any products that you purchase, and beware that cross contamination is a real concern. It may be prudent to purchase supplements from companies that do not, though contamination can originate from the raw materials.

Weight Loss Supplements

Weight loss supplements are surrounded by strong claims and are often purported to speed up metabolism, burn fat, and decrease appetite. Although several ingredients found in weight loss supplements are legal (and ineffective), some weight supplements are banned substances and may be dangerous to use.

Until 2004, the most widely purchased weight loss supplement was ephedra. Because it was the supplement with the highest incidence of reported side effects, the FDA has also banned this substance. Ephedra, or ephedrine or Ma Huang, stimulates the central nervous system and improves appetite control. However, because of its stimulant nature, reported side effects include nervousness, headache, heart palpitations, dizziness, insomnia, and anxiety. Prior to the FDA ban, ephedra was also a banned substance in sport and its use will result in a positive test.

Another banned weight loss supplement with serious safety concerns is phenylpropanolamine (PPA), also known as norephedrine. This product claims to suppress appetite and stimulate metabolism. However, it can also increase the risk of bleeding stroke, and its safety risks far outweigh its effectiveness. The FDA has warned consumers to stop use of a product that contained PPA. In addition to PPA, this dietary weight loss supplement also contained caffeine, another herb called yohimbine, and diiodothyronine, a form of thyroid hormone. The FDA received multiple reports of liver injury or liver failure with use of this product over a 2-week to 3-month period.

Many weight loss supplements are currently marketed as being ephedra-free. However, these supplements may also contain banned products such as citrus aurantium or bitter orange, which is banned by both the NCAA and the IOC, and pseudoephedrine, which is also banned by the IOC. Many other ingredients in weight loss supplements lack a solid research backing. Some weight loss supplement ingredients that you should avoid include caffeine, cola nut, gingseng, and willow bark. Many of these supplements may contain high amounts of caffeine and be strong stimulants, just like ephedra, and can produce potentially dangerous side effects.

Caffeine

One of the oldest known drugs, caffeine belongs to a group of compounds known as methyl-xanthines. Caffeine is found naturally in coffee beans, tea leaves, cocoa beans, and cola nuts. Caffeine-containing foods are a natural part of many athlete's diets from coffee, tea, chocolate, and soft drinks. Many of these products provide 30 to 100 milligrams per serving.

While it appears that caffeine does provide some muscle glycogen-sparing effects, this appears to be limited to the first 15 to 20 minutes of exercise. Researchers are not certain exactly how caffeine produces this effect. The classic theory is that caffeine elevates free fatty acids in the blood, which exercising muscles use for energy, while conserving muscle glycogen. Caffeine may also impact the enzyme that breaks down glycogen. Besides sparing glycogen, caffeine also stimulates the central nervous system (increasing alertness), stimulates blood circulation and heart function, and releases epinephrine, all which could enhance a variety of performance-related functions. Caffeine also stimulates calcium release from the muscle, which stimulates muscular contraction.

Recent, well-designed studies with elite athletes have found that caffeine can effectively enhance performance when consumed in relatively low amounts. Doses as low as 1.5 to 2.0 milligrams per pound (3 to 5 milligrams per kilogram) of weight are effective. The optimal dose appears to be at 2.25 to 2.7 milligrams per pound (5 to 6 milligrams per kilogram). Consuming higher caffeine amounts provides no additional performance benefits and may result in adverse side effects such as rapid heart rate, nervousness, and gastrointestinal discomfort. Most studies have had subjects ingest caffeine one hour prior to exercise.

It is important for you to appreciate that not all athletes react to caffeine in a similar manner. Some individuals may have a performance response to caffeine, while others may not respond to caffeine with improved performance. Caffeine's diuretic effect has long been debated, but it appears that it is essentially insignificant. Studies indicate that caffeine does not increase urine output during exercise. Athletes who wish to use caffeine as an ergogenic aid during competition should experiment during training. The positive effects of caffeine during intermittent high-intensity exercise and power exercise are less defined due to limited data.

MCT Oil

Available for clinical use for several years, MCTs have been promoted to athletes for several years. Because of their smaller size (compared to long-chain triglycerides), MCTs empty from the stomach more quickly and are more easily absorbed. In fact, they are absorbed as quickly as glucose and transported to the liver where they are metabolized. Their ergogenic benefit would result in providing quick fuel during exercise and sparing muscle glycogen during extended training.

Of the several studies conducted with MCT oil, one found a performance improvement, while the others did not. One study did determine that the amount of MCT oil that can be tolerated within the gastrointestinal tract might be limited. GI symptoms ranging from mild to severe can result. Consuming carbohydrate prior to exercise (as is recommended in this book) could also negate the effects of MCT supplementation. MCT oil is also promoted as a metabolism enhancer and fat burner. However, these claims are not supported by research. Overall, this supplement is not recommended to athletes.

» THE NCAA AND NUTRITIONAL SUPPLEMENTS

The NCAA currently has a policy regarding sports nutrition supplements that it is not permissible for an institution to provide any nutritional supplements/ingredients to student athletes unless it is a non-muscle-building product and is included in one of the four classes of permissible supplements. Permissible supplements include vitamins and minerals, energy bars, calorie replacement drinks, and electrolyte replacement drinks. A listing of nonpermissible supplements include amino acids, chrysin, condroitin, creatine and creatine-containing compounds, ginseng, glucosamine, glycerol, HMB, L-carnitine, melatonin, Pos-2, protein powders, and tribulus. However, a supplement that contains protein is permissible if it does not contain more than 30 percent of its calories from protein and falls under one of the four permissible categories.

The NCAA is concerned with the lack of quality control in the production and manufacture of nutritional supplements. Supplements geared toward muscle building have been found to be contaminated with substances currently on the NCAA banned drug list. In one study funded by the International Olympic Committee, approximately 15 percent of 600 over-the-counter supplements were found to contain nonlabeled ingredients that could result in a positive doping test. The NCAA promotes the superiority of a well-balanced diet over nutritional supplements, and it is concerned about the long-term safety of some of these products.

Currently, student athletes wishing to take muscle-building supplements must obtain them on their own. Athletes still require sound nutrition advice from qualified sports nutritionists and information on the scientific data behind these products, rather than advertising claims and professional athlete endorsement. It is not worth risking eligibility to take products that may offer no real benefit beyond nutritional strategies of adequate calorie and protein intake and optimal nutrient timing.

The NCAA encourages students to refer to the Resource Exchange Center (REC), which is sponsored by the National Center for Drug Free Sport, at www.drugfreesport.com/rec.

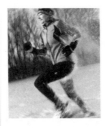

6 Creating the Optimal Winter Performance Diet

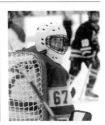

As a dedicated winter sport athlete who strives for optimal energy for training and full recovery, you must translate sound scientific sports nutrition recommendations into everyday food choices. The proper food choices can replenish your body fuel stores, build and repair muscle tissue, promote good health and a strong immune system, and leave you feeling satisfied with your daily diet. Guidelines for meal planning and choosing a diet that is integral to your training program provide a good foundation for making your daily food choices. Focusing on foods that are available and appealing in the winter months and that support a strong immune system also boosts your winter training.

YOUR DAILY MEAL PLAN

Much of the success of your daily eating plan will hinge on consuming adequate calories, carbohydrates, and proteins that match your training program for that day (and for the next day), and on rounding out your meals and snacks with the correct balance of fats. As described earlier, how you time your meal and snacks around your indoor and outdoor training sessions and weight-training workouts is also crucial.

Meal planning is not as complicated as it may sound. In fact, you will be amazed at how quickly you can adopt some new food strategies and incorporate them into your daily life of training and eating once you have a program and some structure in place. You will find that planning and organization makes this part of your life easier and more effective. Just as you plan ahead to ensure that all the necessary equipment and clothing is available for training, you must also plan to ensure that the optimal foods and required sports nutrition supplements are available to support your training program that day.

Table 6.1 summarizes the range of nutritional requirements for calories, carbohydrate, protein, and fat for winter sport athletes based on how hard you measure your training session for that day to be. (Also refer to the guidelines for estimating energy requirements as outlined in Chapter 3.) This table outlines the total calorie, carbohydrate, protein, and fat requirements of both a 130-pound (59-kilogram) and 160-pound (73-kilogram) athlete who has completed some hard training that day.

Of course, your energy needs can vary depending on the intensity of your training, if you are in a serious muscle-building phase, and if you are going to train more than once daily. Your daily energy requirements can also vary not only day to day but during differ-

TABLE 6.1 ›› NUTRITIONAL REQUIREMENTS BASED ON TRAINING INTENSITY

Calories per Pound Weight (cal/kg)	Carbohydrate Grams per Pound Weight (g/kg)	Protein Grams per Pound Weight (g/kg)	Fat Grams per Pound Weight (g/kg)
Mild: 12-14 (26-30) Moderate: 15-17 (33-37) High: 18-24 (40-53) Very high: 24-29 (53-64)	Mild/moderate: 2.25-3.0 (5-6.5) Moderate/high: 3.0-4.5 (6.5-10) High/very high: 4.5-5.5 (10-12)	Moderate: 0.45 (1.0) High: 0.5-0.75 (1.1-1.65) Very High: 0.8-0.9 (1.8-2.0)	> 0.5 g/lb. (1.0 g/kg) depending on energy needs
140-lb. (64-kg) athlete with moderate activity level:			
2,100-2,380 calories	325 g (62% calories)	64 g (12%)	60 g (26%)
160-lb. (73 kg) athlete with high activity level:			
2,800-3,800 calories	560 g (60% calories)	128 g (13% calories)	115 g (27% calories)

ent times of the season. A qualified sports dietitian can assist you in determining your nutritional requirements during different phases of your training program.

After you determine your nutritional needs for training, how these recommended nutrient amounts are translated into specific food choices and serving sizes can initially be one of the most difficult aspects of adopting your optimal high-performance diet. In real life, an individualized plan can differ from athlete to athlete depending on your medical history, age, gender, food preferences, training and life schedule, and culinary skills. But food charts can be very helpful in making carbohydrate servings more accessible, and carbohydrate is often an important theme of your diet for several reasons:

- Running low on liver and muscle glycogen can impair your training efforts long before depletion of other body fuels slow you down.
- Your carbohydrate intake is directly linked to the amount of glycogen you store in your liver and muscles, and these stores are relatively limited depending on your training that day.
- On certain training days you require significant amounts of carbohydrates to replenish your muscle glycogen stores, and if you don't consume these amounts, your muscle glycogen stores may not be adequate to properly fuel your subsequent training efforts.
- Consuming these carbohydrates takes planning as the amounts you require often exceed what is found in an everyday diet, and if you leave your diet to chance, your intake may be inadequate.
- You need to consciously choose wholesome and nutrient-filled carbohydrates among less healthful choices available in the North American food environment.
- Timing of your carbohydrate intake is also essential to your training and recovery.
- During various cycles of your training program, you still need a diet that provides at least 50 percent carbohydrate calories, and needs may increase to 60 percent or perhaps more during various training cycles. This means that the total grams of carbohydrate that you need to consume can fluctuate.
- Many winter sport athletes participate in more than one sport and may participate in several sports year-round as the seasons change, requiring a well-planned sports nutrition diet for much of the year.

Food tables providing 10- to 30-gram carbohydrate portions can make meal planning for your training diet smoother and more effective. You receive carbohydrates from several food groups: the bread, cereal, and grain group; the fruit and fruit juice group; the vegetable group; and the milk, yogurt, and soy group; and of course miscellaneous carbohydrate foods provided by snack items, desserts, and other carbohydrate toppings. You can match up the number of servings you require from these carbohydrate-containing groups to meet your requirements for training and recovery. On days when your carbohydrate needs are especially high, grains and starches are likely to comprise a good portion of your diet. They are concentrated food sources and provide 30 grams of carbohydrate per serving. As discussed in Chapter 1, try to choose lightly processed or whole-grain sources as much as possible. Many items from the grain group, such as pretzels and crackers, also make good snack choices.

Fruits, dried fruit, and fruit juices, which also provide 30 grams per serving, are your next great source of carbohydrate and are excellent food choices for maintaining good health due to the abundant nutrients they supply. Vegetables also provide carbohydrate, though not as high per portion as grains and fruits, at 10 grams per serving. However, few foods can match vegetables for their high nutrient content.

» BENEFITS OF BERRIES

Even during the winter months, focus on deeply colored raspberries, strawberries, and blueberries, as well as the likely less familiar blackberries, boysenberries, and huckleberries. These little fruit powerhouses provide a very generous supply of flavonoid phytonutrients, vitamin C, potassium, and fiber. While not in season during much of the winter, berries do freeze well and retain much of their nutrient profile, except for a slight loss of vitamin C.

But nonvitamin nutrients are among the best reasons for eating berries. Anthocyanins, which are pigments that give berries their deep color, are powerful antioxidants. Ellagic acid, a phytonutrient found in berries, is believed to prevent cancer cell growth. The seeds in berries are a great source of fiber, and the proanthocyanins in cranberries and blueberries can prevent urinary tract infections.

One of only three fruits native to North America (grapes and cranberries are the two others), blueberries are particularly a powerhouse of antioxidant nutrients. A U.S. Department of Agriculture (USDA) study ranked blueberries number one in antioxidant activity over 40 other fruits and vegetables. It makes sense when you consider that one-half cup of blueberries has as much antioxidant strength as several servings of other fruits and vegetables. Bilberry is a species of blueberry grown mainly in Canada and Europe that contains even more antioxidants than the "highbush" blueberry variety grown in Michigan and New Jersey. In addition, blueberries contain resveratrol, another cancer-inhibiting compound.

You can buy frozen bags of blueberries and other berries with no sugar added. Fresh berries can be frozen in freezer bags or airtight containers after washing, making them available all winter for great-tasting smoothies.

» WINTER SQUASH: STAYING IN SEASON

There are many varieties of delicious winter fruits and vegetables available that provide carbo-hydrates, vitamins, minerals, and phytonutrients to your winter training program. While many fruits and vegetables are now available all year, the choices that are in season easily taste the best. Some good winter choices include lycopene-rich tomatoes, bok choy, broccoli, brussels sprouts, potatoes, red grapes, tangerines, apples, and bananas. But winter squash, which includes a wide variety of plants, is hard to beat because of its superior nutritional value.

Winter squashes come in a variety of unusual shapes, colors, sizes, and flavors, including acorn, but-ternut, spaghetti, turban, Hubbard, pumpkin, and banana squash. Winter squashes ripen on the vine and can be held in cold storage throughout the winter months when they taste best.

On average, 1 cup of cut-up winter squash provides 6 grams of fiber, a nice 900-milligram dose of potassium, and even modest amounts of vitamin C and calcium, as well as small amounts of folate and magnesium. But the orange-colored squash varieties (especially butternut) are exceptional sources of potent antioxidant beta-carotene.

Winter squash is easy to keep. It can be stored in a cool dry place for several months (don't refrig-erate—it will hasten deterioration). Once cut up, it can be refrigerated for 1 week. Winter squash can be baked whole or in halves, and it is delicious in soups, mashed or pureed, or mixed with grains and beans. Spaghetti squash can be tossed and topped with tomato sauce.

Dairy milk and yogurt, and other milks such as soy milk and rice milk, are also good sources of carbohydrate, ranging anywhere from 12 to 40 grams per serving. Yogurts can be especially high in carbohydrate when they come mixed with fruit and sugars.

One last source of concentrated carbohydrates are sweets and desserts, which also supply 30 grams per serving. Sweets should not routinely replace more wholesome car-bohydrate choices in your diet, but they are a source of additional carbohydrate. They

» SMOOTHIES TO GO

Even in the winter months, smoothies are a welcome treat. The fact that they are highly nutritious and fit in perfectly with most if not all sports nutrition plans is even better. Because of their basic ingredients, milk- and yogurt-based smoothies are a great source of high-quality protein, calcium, potassium, vitamins C and D, and antioxidants and phytonutrients. Soy-based smoothies also pro-vide healthy isoflavones. Smoothies can be consumed preworkout for a nice steady supply of blood

CONTINUED

SMOOTHIES TO GO (CONTINUED)

glucose. Low-glycemic varieties can be made from skim milk, yogurt, and frozen berries. You can even add a touch of flaxseed oil for some healthy essential fatty acids. In fact, any variety of frozen fruit can be used in your favorite smoothie base, whether dairy milk or soy milk, to obtain lots of important nutrients and even a taste of summer. Try frozen mango or papaya or even add a little kiwi, which is available year-round. Chocolate lovers can add a taste of cocoa powder to their smoothie recipe.

When making your own smoothies, you obviously can control your ingredient choices and portions to design a smoothie that works best for you. If the need for convenience causes you to reach for commercial smoothies, check labels carefully. Many commercial varieties may contain plenty of high-fructose corn syrup and be low on real fruit and 100-percent fruit juice. Some smoothie sources may even be high in saturated fat. Commercially blended smoothies can also be very high in calories, which may or may not suit your nutrition plan. Check not only calories per serving but also the number of servings per container.

» SAVED BY CHOCOLATE

While modern chocolate lovers appreciate the substance for its texture, aroma, and mouth and complex flavor appeal, chocolate's delicious history dates back more than 1,500 years ago when the Mayans of Central America crushed cocoa beans to make a bitter beverage. Brought back to Spain, it became widely popular in Europe, and cocoa trees that supply the cocoa beans to make chocolate now grow in the rainforests of Central America, the Caribbean, and Africa.

Chocolate is produced when cocoa beans are fermented, dried, roasted, and crushed into a thick paste, which contains both cocoa butter and cocoa solids. Cocoa is chocolate paste without the cocoa butter. Chocolate as we know and love it is made from various amounts of chocolate paste, cocoa butter, sugar, and flavorings. The more common milk chocolate contains milk and sugar, while dark and semisweet chocolate are highest in chocolate paste.

Much has been made of the health benefits of chocolate. While two-thirds of the fat in chocolate is saturated fat, one form is stearic acid, which does not raise blood cholesterol. The other fat is healthy monounsaturated fat, which means that chocolate is not harmful in regard to blood cholesterol. Chocolate may even be good for your heart as it contains flavonoids, which can help prevent the oxidation of the harmful LDL cholesterol. But it is important that you choose chocolates high in flavonoids to receive the beneficial effects. Dark chocolate has the highest flavonoid content, whereas cocoa loses some flavonoids, and white chocolate contains no flavonoids.

Health effects aside, chocolate is high in calories, so keep consumption reasonable. Chocolate cravings are also believed to be a true occurrence related to the natural chemicals in chocolate that can produce positive psychological sensations. When checking labels, reach for cocoa that has not been processed with alkali, because it is higher in flavonoids, and dark chocolate with a high content of cocoa solids and chocolate liquor or paste. Sugar should be low on the ingredient list.

offer the advantage of being dense and less filling than some higher-fiber, more whole-some choices, and when your carbohydrate requirements are especially high, these foods are handy choices when your daily needs exceed 500 grams daily. For very heavy training days, you can also consider adding some sports nutrition products high in carbohydrate to your food plan.

But, of course, winter sport and weight-training athletes cannot live—and should not live—on carbohydrate alone. Choosing quality proteins and healthy fats will provide you with essential nutrients and balance out your meals and snacks. Proteins and fats also keep you full longer and even out blood glucose levels during the day. Protein foods are ranked according to their fat content so that you do not exceed healthy limits of total fat and saturated fat in your diet. Plant proteins and milk and dairy sources are emphasized for vegetarian athletes. Fats are also organized according to the types of fat they provide, so that you can choose healthy essential fatty acids and foods high in monounsaturated fat.

Table 6.2 outlines some of the serving recommendations for various calorie levels. This table is intended to be a framework from which you can base your own individual food choices. You may find that you prefer to do a bit of shuffling around with the suggested food groups and number of servings to suit your own health goals and personal tastes. For example, some of the suggested daily plans may be too high in dairy foods for your own tastes. These plans can be modified and the carbohydrate intake maintained by adding the equivalent grams of carbohydrate servings from fruits and juices or perhaps

» GOING CRAZY OVER NUTS

Health experts now tout the benefit of nuts, legumes, and seeds for preventing heart disease thanks to their great nutritional profile. Eating nuts seems to significantly reduce the risk of developing heart disease and even type 2 diabetes, and benefits can be obtained by consuming amounts as small as 1 ounce five times weekly. That's good news because while nuts are tasty and nutritious, they are high in fat (45 to 75 percent of total calories) and consequently a very high-caloric food at 160 to 200 calories per ounce.

Nuts are a great source of nutrients. Brazil nuts are very high in selenium and quercetin, which have anticancer properties. Most of the fat in nuts is rich in olic acid, which can lower bad LDL cholesterol, decrease blood pressure, and protect arteries. Nuts are also a good source of protein, and walnuts have the all-important alpha-linolenic acid. Almonds are rich in vitamin E, as are sunflower seeds. One to 2 tablespoons of nuts daily is reasonable for your fat choice with meals and snacks. You can toss nuts and sunflower seeds on salads, or stir them into your yogurt. Nuts also make a great snack when training outdoors.

TABLE 6.2 » SERVING RECOMMENDATIONS FOR VARIOUS CALORIE LEVELS

Food Group	Calorie needs				
	2,000	2,400	2,900	3,400	4,000
Grains	6	7	8	10	12
Fruits	3	3	4	5	6
Vegetables	2	3	3	3	3
Milk/yogurt/ soy milk	2	2	2 (milk) 1 (yogurt)	2 (milk) 1 (yogurt)	3 (milk) 1 (yogurt)
Proteins	6	6	6	7	8
Fats	3	4	5	6	8
Menu breakdown	315 g carb 84 g protein 45 g fat	350 g carb 112 g protein 60 g fat	450 g carb 114 g protein 70 g fat	550 g carb 120 g protein 80 g fat	650 g carb 150 g protein 89 g fat

by substituting soy milk for dairy milk. You may also wish to have fewer grain servings and increase the number of servings from fruits and fruit juices to match your carbohydrate requirements on certain training days. On some training days, your carbohydrate needs may be less than the proportion outlined in the sample menus. However, regardless of your personalized food plan and preferences, you need to reach the recommended carbohydrate amounts for optimal recovery, so add up the carbohydrate in the manner that best suits you. Of course, the nutrition guidelines presented in Chapter 1 should also direct you in making quality food choices as often as possible.

Food Journals
Tracking Your Intake

One useful tool for helping you determine whether you are meeting your energy and nutrient requirements is a food journal. You may already keep a training program diary and have learned what a good feedback tool a journal provides for fine-tuning your training program. To reap the most benefits from keeping a food journal, it is best if you write down your food choices and portions while eating or immediately after eating. Don't forget to note snacks, supplements, and any fluids consumed. With help from the food lists provided, you can assess a number of items regarding your food intake.

For starters, add up the amount of carbohydrate grams you consume in one day and determine whether your intake matches your training efforts. Note carbohydrate amounts from food labels, and use the food lists provided to estimate carbohydrate amounts per serving. You can also tally your total serving intake from the carbohydrate-containing food lists and see how your choices match up with the meal plans provided. You can determine not only whether your daily totals are adequate but also whether the amount of carbohydrate you consume before and after exercise is appropriate to support your training and recovery efforts.

Record the amount of fluids and carbohydrate that you consume before, during, and after practice. You can learn whether you meet the recommended fluid amounts and are taking ample opportunity to consume fluids and carbohydrates during breaks in training. Note how your energy levels during training may fluctuate depending on your carbohydrate and fluid intake.

Look through the day's intake to ensure that you are consuming adequate sources of concentrated and high-quality lean proteins. If you are vegetarian, check that your portions of plant proteins are full portions so that your body receives all the required amino acids. Check that protein is included in your recovery foods and fluids and that you also consume high-quality protein before and after weight training.

Determine whether the fats you consume are derived from healthy monounsaturated oil, liquid unhydrogenated polyunsaturated oil, and omega-3 fatty acid food choices. Check that you consume good sources of essential fatty acids in your diet.

» TEA TIME

Warm liquids are appealing in the cold winter months, and while you may enjoy a hot cup of your favorite coffee in the morning for its wake-up call of caffeine content, don't underestimate the benefits of another widely consumed hot beverage: tea. While all teas (except for herbal teas, which are not really teas) come from the same plant, there are several types of tea. Green tea is processed directly after picking, while black tea is oxidized for 2 to 4 hours before processing. Oolong tea leaves are only partly oxidized, and white tea is made from young tea leaves for a few days each spring when the buds are beginning to grow. All teas contain polyphenols, which are powerful antioxidants, and a variety of flavonoids. White tea has the highest level of flavonoids because it undergoes the least amount of processing.

Most tea research has focused on heart health, and drinking anywhere from 1 to 5 cups daily can reduce risk factors for heart disease or reduce risk of having a heart attack. The flavonoids in tea may prevent platelets from sticking to the walls of your arteries and decrease the risk of developing atherosclerosis. Other possible health benefits of tea include reduced risk of developing cancer, and green tea consumption may boost metabolism and lower body fat, though more research is needed. Tea may also benefit diabetics because of its capacity to increase insulin activity in fat cells.

Measure your intake of hydrating fluids for the day and before and after training. Make sure that you are well hydrated before exercise and that you consume enough fluid to replace sweat losses after exercise.

Check for hidden fats, such as those found in muffins, pastries, and high-fat crackers. Try to minimize your intake of these foods whenever possible.

Pay attention to your eating patterns. Note if you become too hungry at some times during the day, and adjust your mealtimes accordingly. Pay attention to any eating that may occur due to boredom, stress, and other issues not related to hunger.

Make sure that you are timing your foods appropriately before and after training. Check that you are consuming quality protein with carbohydrate before and after weight training. It is also important that you practice recovery nutrition strategies after intense training with your team.

Tables 6.3, 6.4, and 6.5 are provided for sports nutrition meal planning. Table 6.3 provides serving and carbohydrate amounts for the major foods that can comprise a well-balanced sports nutrition diet. Table 6.4 ranks the protein foods according to fat content so that you may choose the leanest choices available and limit your intake of saturated fat. In Table 6.5, the fats are also grouped according to types of fat, so that you may make the healthiest choices possible.

TABLE 6.3 » CARBOHYDRATE-CONTAINING FOODS

	Food	Serving Size
30-g Carbohydrate Servings for Cereals, Starches, Grains		
Bread	Bagel	½ large or 2 oz. (60 g)
	Bread crumbs	½ c. (120 ml)
	Bread sticks	2 oz. (60 g)
	Bread	2 slices or 2 oz. (60 g)
	Corn bread	1 square or 2 oz. (60 g)
	Dinner rolls	2 oz. (60 g)
	English muffin	1 whole or 2 oz. (60 g)
	Hamburger bun	1 whole or 2 oz. (60 g)
	Pita pocket	1 round or 2 oz. (60 g)
Cereals	Bran cereal	⅔ c. (160 ml)
	Cereal, cold, unsweetened	1.5 oz. (45 g)
	Cream of wheat, cooked	1 c. (240 ml)
	Grits, cooked	1 c. (240 ml)
	Granola, low-fat	½ c. (120 ml)
	Grape-Nuts	⅓ c. or 5 tbsp. (100 ml)
	Oatmeal, cooked	1 c. (240 ml)

CONTINUED

TABLE 6.3 continued

	Food	Serving Size
	Puffed cereal	3 c.
	Shredded Wheat	¼ c. or 1.5 oz. (45 g)
Grains	Barley, raw	¼ c. (60 ml)
	Bulgar, cooked	¾ c. (180 ml)
	Buckwheat, raw	¼ c. (60 ml)
	Muffin, low-fat	3 oz. (90 g)
	Pasta, cooked	1 c. (240 ml)
	Pancakes, 4-inch diameter	3
	Pancake mix, dry	⅓ c. (80 ml)
	Pretzels	1.5 oz. (45 g)
	Rice, cooked	⅔ c. (160 ml)
	Rice milk	1 c. (240 ml)
	Tortilla, corn or flour	2 small or 1 large
	Saltines	8 crackers, 1.5 oz. (45 g)
	Crackers	1.5 oz. (45 g)
Starchy Vegetables	Baked beans, cooked	¾ c. (180 ml)
	Corn, cooked	¾ c. (180 ml)
	Kidney beans, cooked	¾ c. (180 ml)
	Peas, cooked	1 c. (240 ml)
	Potato, baked	1 medium or 5 oz. (150 g)
	Sweet potato, baked	4 oz. (120 g)

30-g Carbohydrate Servings for Fruit

	Food	Serving Size
	Apple	1 ½ medium
	Applesauce, unsweetened	1 c. (240 ml)
	Applesauce, sweetened	½ c. (120 ml)
	Apples, dried	7 rings
	Apricots, fresh	8 medium
	Banana	1 large
	Blueberries	1 ½ c. (360 ml)
	Cantaloupe, raw pieces	2 c. (480 ml)
	Dates, dried	1 fruit
	Figs, dried	3 whole
	Fruit salad	1 c. (240 ml)
	Grapefruit	1 large
	Grapes	30 or 1 c. (240 ml)
	Kiwifruit	3 medium
	Mango	1 medium
	Nectarine	2 small
	Orange	2 medium
	Papaya	1 whole
	Peach	2 medium

CONTINUED

TABLE 6.3 continued

Food	Serving Size
Pear	1 large
Pineapple, fresh, pieces	1½ c. (360 ml)
Plum	3 medium
Raisins	⅓ c. or 3 tbsp. (60 ml)
Raspberries	2 c. (480 ml)
Strawberries	2½ c. (600 ml)
Watermelon	3 slices or 3 c. (720 ml)

30-g Carbohydrate Servings Fruit and Vegetable Juices

Apple juice	8 oz. (240 ml)
Carrot juice	10 oz. (300 ml)
Cranberry juice cocktail	8 oz. (240 ml)
Grape juice	8 oz. (240 ml)
Grapefruit juice	8 oz. (240 ml)
Orange juice	8 oz. (240 ml)
Pineapple juice	8 oz. (240 ml)
Vegetable juice cocktail	24 oz. (720 ml)

10-g Carbohydrate Servings for Vegetables

Artichoke	1 medium
Asparagus, boiled	1 c. (240 ml)
Beans, green, boiled	1 c. (240 ml)
Beet greens, cooked	1¼ c. (60 ml)
Broccoli, boiled	1 c. (240 ml)
Broccoli, raw	2 c. (480 ml)
Brussels sprouts, boiled	¾ c. (180 ml)
Cabbage, cooked	¾ c. (180 ml)
Carrots, raw	2 medium
Carrots, cooked	⅔ c. (160 ml)
Cauliflower, cooked	¾ c. (180 ml)
Kale, boiled	1¼ c. (300 ml)
Mushrooms, cooked	1 c. (240 ml)
Mustard greens, cooked	1½ c. (360 ml)
Peppers, sweet, raw	2 c. (480 ml)
Summer squash, cooked	1 c. (240 ml)
Spinach, boiled	1½ c. (360 ml)
Tomato, raw	2

12- to 50-g Carbohydrate Servings for Milk and Yogurt

Milk, buttermilk, 1%	8 oz. (240 ml)
Milk, nonfat	8 oz. (240 ml)
Milk, 1%	8 oz. (240 ml)
Milk, 2%	8 oz. (240 ml)
Yogurt, nonfat	8 oz. (240 ml)

CONTINUED

TABLE 6.3 continued

Food	Serving Size
Yogurt, low-fat	8 oz. (240 ml)
Yogurt, with fruit	8 oz. (240 ml)

30-g Carbohydrate Servings for Sweet and Baked Goods

Food	Serving Size
Angel food cake	$1/12$ whole
Chocolate milk	8 oz. (240 ml)
Cake	$1/12$ whole
Cookie, fat-free	4 small
Fruit spreads, 100% fruit	2 tbsp. (40 ml)
Gingersnaps	6 cookies
Graham crackers	6 squares
Granola bar, low-fat	1 bar
Honey	2 tbsp. (40 ml)
Ice cream	1 c. (240 ml)
Jam or jelly	2 Tbsp. (40 ml)
Pie	$1/8$ whole
Pudding, regular	$1/2$ c. (120 ml)
Sherbet	$1/2$ c. (120 ml)
Sorbet	$1/2$ c. (120 ml)
Syrup, regular	2 tbsp. (40 ml)
Vanilla wafers	10
Yogurt, frozen, low-fat	$2/3$ c. (160 ml)
Yogurt, frozen, fat-free	1 c. (240 ml)

TABLE 6.4 » FAT CONTENT OF PROTEIN CHOICES

Very Low-Fat Proteins (<2 g fat/oz. or 30 g)	Low-Fat Proteins (3–4 g fat/oz. or 30 g)	Medium-Fat Proteins (4–5 g fat/oz. or 30 g)	High-Fat Proteins (6–8 g fat/oz. or 30 g)	Very High-Fat Proteins (>8 g fat/oz. or 30 g)
Fish White fish: Grouper, Tuna Haddock Sole, Halibut Bass Shellfish: Crab, Shrimp Lobster, Clams	Dark fish: Salmon Mackerel Sardines	Tuna and salmon packed in oil		Any fried fish product

CONTINUED

TABLE 6.4 continued

Very Low-Fat Proteins (<2 g fat/oz. or 30 g)	Low-Fat Proteins (3–4 g fat/oz. or 30 g)	Medium-Fat Proteins (4–5 g fat/oz. or 30 g)	High-Fat Proteins (6–8 g fat/oz. or 30 g)	Very High-Fat Proteins (>8 g fat/oz. or 30 g)
Cheese Fat-free cheese Cottage cheese, 1% Cottage cheese, 2%	Low-fat cheeses	Feta cheese Mozzarella, part skim Grated Parmesan	Mozzarella Neufchatel	American, processed Cream cheese Brie, Cheddar Edam, Monterey Muenster Limburger, Swiss
Beef Round, choice, 90% lean	Round, choice, 85% lean Rib-eye, choice Flank steak, choice Porterhouse, choice	Round, choice, 73% lean Round, choice, 80% lean	Roast beef Meatloaf	Short ribs Corned beef Prime cuts
Pork Ham, lean, 95% fat-free Pork tenderloin Boneless sirloin chop Top loin chop	Sirloin roast Center loin chop Boneless rib roast Center rib chop Blade steak Canadian bacon	Pork butt	Italian sausage	Pâté Pastrami Bacon Pork sausage
Lamb Leg, top round Leg, shank, half	Loin chop Loin roast Rib chop	Roast lamb		Ground lamb
Legumes (per c. or 240 ml) Black beans Kidney beans Lentils, Lima beans, Pinto beans	Chickpeas	Tofu	Soybeans	
Poultry Turkey breast Chicken, white, no skin Turkey, dark, no skin	Chicken, dark, no skin Chicken, dark, w/skin Turkey, dark, w/skin Duck, roasted, no skin	Ground turkey, mixed meat/skin	Duck, roasted, w/skin	

CONTINUED

TABLE 6.4 continued

Very Low-Fat Proteins (<2 g fat/oz. or 30 g)	Low-Fat Proteins (3–4 g fat/oz. or 30 g)	Medium-Fat Proteins (4–5 g fat/oz. or 30 g)	High-Fat Proteins (6–8 g fat/oz. or 30 g)	Very High-Fat Proteins (>8 g fat/oz. or 30 g)
Other 95% fat-free lunch meat Egg whites Egg substitute	86% fat-free lunch meat Egg substitute	Eggs	Lunch meat: Bologna Turkey/chicken Hot dogs Salami	Knockwurst Bratwurst Beef/pork hotdogs Peanut butter

TABLE 6.5 » SOURCES OF FAT

Polyunsaturated Fat, 5-g Serving	Monounsaturated Fat, 5-g Serving	Saturated Fat, 5-g Serving
Margarine, stick, tub, or squeeze, 1 t. (6 ml)	Avocado, medium, ⅛	Bacon, cooked, 1 slice
Margarine, lower-fat, 1 tbsp. (20 ml)	Oil, canola, olive, peanut, 1 t. (6 ml)	Butter, stick, 1 t. (6 ml)
Mayonnaise, regular, 1 t. (6 ml)	Olives, black, 8 large	Butter, whipped, 1 t. (6ml)
reduced-fat, 1 tbsp. (20 ml)	Nuts:	Butter, reduced fat, 1 tbsp. (20 ml)
Nuts, walnuts, 4 halves	Almonds, cashews, 6 nuts	Cream, half-and-half, 2 tbsp. (40 ml)
Oil: corn, safflower, soybean, flaxseed, walnut, 1 t. (6 ml)	Peanuts, 10 nuts	Shortening or lard, 1 t. (6 ml)
Salad dressing, regular, 1 tbsp. (20 ml)	Pecans, 4 halves	Sour cream, regular, 2 tbsp. (40 ml)
Sunflower seeds, 1 tbsp. (20 ml)	Peanut butter, 2 t. (12 ml)	Sour cream, reduced fat, 3 tbsp. (60 ml)
Pumpkin seeds, 1 tbsp. (20 ml)	Sesame seeds, 1 tbsp. (20 ml)	
	Tahini paste, 2 t. (12 ml)	

PLANNING YOUR DAILY MEALS

Meal planning does not need to be a frustrating experience for dedicated winter sport athletes. The tools that are needed depend on who is responsible for preparing your meals and what types of food choices are presented to the athlete. Of course, younger athletes require their parents' support in providing healthy food choices for their growth and training program. High school athletes can take responsibility for their food choices away from home, including lunches and snacks at school, as well as when eating out with friends. Collegiate athletes often have a wide range of choices available at the dorm food service, and many schools now support their athletes with a training table. Athletes living on their own can shop for and prepare their own healthy meals, and it isn't necessary to employ your own personal chef for quick, gourmet meals, though professional athletes may do just that. Regardless of your living situation and resources, like your training program, meal planning does require forethought, organization, and flexibility. With practice, your meal-planning skills will become second nature.

Some of the fundamentals of meal planning when preparing your own meals are as follows:

Have a well-organized, well-equipped kitchen. Make sure that you have all the convenience items that you need, including a microwave, steamer, toaster oven, microwave-proof cookware, and a slow cooker. Other handy items include a large stove-top skillet or wok, a rice cooker, a lasagna dish, and sharp knives. Knowing where all your items are located and feeling comfortable in your kitchen will make putting together quick and easy meals that much easier.

Have a stock of some foods and snacks and use what limited cooking resources are available if applicable. For collegiate athletes, keeping some dry snack items and sports nutrition products on hand can be useful and supplement on-campus food appropriately. You should be able to keep some perishable items refrigerated in your room, and some dorms have limited cooking facilities on the floor.

Plan out your week's meal ideas beforehand. Think ahead to what meals you will need to cook, pack, or eat out based on that week's schedule. Determine how many dinners you will cook that week, and leave room for healthy takeout, eating out, and leftovers. Think about where you will be for lunch. Do you need to pack a full lunch or some extras like whole-grain crackers and fruit? Determine whether your training schedule requires you to have energy bars or carbohydrate drinks on hand. Perhaps you require quick recovery nutrition items to tie you over until your next full meal. You may want to be very specific and have certain days of the week designated for specific types of meals. For example, Monday night could be chicken, Thursday is fish, and Friday is stir-fry. Try to vary the types of vegetables and sides you consume. Sometimes it is easier to obtain variety when dinner is prepared for an entire family. When cooking for just one to two persons, try to obtain variety on a weekly basis, switching the grains, fruits, and vegetables you consume.

Understand the choices available to you in your food environment. Just as people purchasing food and preparing their own meals can plan ahead, you can also be aware of the healthier food choices offered at your work, school, and various locations on campus. Have a strategy for choosing lower-fat items and making healthy choices. Look ahead to menus that may be posted regarding main courses. Have a list of backup healthy meals that are offered on a regular basis. Pack snacks to consume between classes and before training as needed.

Keep nonperishable stock food items amply supplied. Having a well-stocked cupboard of items such as rice, pasta, whole grains, instant couscous, and other dry items can save you in a pinch when fresh food supplies run low or during busy training weeks. Some quick meals made from these ingredients include black bean burritos (freeze the tortillas), pasta and tomato sauce, stir-fry made from frozen chicken, instant rice, frozen vegetable mixes, and canned chili with bread or crackers. A suggested stock list is provided in the sidebar. Choose the items that best suit your training diet and food preferences. College athletes can keep a stock of healthy snacks in their room.

Go grocery shopping every week for fresh items. Have a designated grocery shopping day and time, and make it part of your weekly schedule. Based on your food plan for the week, put together a shopping list. Don't wait to shop when it is convenient, as it may never be convenient! You also don't want to set yourself up for several quick trips to the store to grab a few needed items. In the long run, this habit will cost you more time. Try to find a supermarket that can supply all the items you need. You will know where all your regular items are located and save time. Go during off-peak times to avoid crowds, and don't mull over items that are not on your shopping list. If you can't make it to the supermarket some weeks, try an increasingly popular alternative and find a grocery store or online grocery system that accepts phone, fax, or Internet orders and delivers.

Keep a running list of items that need to be replenished. Have a pad and pen handy. When you notice that items are running low or are used up, add them to your list. Trying to remember everything you need while shopping at the grocery store may not be the best strategy for a busy athlete.

Batch-cook meals, make extra portions, and freeze single servings. This strategy can be a great time-saver. You can set aside a lighter training day to cook items such as soups, chilies, and lasagnas. When cooking regular meals, making an extra one to two portions for the next day can save dinner preparation time or provide you with a nice midday meal. Freeze single-item portions in plastic containers for future heavy training days.

Pack meals, snacks, and food supplements for the next training day the night before. If your next day's schedule is full, consider packing your foods and snacks the night before. Having some portioned items and fresh food in the fridge will make this task as simple as possible. Plan snacks that can be eaten on the run.

Acquire a repertoire of quick and easy to prepare meals. Anyone can become a proficient cook, and it does not have to be a time-consuming project. Be on the lookout for quick and simple recipes. Ask friends for some of their quick meal ideas. Focus on recipes like stir-fry, risotto, burritos, and pasta ideas.

Take advantage of food shortcuts. You can purchase chicken tender strips, beef stir-fry strips, and frozen precooked shrimp, and rotisserie chickens. Try frozen vegetable stir-fry mixes, precut fruits, preseasoned and cut tofu, ready-to-heat soups, instant couscous mixes, fresh pastas (you can freeze them), and canned beans, chickpeas, and other legumes.

While you may not always have access to full kitchen facilities in college, some options are available for storage in your dorm room. Often a small refrigerator or hot plate

» SIMPLE SUGGESTIONS FOR STOCKING YOUR PANTRY

For the Freezer

Chicken tenders	English muffins
Cooked shrimp	Muffins
Lean ground beef	Tortillas
Lean pork fillets	Frozen vegetables
Cubed meat for stir-fry	Stir-fry mixes
Soy and garden burgers	Sorbet
Textured vegetable proteins	Frozen fruit
Variety of breads	Precooked pasta and rice
Waffles	Egg substitute

For the Refrigerator

Fresh fruit	Mini carrots
Fresh vegetables	Oranges, apples, bananas
Juices	Lean deli meats
Milk	Fresh pasta
Yogurt	Soy and rice milk
Eggs	Sauces and condiments
Reduced-fat cheese	Salsa
Prewashed salad greens	Tub margarine

For the Cupboard

Pasta	Low-fat crackers
Rice	Cold cereal assortment
Couscous	Oatmeal and farina
Quinoa	Dried fruit
Pilaf	Granola bars
Tabouleh	Canned soup
Canned beans and chickpeas	Nuts and sunflower seeds
Canned Tuna	Pretzels
Peanut butter	Instant soup and grains
Instant stuffing mixes	Fig Newtons
	Seasoning mixes

is available. Some items that you can keep on hand are peanut butter, whole-grain bread, jam, instant soup and grain cups, fresh fruit, and granola bars. Stocking up your dorm room with healthy foods can mean making good choices when snacking in the evening and packing healthy snacks for between meal eats during the day.

Breakfast, Lunch, and Snacks

Breakfast is one of the most important meals of the day. It revs up your body's metabolism and fills up liver glycogen stores that have become depleted overnight. It may even be an important recovery meal after a solid early-morning practice session. By skipping breakfast, eating a medium-size lunch, and feasting at dinner, you may not only be compromising your recovery but also be cheating your body of important nutrients. Skipping breakfast is also a terrible weight management strategy that can set you up for increased hunger and overeating later in the day.

Breakfast will keep your digestive juices flowing, but it may keep you feeling satisfied for only three hours or so until you are hungry again. If this occurs, place a midmorning snack into your eating plan. If your energy needs are high, try to have a substantial breakfast. Eat up on calorically dense cereals such as granola and muesli. A large glass of juice will also add a substantial amount of calories and carbohydrates. Adding some protein to your breakfast can do a nice job of keeping you comfortably full until the next meal. Depending on your schedule, you may consume breakfast on the fly. Quick choices can include a fruit smoothie made with yogurt and granola. Quick-packs include yogurt, bananas, dried fruit, bagels, and muffins. See the sidebar for some breakfast ideas.

» BREAKFAST IDEAS

Cooked oatmeal with raisins, cinnamon, and low-fat milk

Open-face English muffin halves with broiled cheese and fruit

Egg substitute omelet with vegetables, toast, juice, and milk

Yogurt with fresh fruit and a low-fat muffin

Whole-grain cereal with milk and fruit

Fruit smoothie made with yogurt, fresh or frozen fruit, and granola

Whole-grain bread with peanut butter, banana, and honey

Any leftovers that sound appealing

» HOT CEREALS

Hot cereal can be one of the most warming ways to start your day on a chilly winter morning, and it fits very well into your sports nutrition plan. A bowl of hot cereal is a great source of carbohydrate, often an excellent source of fiber, and low in sugar. You can make or top your favorite hot cereal with dairy or soy milk and top it with fresh and even frozen fruit that would normally be out of season. Other hot cereal toppings include nuts, raisins, sunflower seeds, and wheat germ. One warm weather classic is oatmeal, but you can also try cream of wheat, cream of rice, and a wide variety of other hot cereals. Some choices include hot wheat bran cereal, oat bran, hot barley cereal, and a variety of hot cereal mixes. Do watch out for varieties that may be as high in added sugar as some cold cereals. Usually the most convenient cereal (shake contents out of packet and add hot water) have the most calories, fat, and sugar, and the least amount of fiber.

For many athletes, lunch will be brought from home, purchased at a restaurant or fast-food establishment, or chosen from a cafeteria-style menu. Like all your meals and snacks, lunch should provide some quality carbohydrates and be balanced out with protein and fat. Eat lunch when hunger first sets in, as this is a sign that your body needs fuel.

Packing a lunch takes a little extra time and planning but is well worth the effort. You can ensure that you have lean proteins and the right type and amount of fats. Sandwiches are always a good place to start when last night's leftovers seem too repetitive. Some good protein options are lean beef, hummus, turkey or chicken, tuna, and low-fat cottage cheese. Liven up that same old turkey sandwich with add-ons such as avocado, lettuce leaves, cucumber and tomato, sprouts, and low-fat cheese. High-carbohydrate items that

» SMART SNACKS TO KEEP YOUR TANK TOPPED OFF

Cereal, with or without milk	Bowl of soup with crackers
Peanut butter and jelly sandwich	Pasta or bean salad
Hard and soft pretzels	Fresh fruit, low-fat cheese, and nuts
Baked potato with low-fat cheese	Cottage cheese and fruit
Crackers with peanut butter	Instant breakfast mix and fruit
Muffins or bagels with jam and	Tuna salad and crackers
low-fat cream cheese	Hummus and crackers or pita bread
Sports bars or breakfast bars	Fruit smoothie
Yogurt with fruit	Milk chug and fruit

you can include with your lunch are fruits, whole-grain crackers, raw vegetables, yogurt, low-fat chips, low-fat crackers, and vegetable and bean soups.

Snacks are also a very important part of an athlete's diet. When your energy needs are high, snacks give you a nice calorie boost. They also provide some fuel before training sessions and keep hunger at bay until you can sit down for a full meal. Many athletes swear by snacking. Plan some serious snacking into your diet. If there is a particular time of day when you experience an energy low or hunger, snacking may make all the difference. The sidebar lists some tasty snack ideas.

LABEL-READING TIPS

Nutritional information on labels can help you determine the nutritional breakdown of foods. First check the ingredient list. You may want to include more whole-wheat flours and other whole grains into your diet. Ingredients are listed in the labels by weight from the most to the least.

Pay attention to the serving size on the label and compare it to the amount that you actually eat. Portions you consume may be double those on the package, and you should adjust the nutrition information accordingly. You can also use the label to evaluate if a food will significantly impact your carbohydrate intake by checking the total grams of carbohydrate listed. You can then determine what portion of that particular food would provide 30 grams or more of carbohydrate to help you meet your training requirements.

Total fat grams, as well as calories from fat, are also listed. To determine the percentage of calories from fat, divide the fat calories per serving by the total calories per serving and multiply by 100. Keep higher-fat foods in perspective. Your fat intake needs to be considered in the context of an entire day. Your total day's intake should provide 20 to 25 percent fat calories, which allows for some healthy foods that may be a bit higher in fat. Some foods such as dried pasta will be very low in fat, while others such as margarine provide a high amount of fat.

The Daily Values for various vitamins and minerals provided on the nutrition label are based on a 2,000-calorie intake. The percentage of Daily Values can tell you whether a food is high or low in a nutrient such as calcium, fiber, iron, or vitamin C. A food is considered to be a good source of a nutrient if it provides 20 percent of the Daily Values. Besides increasing your intake of foods high in specific nutrients, you can also use the Daily Values to avoid excess fat, saturated fat, and cholesterol.

EATING OUT

Like many North Americans, chances are that you eat out several times weekly. Lunch is the meal most frequently eaten away from home, followed by dinner, and then breakfast.

Currently, more than 45 percent of money spent on food in the United States goes to restaurant meals and other foods purchased away from home. You may eat out at restaurants, in a cafeteria, on campus, at work, and even in the car.

Regardless of where you eat your meal out, the basic strategies are the same. Watch out for hidden and added fat, and keep a close eye on the portions. Despite your high energy requirements for endurance training, not all restaurant meals fit nicely into your nutrition plan. They may be too high in fat to become a frequent indulgence, and they may not provide the healthy ingredients that you require. It is important to learn what healthy food choices are available at your favorite restaurants. Ask questions about how foods are prepared, and don't hesitate to request modifications or changes. Often you can creatively outsmart the menu and enjoy your meal as well.

Fast Food

Fast food can provide excessive amounts of protein and fat through supersize burgers and grease-laden French fries. But it is possible to make choices that fit into a sports diet at some fast-food establishments. Have the small hamburgers that provide only 2 to 3 ounces of meat. Order baked potatoes over French fries whenever possible. Broiled chicken sandwiches are decent choices, while chicken pieces are generally fried. The same goes for fish sandwiches, as they come dripping with plenty of unwanted oil. Order skim milk when possible, and juice is often available as well. Salads and vegetables may be on the menu, but watch out for dressings. Limit sauces and toppings whenever possible.

Many fast-food establishments now provide good sandwich choices. You can choose lean roast beef, ham, turkey, or chicken and limit oils, mayonnaise, and cheese. Go for baked chips and pretzels when offered. Chicken fajitas or tacos make some good lower-fat choices. You can also choose frozen yogurt and low-fat milkshakes.

Other fast-food choices that can fit into your sports nutrition plan include vegetarian thin-crust pizza. Some establishments also have a soup and baked potato bar. Bean burritos and soft tacos are also available, as are chili, bagels, English muffins, waffles, pancakes, and cereals. The sidebar reviews some health strategies at fast-food establishments.

Ethnic Cuisine

Chances are that if you eat out frequently, you enjoy the many types of ethnic cuisine that are increasingly popular and available. These cultural edibles can fit into a healthy training diet if you know what choices to make and avoid consuming hidden fat.

Italian Cuisine

Italian food is a popular favorite and can be consumed at a variety of settings—upscale, family style, pizza, or fast food. With an emphasis on grains and vegetables, Italian eating

» NAVIGATING THE FAST-FOOD LANE

Most fast-food choices tend to be high in calories, fat, and sodium, while being low in fiber and vitamins A and C. Menus tend to be high in protein choices and lacking in fruits and vegetables. Here are some fast-food tips for athletes who want to make the best choices possible. Always avoid the largest sizes of sandwiches, burgers, fries, and drinks. These portions are too large to regularly be part of a healthy sports diet. Order smaller versions of these items.

Chicken and fish are only good choices if grilled, broiled, or baked. Often these proteins are breaded and deep-fried and can contain more fat than a burger.

Fast-food establishments that offer lower-fat sandwiches are likely to be your best choice.

Portion distortion has become a big part of our fast-food culture. Choose the smaller items on the menu. Often they provide all the protein and calories that you need for your training diet.

Dairy Products:
Choose low-fat milk, frozen yogurt, and low-fat milkshakes. Avoid whole-milk products and hard ice cream.

Starches and Grains:
Choose the small order of fries, low-fat muffins, bagels, cereals, baked potatoes, and pancakes and waffles. Avoid large fries, croissants, hash browns, and pastries.

Meats and Main Dishes:
Choose grilled chicken, plain small hamburgers, chicken fajitas, bean burritos, bean chili, vegetable pizza, and chicken, turkey, vegetarian, and ham sandwiches. Avoid fried chicken and fish sandwiches, large hamburgers and cheeseburgers, fish or chicken nuggets, and pizza with meat toppings.

Salad Bar:
Choose lettuce, pasta with marinara, raw vegetables, low-fat dressing, vegetable soups, fresh fruit, and baked potatoes with vegetable toppings. Avoid cream soups, high-fat dressings, potato salad, and tuna salad.

Sauces:
Choose ketchup, mustard, and barbecue sauce. Avoid mayonnaise and cream sauces.

can be healthy. Some lighter, lower-fat choices would be starches such as spaghetti (not cheese filled), risotto and polenta (prepared low-fat), vegetable choices such as tomato-based sauces, zucchini, and other vegetables prepared without fat, and lean meats such as skinless chicken, veal, shrimp, and grilled fish. You can also try condiments including herbs, cooking wines, vinegar, garlic, and crushed red peppers. Fill up on minestrone soup, and top pasta with marinara or red clam sauce. Order your dressing on the side, and have

Italian ice for dessert. You can also make some special requests, including removing the olive oil from the table and having the skin taken off chicken.

Plenty of heavier choices are offered at Italian restaurants, too. Starches such as garlic bread and focaccia contain fat, as do fried vegetables and meats such as salami, prosciutto, and sausage. Watch out for high-fat cheeses and dishes prepared with cream, butter, and even olive oil, which still contains plenty of fat calories. Go easy on the antipasto plate and the olive oil served with bread. Alfredo sauce, Italian sausage, lasagna, and parmigiana dishes are all high in fat because of the ingredients and methods of preparation.

Mexican Cuisine

Mexican cuisine may also be on your list of ethnic favorites. Like Italian food, this cuisine contains both light and heavy choices. Many staples of Mexican cuisine can be considered low-fat items such as whole beans, refried beans prepared without oil, tortillas, rice cooked without oil, grilled vegetables, and salsa. Grilled proteins such as shrimp, fish, or chicken are good choices, as are whole black beans. You can also fill up on gazpacho, marinated vegetables, and burritos (easy on the cheese).

Some heavier choices at Mexican restaurants would be tortilla chips, chimichangas, and taco shells. Avocados (guacamole), olives, sour cream, and cheese are also high in fat. You should also watch out for chorizo, cheese, sour cream, and oil used in cooking as they may contribute a significant amount of fat and saturated fat to your diet.

Chinese Cuisine

Chinese cuisine, providing a variety of regional cooking styles, is a frequent favorite at mall eateries and small neighborhood restaurants. While there are light choices in Chinese cooking, there are also many high-fat pitfalls. To keep your meal on the light side, look for stir-fried vegetables. You have a variety to choose from like peapods, bamboo shoots, water chestnuts, cabbage, baby corn, and broccoli.

Lean proteins that are found in Chinese dishes include vegetable dishes with shrimp, chicken, tofu, and lean cuts of beef and pork. Dishes may also contain low-fat fruits such as pineapple and orange sections. Condiments like mustard, soy sauce, ginger, sweet sauce, and garlic will not increase the fat content of your meals.

Chinese cuisine also contains plenty of high-fat choices. Everyone is familiar with the fatty breaded and fried sweet-and-sour dishes. Fried rice has twice the calories as steamed rice, with all the additional calories coming from oil. Fried noodles and egg rolls can also up your fat intake. Try to stay away from fried seafood, pork, spare ribs, and duck with skin. Stir-fry dishes that contain nuts and peanuts will also be much higher in fat, as will any choices in which oil is used heavily. Request that your dish be prepared with as little oil as possible, and try to split entrées with a friend because portions are often large.

Thai Cuisine

Thai food is quickly becoming one of the most popular and frequented types of Asian restaurants. Besides being hot and spicy when desired, you can make healthful low-fat choices at a Thai restaurant, and be aware of special menu requests that keep down the fat content of the dishes.

Thai tends to be a healthier food choice than Chinese cooking and does employ similar cooking techniques such as stir-frying. Ingredients are also similar, with an emphasis on rice and noodles and certain vegetables and proteins. It is very important to gravitate toward leaner proteins that are cooked stir-fry-style, such as chicken, shrimp, and even thin strips of pork or beef. Sometimes proteins are prepared by deep-frying, so ask questions and make sure that you understand what is on the menu. However, dishes are usually stir-fired, steamed, or braised. You can also request that dishes be prepared light on the oil. Vegetable oil is usually used, but coconut oil is more traditional. Large portions can also be shared family-style. Nuts and peanuts can be added to dishes in small amounts. Soups at Thai restaurants can be vegetable based and filling. Some menu items may load up on vegetables and use light sauce for cooking. Tofu or bean curd dishes are also widely available.

At Thai restaurants, try to avoid fried or deep-fried items, crispy noodles, coconut milk soup, and duck meat. Dressing can be requested on the side, inquire about the type and amount of oil, and choose leaner proteins.

Middle Eastern Cuisine

Middle Eastern food fare is distinguished by such tasty dishes as hummus, tabouli, baba ganoush, and shish kebabs. Some central ingredients include chickpeas, olives, wheat and pita bread, grains such as rice and couscous, legumes, tomato, and onion. Stuffed dishes, either meat based or vegetarian, are common, and olive oil is the predominant oil used. Common protein-containing foods include yogurt, lamb, beef, and eggs. Foods can be grilled, fried, or stewed.

Middle Eastern food can be a good match with a healthy sports diet. There are plenty of carbohydrates to choose from, protein portions can be kept to reasonable levels, and vegetables fill the menu. As with many other cuisines, you need to watch out for hidden fats. Watch out for excess olives, olive oil (though it is a healthy type of fat), salad dressings, marinades, and sauces. Try to avoid fried foods such as falafel, and of course desserts, such as baklava, which are high in fat. Tahini, which is ground sesame paste, is full of unhealthy fat.

Typically, you have many health salads to choose from; just ask for dressings on the side. You may find healthy lentil soup on the menu. You can also order a series of appetizers and even split some larger entrées. Look for lower-fat items such as chickpeas, tomatoes, onions, and green peppers; grilled meat or kebabs; and charbroiled or stewed items. Go easy on cheeses and oils, and fried items.

Pizza

Pizza is a popular and inexpensive meal out or easily ordered in for lunch, dinner, or a late-night snack. Cold leftover pizza is also good the next day. Pizza starts with dough, then tomato sauce, and then usually high-fat cheese. Vegetables offer a variety of toppings, as do fatty meats such as pepperoni and sausage. It is unlikely that you will find low-fat cheese at most pizzerias, though some gourmet varieties may use a variety of cheese and even leaner proteins such as chicken. Overeating is one of the biggest problems with pizza. It is easy to have more than two slices, and some varieties offer a thick-crust version or the extra cheesy deep-dish variety.

Besides portion control, you can also make special requests when ordering your pizza. Ask for half the cheese, or even cheeseless pizza. You can also ask for extra vegetable toppings and tomato sauce. A sprinkle of cheese such as grated Parmesan can go a long way to adding flavor and not many calories on a cheeseless pizza. Try to avoid fatty proteins such as sausage whenever possible. When ordering salad at pizzerias, ask for dressing on the side.

Seafood

Seafood restaurants are everywhere, and fish is served in a wide variety of restaurants from some of the most pricey to greasy fast-food fare. With this range of restaurants offering fish, a range of choices from the low-fat, such as mesquite grilled, to the ultra-fat-laden Lobster Newberg is available. Of course, the fast-food varieties that are breaded and deep-fried are filled with fat as well. All fish prior to preparation is relatively low-fat, even the "fattier" varieties that are full of the healthy omega-3 fatty acids. When choosing fish on the menu, it all comes down to preparation.

Common good appetizer selections, if they are not breaded and deep-fried, include oysters, sushi, shrimp cocktail, and clams and mussels. Blackened fish tends to be low-fat. Inquire about the sauces used to prepare the fish, and avoid cream sauces. Request that the chef go easy on clear sauces that contain oils. Marinated and stir-fried varieties are usually good menu choices, as are teriyaki and any steamed variety. Fish can come with rice or potatoes, prepared low-fat or high-fat. Again, make menu inquiries and make substitutions as needed.

Lunch Spots

Lunch is the meal consumed out most frequently, mainly due to timing and convenience. Aim for low-fat items, such as clear, noodle, or vegetable-based soups. Request salads easy on the cheese, with dressing on the side. Look for roasted or grilled chicken items, and request sandwiches to order whenever possible. Watch out for fatty sides such as French fries or onion rings, and fatty potato and macaroni salads. Pretzels are lower-fat, as are fruit sides and low-fat yogurts.

Salad Bars

Visits to the salad bar are often well intended but can result in surprisingly high-fat meals. Besides those healthy raw vegetable items like spinach, tomatoes, broccoli, and green peppers, there are plenty of items mixed with fat or sitting in oil. Some of the less healthy choices include pasta salad, potato salad, marinated vegetables, cheeses, and bean salads made with oil. Go easy on portions of these items. Of course, try to keep salad dressing portions reasonable.

Salad bars have plenty of carbohydrates and fiber that can help you keep your protein portions low and reasonable. Obviously fresh greens and plain raw vegetables are your best choices. Starches on the salad bar may include chickpeas, kidney beans, green peas, crackers, and pita bread. Lean protein salad bar choices include plain tuna, cottage cheese, egg, ham, and feta cheese. Try to avoid most cheeses and pepperoni. Keep marinated vegetable portions small, and especially watch out for tuna, chicken, seafood salad, and macaroni and potato salads that can contain plenty of mayonnaise. High-fat items, such as peanuts, sesame seeds, and sunflower seeds, provide good fats and can be used in small amounts.

» PROTEIN AND THE VEGETARIAN ATHLETE

Winter sport athletes do have increased protein requirements, and vegetarian athletes should appreciate that a portion of a quality plant is not as concentrated a source of protein as an animal protein. The key to obtaining enough protein in your diet is to first consume enough calories, so that the protein you do consume is not processed for energy. Second, an emphasis must be placed on high-quality and concentrated plant protein sources. Certain grains, dried peas and beans, lentils, and nuts and seeds are some of the best sources. Soy products such as tempeh and tofu are one plant protein essentially equivalent to animal protein.

Although it is not necessary to combine or complement various plant proteins at the same meal as was once thought, you should make a concerted effort to obtain adequate plant proteins in your diet

CONTINUED

PROTEIN AND THE VEGETARIAN ATHLETE (CONTINUED)

throughout the day. The body will make its own complete proteins over the course of the day, if you consume enough calories. If your calorie intake falls short, some of the protein you do consume may be processed for energy, rather than be utilized for important protein functions. Table 6.6 lists some good plant protein sources.

TABLE 6.6 » PROTEIN CONTENT OF PLANT FOODS

Food	Serving Size	Protein (g)
Tempeh	1 c. (240 ml)	39
Soybeans, cooked	1 c. (240 ml)	29
Seitan	4 oz. (120 ml)	21
Tofu, firm	4 oz. (120 ml)	20
Lentils, cooked	1 c. (240 ml)	18
Kidney beans, cooked	1 c. (240 ml)	15
Lima beans, cooked	1 c. (240 ml)	15
Chickpeas, cooked	1 c. (240 ml)	15
Black beans, cooked	1 c. (240 ml)	15
Pinto beans, cooked	1 c. (240 ml)	14
Quinoa, cooked	1 c. (240 ml)	11
Soy yogurt	1 c. (240 ml)	10
Soy milk	1 c. (240 ml)	10
Tofu, regular	4 oz. (120 ml)	10
Peanut butter	2 tbsp. (40 ml)	8
Sunflower seeds	¼ c. (60 ml)	8
Peas, cooked	1 c. (240 ml)	8
Bulgar, cooked	1 c. (240 ml)	6
Bagel	1 medium	6
Pasta or grain	1 c. cooked (240 ml)	6
Almonds	¼ c. (60 ml)	5.5
Brown rice, cooked	1 c. (240 ml)	5
Bread, whole wheat	2 slices	5
Potato	1 medium	4.5

Protein Tips for Vegetarians

Include a protein-rich food at all meals and snacks.

Add milk or fortified soy milk or the yogurt equivalent to every meal or snack.

Use nuts butters, hummus, and low-fat cheeses (soy and regular) for toppings on breads, bagels, and crackers.

Add nuts and seeds to a fruit and yogurt snack.

Make tofu and tempeh stir-fry.

Experiment with quick and easy bean recipes such as burritos, casseroles, and salads.

Make thick soups and stews with beans and lentils.

Experiment with all the meat replacement soy products on the market such as tofu dogs and burgers.

Make casseroles, lasagna, and stuffed shell recipes with tofu.

Meal-Planning Tips for Vegetarians

The health food section of many supermarkets and most health food stores provide a wide selection of vegetarian food choices and convenience items.

The number of textured vegetable protein products has increased significantly in the past several years. You can now buy products that resemble and taste like hot dogs, burgers, and breakfast sausage, and make quick and easy lunch ideas.

Tofu can be substituted for chicken in most recipes. Seasoned tofu is available, and you can also season the recipe to spice up tofu's milder taste.

You can substitute vegetable broth when recipes call for beef or chicken stock. Vegetable broth is available in many supermarkets and most health food stores.

Canned lentils, chickpeas, and beans are a quick and nutritious vegetarian option. When time allows, soak the dried lentil and bean versions. Many bean and lentil recipes can be batch-cooked and frozen for later use.

If you need assistance, find a vegetarian cookbook with meal ideas suited to athletes.

Include protein-rich foods at each meal. Because vegetarian options are not as concentrated in protein as animal protein, you need to include adequate portions at most meals and snacks.

Purchase calcium-fortified soy and rice milks if you drink these products instead of dairy milk.

Purchase iron-fortified cereals, and consume them with products high in vitamin C such as orange juice.

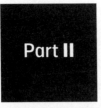

Part II

Sport-Specific Nutrition

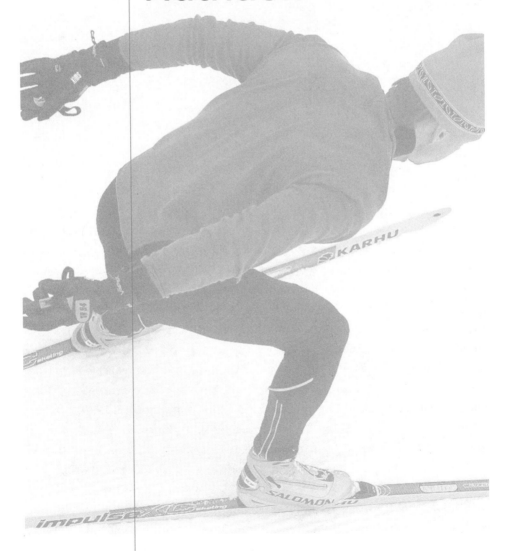

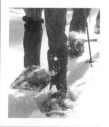

7 Nutrition for Cross-Country Skiing and Snowshoeing

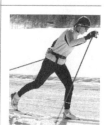

Cross-country skiing and snowshoeing are popular endurance sports whose histories date back thousands of years. Cross-country skiing originated in Scandinavia more than 4,000 years ago, as a practical method of transportation. Snowshoeing is a rapidly growing endurance sport and was practiced in central Asia some 6,000 years ago. It is believed that the ancestors to the Inuits and Native Americans brought snowshoes with them after crossing the Bering Strait by foot. Europeans adapted the snowshoe in North America for exploring, surveying, and trapping.

Both sports have evolved greatly beyond the practical and effective methods of transportation that they offer. Cross-country skiing is now a popular recreational sport and competitive at the high school and collegiate levels. Adult competitors can compete at many levels, and cross-country skiing is a popular winter sport among many endurance athletes who participate in cycling, triathlon, and other sports during the warmer months. One-third of all Winter Olympic Game medals are awarded in cross-country skiing and related Nordic sports. Cross-country skiing is divided into two competitive styles. Classic or traditional skiing involves a straight-ahead gliding motion, and ski skating or freestyle skiing involves a V-style glide and edge motion similar to inline skating.

Cross-country skiing is one of the most demanding endurance sports around and ideal for improving your fitness level. This sport develops both upper- and lower-body strength, while stressing and enhancing both the aerobic and anaerobic energy systems. Just about anywhere that there are groomed trails and snow, there are cross-country ski competitions. Small races may attract several dozen local skiers, while the largest events attract tens of thousands of racers and elite racers from foreign countries. Races can range in distance from one to several kilometers for the youngest competitors, to 5K, 10K, 15K, and 20K races in collegiate and age-group racing. Endurance cross-country ski races can extend to 30K and more than 50K in distance. Some races may include relay teams. Elite racers may ski in endurance events from 1 to 3 hours or more depending on the length of the race. The rest of the pack may take twice to three times as long to finish the race. Training commitments can extend to anywhere from 7 to more than 15 hours weekly, depending on the level and competitive goals of the athlete.

Elite cross-country ski racers are renowned for their astounding fitness as evidenced by their high VO$_2$max, low levels of body fat, and low resting heart rates. Cross-country ski training consists of steady endurance, hill, and interval training, as well as development of skill and technique. Training often follows periodized cycles during specific times of the season when training incorporates off-season workouts such as roller skiing, in-line skating, hiking with poles, running, cycling, mountain biking, and weight training.

Snowshoeing is an easy and fun way to walk or run through powdery terrain, thanks to much recent development in modern snowshoe technology and materials. The first large-scale productions of snowshoes began in the mid-1800s, but the more modern versions were not developed until the 1950s. Current snowshoe models are aluminum and lightweight, and they have easy-to-use bindings that make snowshoeing fun on the first try.

The versatility of snowshoeing is endless, and snowshoe activity level includes walking and recreation, training and racing, and back-country mountaineering and camping. Half of all snowshoers are women.

Snowshoe clubs were first developed in the mid-1800s, and in the early 1900s, races were offered on oval tracks with specific distance. Race lengths varied in distance, ranging from 100 yards (91 meters) to 6 miles (9.7 kilometers). Today snowshoe racing is popular among runners and marathoners who continue their endurance training and competition into the winter months. Snowshoeing is also part of multisport racing such as winter duathlons and triathlons, and it may be combined with cross-country skiing or mountain biking on the racecourse. Courses vary among regions and can consist of hill climbs and untracked trails, or prepared and groomed courses.

The United States Snowshoe Association (USSSA) has established rules for sprint racing and distance racing on snowshoes. Nordic sprint races are held on a 300-meter oval and races may be 100, 200, or 300 meters in length. Race categories for men and women are available at the junior, open, masters, senior, and veteran levels. Distance races are typically 5K and 10K in length, with a smattering of some 20K and ultradistance races. For the 2004 to 2005 season, more than 100 races were held from December through March in the United States and Canada, with even more races held in Europe. Many top finishers in the annual U.S. championships are also top athletes in other sports including mountain running, ultrarunning, and XTERRA triathlons, and races are becoming more and more competitive. The very first USSSA snowshoe championships were held in 2001 for the 5K and 10K distances.

NUTRITIONAL DEMANDS OF ENDURANCE TRAINING

Whatever the level of training for the competitive cross-country skier or snowshoer, these endurance athletes can benefit greatly from meeting their energy needs, matching carbohydrate requirements to training, staying adequately hydrated, and timing meals and snacks properly for optimal recovery. Recreational participants in both sports also need to be aware of their nutritional needs and can burn moderate amounts of muscle glycogen during training.

Energy Requirements

Average daily expenditures for cross-country skiers are high. One study estimated that female skiers burned about 3,500 calories daily, and male skiers about 5,000 calories daily when at the peak of training. For example, a 140-pound (64-kilogram) female cross-country skier exercising steadily at 5 miles per hour (8 kilometers per hour) would burn 10.8 calories per minute. During a 2-hour training session, she would burn almost 1,300 calories in that one training session. These training calories are burned on top of her daily energy needs estimated at 1,800 calories or more, for a total daily minimum energy expenditure of 3,100 calories. Longer training sessions would necessitate even higher energy intakes.

Male cross-country skiers, generally at higher body weights, also have very high energy needs. A 170-pound (77-kilogram) male training for 2 hours would burn up to 1,600 calories at 13.1 calories per minute. Daily energy expenditure when not training is estimated at 2,200 calories or more, for a total minimum energy requirement of 3,500 calories. Of course, energy expenditure during training for both men and women is affected by snow conditions and the skier's training level and technique.

While cross-country skiing utilizes both aerobic and anaerobic energy pathways, testing indicates that the majority of a 2-hour workout would be fueled by the aerobic energy system, with a predominant use of Type I muscle fibers. Type I muscle fibers predominate among elite-level skiers at about 67 percent of total muscle fibers, with the rest being mainly Type IIa muscle fibers, possibly to adapt to varying terrain and exercise intensities. Steady state endurance athletes, such as marathoners, have an even higher percentage of slow-twitch fibers. The superfast Type IIb fiber is practically nonexistent in cross-country skiers, as it is in most endurance athletes. Cross-country skiing is also distinguished from other endurance sports by the importance of upper-body power for performance.

Data on snowshoeing are more limited than that of cross-country skiing, but more physiology data should become available in the coming years as this is a rapidly growing and highly popular winter sport with relatively simple equipment and clothing requirements. A number of factors can affect the energy expended during snowshoeing workouts. Obviously the sport takes place in cold weather like any other winter sport, which raises energy expenditure. Snowshoers can also climb, walk, or run over varying terrain, and the speed at which they train can affect the amount of calories burned, as can climbing uphill. Snow conditions can also affect energy expenditure, with unpacked snow requiring more effort and calorie expenditure than packed snow. Snowshoers may or may not carry a pack, but the weight of any load will also increase the calories expended. Heavier-weight snowshoes will also increase energy output when both walking and running across the snow. When compared to walking on groomed snow, snowshoeing expends more energy, and the calorie expenditure data currently available indicate that snowshoeing is a great endurance workout.

BODY COMPOSITION

While Olympic cross-country skiers are extremely lean endurance athletes and much leaner than the average male and female, ideal body fat levels are individual to the skier. This is also true of competitive snowshoers who often compete in cycling, triathlon, and running in the warmer training months. Body fat contributes no strength or endurance advantage and must be carried across the snow, possibly limiting speed and endurance if levels are too high for the individual athlete. Endurance-focused winter sport athletes should follow a well-formulated training program and match energy and nutrient intake through the various training cycles to arrive at their healthiest and, if appropriate for their goals, most competitive body composition.

When in full training, losing body fat should be done carefully, and endurance athletes should not restrict more than 200 to 300 calories daily. It is best if more intense weight loss efforts occur before training loads are very high, and a substantial part of body composition change can be accomplished in the off-season and early preseason. Refer to Chapter 5 for safe and appropriate weight loss guidelines.

Training Diet Composition

Cross-country skiers and snowshoers deplete muscle glycogen stores to varying degrees depending on the intensity and duration of the training session. Significant muscle glycogen depletion can occur during one training session, or it may occur more gradually over several days or a weeklong cycle of training. Pay close attention to meeting your total carbohydrate requirements for the day, as well as recovery nutrition immediately after intense training. A full day's training, followed by another demanding day of exercise, requires that you replenish stores to train again the next day.

Periodizing Your Nutritional Intake

Many endurance athletes, such as those who participate in cross-country skiing and snowshoeing, follow a training program that consists of specific training cycles. These cycles can be designed to assist you in peaking for winter races and may also include training cycles during the warmer months specific to cross-country skiing or snowshoeing, but they often focus on another endurance sport. Generally training cycles for endurance training include the *preparation or base cycle*, the *build or competition cycle*, and the *transition or recovery cycle*. These cycles are designed to build endurance, strength, and then speed. Cross-country ski racing and snowshoe racing require a blend of endurance and speed. Regardless of your goals, you likely will have some variety in your training as dictated by weather and snow conditions, including long, slow workouts, recovery training, interval training, and weight training.

Base Training

Base training generally starts with lower-intensity training that gradually increases and moderate training volume that progresses over the course of the cycle. During this cycle while you are building aerobic endurance and muscular strength, your nutritional requirements progress as well. As described in Chapter 3, carbohydrate intake should especially match your training program. For low-intensity training several hours long or moderate-intensity training of 1 hour, try to consume 2 to 3 grams of carbohydrate per pound of body weight (5 to 7 grams per kilogram). As your training increases in intensity and volume, aim for 3 to 4.5 grams of carbohydrate per pound of body weight (7 to 10 grams per kilogram). Moderate workouts longer than 4 hours duration require 4.5 to 5.5 grams of carbohydrate per pound of body weight (10 to 12 grams per kilogram).

Protein requirements during this training cycle are about 0.45 to 0.75 grams per pound of body weight (1.0 to 1.6 grams per kilogram); aim for the higher end of the protein range for longer training days. You should also consume 0.4 to 0.5 grams fat per pound of body weight (0.8 to 1.0 gram per kilogram), to obtain additional calories after eating enough carbohydrates and protein during this particular training cycle.

Recovery nutrition—more specifically, consuming the correct amounts of carbohydrate, protein, and fluid in the 4 hours after training—is an important nutrition strategy during the base training phase. Immediately after moderate training lasting longer than 75 to 90 minutes, consume 0.5 to 0.7 grams of carbohydrate for every pound of weight (1 to 1.5 grams per kilogram), and for sessions over 90 minutes, consume 10 to 15 grams of high-quality protein. Many times this carbohydrate can be in liquid form, as you also need to consume 20 to 24 ounces of fluid (600 to 720 milliliters) for every pound (0.5 kilogram) of weight lost during training. The same amount of carbohydrate and protein can be consumed again in 2 hours to continue the recovery process.

Precompetition or Building Phase

During this training cycle, training intensity increases as volume decreases. Training sessions have a specific focus in sport-specific strength and speed. Sessions typically consist of high-intensity repeats, specific interval sessions, an emphasis on sport-specific explosive power, and increased weights during weight-training sessions. Overall, volume is moderate to allow for quality strength and speed training, with adequate recovery between sessions. Calorie and carbohydrate needs can be fairly high during specific training sessions due to the high intensity of the exercise.

Aim for higher amounts of carbohydrate on speed days where muscle glycogen is the most important fuel source, with 3 to 4.5 grams per pound of body weight (7 to 10 grams per kilogram) meeting your carbohydrate needs. Superhard training days may even require 4.5 to 5.5 grams per pound (10 to 12 grams per kilogram). You may need less carbohydrate on the recovery days built into this training cycle. Protein needs are also on the higher end for high-intensity training, but, again, amounts are easily met with good foods and good planning. Aim for 0.65 to 0.9 gram per pound of body weight (1.4 to 2.0 grams per kilogram) to recover from the higher stress placed on your muscles. Fat intake should be around 0.5 to 1 gram per pound of body weight (1 to 2 grams per kilogram).

Immediate recovery needs are essential to start the glycogen resynthesis process. Aim for 0.5 to 0.7 gram of carbohydrate for every pound of weight (1 to 1.5 grams per kilogram) and 10 to 15 grams of high-quality protein. Consume 20 to 24 ounces (600 to 720 milliliters) of fluid for every pound (0.5 kilogram) of weight loss.

Recovery Cycle

When you are in a recovery cycle after an important race, both your training intensity and volume have significantly decreased. As you rest, you will also need to decrease your caloric intake while maintaining a healthy, nutrient-dense diet high in fruits and vegetables.

Carbohydrate requirements decrease to 2.5 to 3 grams per pound of body weight (5.5 to 7 grams per kilogram), protein needs are at 0.5 to 0.6 gram per pound (1.2 to 1.4 grams per kilogram), and fat intake should not exceed 0.5 gram per pound (1 gram per kilogram). Stick with lean proteins and healthy fats to round out your diet. Snacking should be light and consist mainly of fresh fruit, and of course always maintain good hydration levels before, during, and after training. The sidebar below presents some meal plans for training.

Carbohydrate and Fluid Intake Before and During Training

As endurance athletes, cross-country skiers and snowshoers should focus on proper carbohydrate and fluid intake before and during training to improve the quality of their

» MEAL PLANS FOR TRAINING

Cross-country skiing or snowshoeing

■ **Training plan for 2-hour afternoon endurance workout**
Breakfast
Oatmeal, cooked, 1 c. (240 ml)
Dairy or soy milk, 8 oz. (240 ml)
Raisins, 2 tbsp. (40 ml)
Orange juice, 8 oz. (240 ml)
Toast, whole-grain,
2 slices (60 g)
Jam, 2 tbsp. (40 ml)

Lunch
Tuna salad, low-fat, 3 oz. (90 g)
Bread, 2 slices (60 g)
Lentil salad mix, 1 c. (240 ml)
Water, 12 oz.

Pre-exercise snack
Banana, 1 medium
Yogurt, 6 oz.
Whole-grain crackers, 12

During training
16 to 24 oz. sports drink
per hour

Recovery smoothie:
Dairy or soy milk, 12 oz.
(360 ml)
Whey protein, 1 scoop
Frozen berries, 1 c.
(240 ml)

Dinner
Fish, 4 oz. (120 g)
Sweet potato, 1 medium
Broccoli, steamed,
1 c. (240 ml)
Salad, mixed greens,
2 c. (480 ml)
Salad dressing, light,
4 tbsp. (80 ml)

2,900 calories
450 g carbohydrate
130 g carbohydrate
64 g fat

■ **Aerobic conditioning and strength training morning workout**
Preworkout
Dairy or soy milk, 12 ounces
(360 ml)
Protein powder, 1 scoop
Bagel, 2 ounces (60 g)
Jam, 1 tbsp. (20 ml)
Peanut butter, 2 t. (14 ml)

**Resistance training,
30 minutes**
**Aerobic cross-training,
45 minutes**
Sports drink, 24 oz
(720 ml)

Recovery breakfast
Cereal, 2 oz. (60 g)
Dairy or soy milk, 12 oz.
(360 ml)
Banana, 1 large

Lunch
Turkey, 3 oz. (90 g)
Bread, whole-grain,
2 slices (60 g)

training sessions. Follow the pre-exercise eating and fluid guidelines described in Chapter 4. Generally, you can eat closer to training times for lower- to moderate-intensity sessions when blood flow to your gastrointestinal system is moderate. Push carbohydrate portions to your maximum tolerance for longer duration workouts to stock up on pretraining fuel. Allow a wider digestion time before speed training when blood flow to the gut is lower and your stomach may be more sensitive. You can also prehydrate before training with water or even a sports drink for additional and easily digested carbohydrates. Gels and energy bars are both a quick, well-tolerated snack before training and can also provide a well-tolerated carbohydrate boost for more strenuous workouts. Pay attention to pre-exercise eating as described in Chapter 4 to maintain blood glucose

Avocado, 2 slices
Bean soup, 1 c. (240 ml)
Raw vegetables, 1 c.

Snack
Apple, 1 medium
Yogurt, 6 oz. (180 ml)

Dinner
Stir-fry:
  Shrimp, cooked, 6 oz. (180 g)
  Mixed vegetables, 1 c. (240 ml)
  Rice, cooked, 1 ½ c.
  (360 ml)
  Sesame seed oil, 3 t.
  (20 ml)

Snack
Frozen yogurt, 1 c. (240 ml)
Frozen berries, 1 c. (240 ml)

2,700 calories
410 g carbohydrate
160 g protein
45 g fat

■ **Meal plan for high-intensity interval training**
6:00 p.m. interval workout
Breakfast
Waffles, low-fat, 2 small
Syrup, light, 2 tbsp. (40 ml)
Yogurt, 6 oz. (180 g)
Frozen berries, 1 c. (240 ml)

Snack
Almonds, 12
Pear, 1 small

Lunch
Wrap:
  Turkey, 3 oz. (90 g)
  Rice, cooked, ⅔ c.
  (160 ml)
  Hummus, 2 tbsp. (40 ml)
  Salsa, ½ c. (120 ml)
  Assorted vegetables,
  ½ c. (120 ml)
  Avocado, 2 slices
  Tortilla, 1 large

Pretraining snack
Soy smoothie:
  Soy milk, 12 oz. (360 ml)
  Banana, 1 large

During training:
Sports drink, 16 to 24 oz.
per hour (480-720 ml)
Carbohydrate gel,
1 packet midworkout

Recovery snack
Carbohydrate-protein
recovery drink, 16 oz.
(480 ml)

Dinner
Fish, 4 oz. (120 g)
Sweet potato, 1 large
Steamed asparagus, 1 c.
Bread, whole-grain,
2 slices (60 g)
Olive oil, 3 t. (20 ml)

2,800 calories
420 g carbohydrate
112 g protein
75 g fat

levels during training. Start all training sessions adequately hydrated by enjoying fluids in the 2 hours before a training session. Remember to allow time for a bladder break
before trekking across the snow.

Your fluid losses when training in the cold can be significant and warrant fluid replacement during training. For sessions lasting longer than 75 to 90 minutes, a sports drink
that also provides carbohydrate is recommended. Sports drinks may also result in less urine
production than water can create, a helpful tip when training out in the cold. Carry
squeeze bottles with a warmer temperature mix, or use a winter hydration system for long

TABLE 7.1 » NUTRITION STRATEGIES FOR TRAINING CYCLES

Training Cycle	Nutritional Strategies

Base Training
Starts with low intensity that increases
Volume builds through cycle
Muscular endurance training
	Match carbohydrate to training intensity and volume
	Aim for 2-3 g carbohydrate per pound (5-7 g/kg) for long duration, low intensity
	Increase to 3-4.5 g carbohydrate per pound (7-10 g/kg) as volume and intensity increase
	For moderate intensity greater than 4 hours duration increase to 4.5-5.5 g carbohydrate per pound (10-12 g/kg)
	Consume 30-60 g carbohydrate per hour during exercise
	Protein requirements at 0.45-0.75 g/lb. (1.0-1.6 g/kg)
	Practice recovery nutrition immediately after training and again in 2 hours for longer efforts:
	    0.5-0.7 g carbohydrate/lb. (1-1.5 g/kg)
	    10-15 g protein
	    200-300 mg sodium
	    20-24 oz. (600-720 ml) fluid for every pound (0.5 kg) weight loss

Precompetition or Build Phase Training intensity increases Volume decreases Session focus on sport-specific strength and speed	Calorie and carbohydrate needs are high with higher-intensity training. Aim for 3-4.5 g carbohydrate per pound (7-10 g/kg) on speed days Increase to 4.5-5.5 g carbohydrate per pound (10-12 g/kg) on super-hard training days. Carbohydrate requirements are lower on recovery days Aim for 0.65-0.9 g/lb. (1.4-2.0 g/kg) of protein Pay attention to recovery nutrition as described for the base cycle
Recovery Phase Training intensity and volume decrease significantly	Decrease carbohydrate intake to 2.5-3 g/lb. (5.5-7 g/kg) Protein needs are 0.5-0.6 g/lb. (1.2-1.4 g/kg) Focus on a high-quality diet

outdoor workouts. Gel products can supply carbohydrate; carry them close to your body to keep them from freezing. Table 7.1 summarizes nutritional guidelines for your endurance training program cycles.

Competition Nutrition

Whatever the length of the ski or snowshoe race in which you are competing, it is important that you are well fueled and well hydrated (see Table 4.4 for optimal meal-timing portions). Practice with food choices and portion before higher-intensity training sessions that will be similar to your race conditions. Skiers and snowshoers should also reduce the fiber content of their meal before competition in anticipation of pre-race nerves.

Precompetition Nutrition
Shorter Events

Skiers and snowshoers competing in shorter events such as 5K and 10K races at higher intensities should take extra care to allow for adequate digestion time. Races with later start times may be preceded by a larger breakfast and a light, high-carbohydrate meal or snack 1.5 to 2 hours before the race. Small amounts of easily digested protein can be incorporated into the early meal. Your pre-race meal should prevent hunger during the warm-up and race, leave the stomach feeling settled and the athlete satisfied, and maintain steady blood glucose levels. Hydrate well before a race, as some degree of dehydration can occur during your warm-up.

Longer Races

Preparation for events that will last longer than 90 minutes for the individual skier or snowshoer requires paying close attention to nutrition in the 48 hours leading up to the event. For cross-country ski events longer than 30K and snowshoe events longer than 20K, tapering and fueling up on carbohydrates for 48 to 72 hours before the event can improve performance. Calorie needs decrease somewhat during a taper, but carbohydrate requirements are generally from 3 to 5 grams per pound of body weight (7 to 10 grams per kilogram) to fully load muscle carbohydrate stores. Pay constant attention to hydration during the days leading to the race.

The night before the race, consume a high-carbohydrate meal. Some well-tolerated choices can include pasta, rice, potatoes, cooked vegetables, and breads. Emphasize lean proteins like poultry and fish. Stick with relatively bland and plain foods, and avoid any items that are spicy, unusual, or high in fiber. Go easy on the fats, and have just enough to provide flavor.

The morning of the race emphasize carbohydrates and easily digested low-fat protein. Aim to consume 1.5 grams of carbohydrate per pound of body weight (3 grams per kilogram) 3 to 4 hours before the race start. Small amounts of fat may improve cold tolerance and keep hunger at bay. Warm foods are also appealing before racing out in the cold, but liquid carbohydrates are also easily tolerated and hydrating. (See page 221 for more specific ideas on meal plans for competition.)

During the Race

Race times of an hour or longer are affected by hydration and fuel levels, so what you consume during the race is just as important as what you consume before the race. Of course, you are focused on finishing the race in the shortest time possible, but topping off your fluid stores with a sports drink along the way maintains a supply of fluid and carbohydrate. Attempt to stay as well hydrated as possible with the assistance of aid stations on the course. Cold weather may dull your sense of thirst, and drinking during a race may be inconvenient, but paying close attention to your fluid needs ultimately improves your performance. If you plan to carry your own sports drink, it can be warmed up prior to the race. You may want to carry a bladder system designed for cold weather or wear an insulated bottle around your waist. When glucose stores run low, a carbohydrate gel carried close to your body can provide a quick carbohydrate boost. Pay close attention to symptoms of low blood glucose levels, such as poor concentration, shivering, and hunger. Extra cold weather and high-intensity efforts such as hill climbing may push up your carbohydrate requirements and increase your risk.

Cross-country skiers and snowshoers need to practice drinking during training so that hydration and fueling skills are fine-tuned during races. Start drinking 15 minutes into the race as you settle into a rhythm. Racing at a slight downhill, in the middle of the pack, or when drafting off other racers presents a good opportunity to drink. Try to slow down and drink at any feed stations. Bend the cup to form a spout and drink fluid quickly. Some solid items that may be provided at feed stations include energy bars, cookies, brownies, and gels. Warmer items may include soup and hot chocolate. Save fluids that you carry for consumption between feeds.

Refueling after the race is also part of your race day strategy. Consume plenty of liquids and 0.5 to 0.7 gram of carbohydrate per pound of weight (1 to 1.5 grams per kilogram) within 15 minutes after racing, and again in two hours. If available, 10 to 15 grams of protein can also be consumed after racing. You may have to plan ahead to have post-race foods and fluids available to start the nutritional recovery process. Consume this amount of carbohydrate and protein again in two hours to continue the recovery process. Continue to rehydrate after the race.

» MEAL PLANS FOR COMPETITION

Competition day

■ 10:00 a.m. race start
Breakfast (7:00 a.m.)
High-carbohydrate energy
drink (80 g carbohydrate),
12 oz. (360 ml)
Toast, 2 slices (60 g)
Jam, 2 tbsp. (40 ml)
Cereal, 1.5 oz. (45 g)
Almond milk, 8 oz. (240 ml)

Warm-up
Sports drink, 32 oz. (480 ml),
consumed in the hours
leading to the race

Pre-race (60 minutes)
Carbohydrate gel, 1 packet
Sports drink, 16 oz.

During race (10K)
Sports drink from aid stations

**Post-race recovery (within
30 minutes)**
Carbohydrate/protein
recovery drink, 12 oz. (360 ml)
Banana, 1 large

**Lunch (within 2 hours
of race finish)**
Pasta, cooked, 3 c. (720 ml)
Marinara sauce,
1 ½ c. (360 ml)
Lean beef or poultry,
4 oz. (120 g)
Bread, 2 slices (60 g)

Snack
Apple, 1 medium
Almonds, 12

Dinner
Rice and vegetable
stir-fry,
2 c. (480 ml)
Salad, 2 c. (480 ml)
Salad dressing, light,
4 tbsp. (80 ml)

3,300 calories
570 g carbohydrate
100 g protein
66 g fat

■ 8:00 a.m. start time
Breakfast (5:30 a.m.)
Smoothie:
  Soy milk, 12 oz. (240 ml)
  Yogurt, 6 oz. (180 ml)
  Fruit, 1 c. (240 ml)
  Juice, 12 oz. (360 ml)
  or high-carbohydrate
  energy drink,
  12 oz. (360 ml)

**Warm-up/Precompetition
(6:30–7:00 a.m.)**
High-carbohydrate gel,
1 packet sports drink,
16-24 oz. (480-720 ml)

During race
16 oz. (480 ml) or more as
tolerated sports drink per hour

**Recovery snack (30–60
minutes post-race)**
Granola bar, 1 medium
Peach, 1 medium
High-carbohydrate protein
recovery drink, 12 oz.

**Recovery lunch (2–3 hours
post-race)**
Turkey, 3 oz. (90 g)
Bread, whole-grain,
2 slices (60 g)
Vegetable or noodle soup,
1 c. (240 ml)
Apple, 1 medium

Dinner
Beef strips, lean, 4 oz. (120 g)
Rice noodles, cooked,
2 c. (480 ml)
Stir-fry vegetables, 1 c. (240 ml)
Sesame seed oil, 4 t. (25 ml)

Dessert
Sorbet, 1 c. (240 ml)
Berries, frozen, 1 c. (240 ml)

2,900 calories
445 g carbohydrate
110 g protein
77 g fat

Sodium and Winter Endurance Athletes

Several studies have looked at the effect of ultraendurance racing in the warmer months on blood sodium levels. Endurance athletes who train and compete in hot and humid weather, as many winter athletes do in their off-season, may have had the experience of lowered blood sodium levels during long training sessions and competition. While this condition of hyponatremia can be dangerous and even fatal, many endurance athletes can experience mild to severe degrees of lowered blood sodium. The lower blood sodium levels drop, the more serious and life-threatening the symptoms. At the very least, this condition can slow down the competitive efforts of the endurance athlete and is best prevented.

While the causes of hyponatremia are many and varied, the main instigators are excess fluid intake, exacerbated by a high rate of sodium loss from sweating. Drinking too much before and during long efforts such as competition, especially in warm and humid climates, also increases the risk for developing hyponatremia. Some endurance athletes sweat more than others every hour and have a higher concentration of sodium in their sweat. When you exercise, urine production decreases and the sodium content of sweat increases, raising the risk of developing hyponatremia. Endurance athletes with longer finishing times have more time to sweat and drink, placing them at greater risk for fluid overload.

We know less about hyponatremia and cold-weather training and racing. Two studies have looked at sodium and cold-weather ultraendurance multisport racing. Subjects were tested during a 100-mile (161-kilometer) ultraendurance race in Alaska. Athletes developed a lowering of blood sodium, with some reaching lowered levels classified as hyponatremia. Hyponatremic athletes consumed a greater amount of fluid per hour at 16 ounces versus 13 ounces (0.5 liter per hour versus 0.4 liter per hour) and consumed less sodium per hour (235 versus 298 milligrams per hour) than subjects who did not develop hyponatremia. Even lowered blood sodium (versus hyponatremia) was related to fluid overload related to excessive fluid consumption of 6 to 13 ounces per hour (200 to 400 milliliters per hour), and sodium intake averaging 310 milligrams per hour. Overall it appears that fluid consumption in cold weather during ultraendurance exercise may need to be less than the recommended 16 to 32 ounces per hour (500 to 1,000 milliliters per hour). During the race participants consumed sports drinks, soda, and water for fluid and also refueled with energy bars, gels, sandwiches, soups, bagels, and cookies.

While more data are needed regarding fluid balance and sodium intake in cold-weather ultraendurance racing, we can say that fluid intake needs to match fluid losses, with adequate sodium consumed during the race. Check your weight before and after cold-weather training. Weight gain indicates that you are consuming fluid in excess of your sweat losses. A weight loss of 2 to 5 pounds (0.9 to 2.25 kilograms) indicates that fluid intake needs to increase during training. Winter sport ultraendurance athletes need to gauge their fluid losses during training in cold weather and be aware of how fluid losses can change during the season.

» DO NUTRITIONAL NEEDS BETWEEN MALES AND FEMALES DIFFER?

Despite the well-established physiological differences between female and male athletes, female athletes are routinely prescribed sports nutrition recommendations based on male-subject-derived scientific data. Fortunately, the past decade has seen increased scientific focus and study of nutritional requirements unique to female athletes. Although much of this research has focused on endurance exercise, rather than the type of training programs practiced in other winter sports, a few key points can be considered by female athletes, particularly those partici-pating and competing in cross-country skiing and snowshoeing.

A full body of research on solely female ath-letes that can be compared to the existing data on men is lacking, but emerging data do provide some practical gender-specific considerations for carbohydrate loading, nutritional intake dur-ing training, and recovery strategies.

Consuming adequate carbohydrate to opti-mize body glycogen fuel stores when resting or decreasing training prior to competition is an im-portant nutritional strategy for female athletes, just as it is for their male counterparts. In order to glycogen-load effectively, women need to consume an adequate number of grams of car-bohydrate, but they appear to glycogen-load only to about 50 percent of the magnitude of men. Female endurance winter sport athletes should still taper and carbohydrate-load for ex-tended competition, but they may derive less benefit than their male counterparts.

Researchers have also studied gender dif-ference regarding carbohydrate consumption during exercise with useful results. Because fe-male athletes do not respond as robustly as men

to carbohydrate loading, the consumption of a sports drink appears to be one place they can make up this difference. Subjects cycled at 60 percent VO_2max for 90 minutes while consum-ing an 8 percent carbohydrate beverage (1 gram carbohydrate per kilogram body weight). This study demonstrated that when female athletes performing endurance exercise were provided with sports drinks during exercise, they oxidized or burned more of the sports drink than males. Overall, however, women still burn more fat than carbohydrate during exercise when compared to men. Carbohydrate consumption during higher training intensities would also be expected to benefit female athletes.

Consuming carbohydrate immediately after training improves muscle glycogen resynthesis and recovery. Female athletes benefit from this strategy as much as their male counterparts. Research indicates the males and females ap-pear to store glycogen at similar rates when carbohydrate is given immediately after endur-ance exercise. Future research can determine how this nutritional recovery strategy affects training programs specific to winter athletes.

Another recent study also points to the need for more data to fine-tune the unique daily nu-tritional requirements of female athletes and the effect of diet manipulations on perform-ance, particularly for carbohydrate intake. Re-searchers had well-trained female triathletes and cyclists consume a low-carbohydrate diet of 1.4 grams per pound (3 grams per kilogram body weight), a moderate-carbohydrate diet of 2.25 grams per pound (5 grams per kilogram), and a high-carbohydrate diet of 3.5 grams per pounds (8 grams per kilogram). Subjects cycled to

CONTINUED

exhaustion. Interestingly, subjects had difficulty consuming the prescribed amount of carbohydrate on the high-carbohydrate diet.

When completing a time trial after cycling at 70 percent VO$_2$max, no significant performance differences were found between the diets. More research and performance testing on various carbohydrate dietary levels in female athletes are needed. Past studies have demonstrated a difference in fuel metabolism between men and women. In the future, it is expected that nutritional recommendations are to be more sex-specific.

Women have a greater increase in core temperature given similar heat exposure when compared to men. The onset of sweating may occur at higher body temperatures, and sweat rates may be lower. However, there are likely more differences in sweat rates among individual women athletes than between men and women. Female athletes should consume fluid during exercise to attempt to match their fluid losses, while staying within their gastrointestinal tolerances. One study indicated that replacing body fluid after exercise is not affected by the phase of the menstrual cycle.

Although protein needs of female athletes are higher than the general population, there appear to be no significant differences between men and women at this time. Recommendations are based on body weight and specific training programs, and they can vary with the amount of calories and carbohydrate consumed. Of course, adequate caloric intake allows for more optimal utilization of the protein consumed.

With a greater number of female athletes reaching lower body fat levels, and women having to work harder to achieve the same level of leanness as men, health could be compromised. When a female athlete's caloric intake is inadequate, her body may be more prone to defend or maintain her current weight than would men. Recent data indicate that inadequate caloric intake is the main trigger for hormonal imbalances, absence of menstruation, and subsequently compromised bone health.

Although more specific nutritional training recommendations for women need to be tested and formulated, women athletes should practice some focused strategies to ensure optimal performance. Consistently practice optimal recovery nutrition following hard training, glycogen-load in combination with adequate caloric intake, and practice techniques for consuming enough carbohydrate during training and competition.

Recreational Touring

Snowshoeing and cross-country skiing are not especially dangerous as far as the risk of injury, but if you plan to spend several hours outdoors in the winter weather, you need to be prepared nutritionally to prevent problems with dehydration and inadequate fuel.

Spending several hours trekking across the snow can put you at significant risk for developing dehydration and overheating your body. Always bring your own fluids with you so that you can drink and keep up with sweat losses as much as possible. Winter hydration systems that prevent valves from freezing and clogging are essential. Insulated bottles can also be carried close to your body. Sports drinks can be warmed, as can other carbohydrate-containing hot drinks such as tea with honey. But pack plenty of solid items for regular consumption to maintain blood glucose levels and fuel muscles. Pack items such as trail mix, cut-up toaster tarts, gummy bears, and any other tasty carbohydrate items. Pack them close to your body to keep items from freezing up, and aim for a carbohydrate consumption of 30 to 60 grams per hour or more for very strenuous efforts. Pay attention for symptoms of dehydration and lowered blood glucose levels.

» NUTRITION AND YOUR IMMUNE SYSTEM

Periods of heavy training are associated with a depressed immune function, and compromised immune function can be further aggravated by inadequate nutrition. Combining training with school and/or work can overtax an athlete's resources, stress your body, and compromise your ability to fight infection. A strong immune system should result in fewer colds or viruses, and if the athlete does get sick, recovery should be quicker.

Dedicated winter athletes don't want to encounter an unwanted halt to their training program due to illness. Specific foods can strengthen your immune system.

One of the nutrients most commonly associated with preventing colds is vitamin C, which has a widespread reputation as an immune system booster. While a daily multivitamin mineral supplement may contain the Daily Value of vitamin C, don't underestimate the importance of ample food sources of this nutrient. Athletes can consume more than three servings of fresh fruit daily and up to 2 cups of cooked vegetables daily for ample amounts of dietary vitamin C. High doses of vitamin C have not been shown to protect the immune system—250 milligrams is adequate to saturate body stores.

Fruits and vegetables also contain hundreds of phytochemicals that provide many preventative health benefits and are also excellent sources of carotenoids that boost the activity of white blood cells called lymphocytes. Beta-carotene can also be converted to vitamin A, an important nutrient for the immune system.

Other nutrients important for a strong immune system include adequate intakes of zinc, iron, and vitamins B6 and B12. A good daily multivitamin mineral supplement providing 100 percent of the Daily Values ensures adequate nutrient intake. Megadosing with vitamins and minerals can compromise the immune system, and excessive intakes of iron, zinc, and vitamin E are not advised.

Consuming adequate calories is not only beneficial for an athlete's recovery and energy levels but also important to maintaining a healthy immune system. Falling short of your calorie requirements can compromise your immune system, as can poorly planned and low-calorie diets low in protein. Diets too low in energy can result in inadequate intake of vitamins and minerals, which also decreases immunity.

Training with optimal stores of carbohydrate not only provides fuel for your workouts but also boosts your immune system. Athletes who train in the carbohydrate-depleted state experience greater increases in the stress hormones that go up during exercise. Consuming carbohydrate during exercise also seems to diminish some of the immunosuppressive effects of intense training. Overall, good carbohydrate replacement supports your immune system.

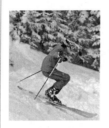

8 Nutrition for Alpine Skiing and Snowboarding

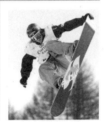

The origins of alpine skiing can be traced back to a version of skiing in Sweden that is more than 4,000 years old. Later, the people of the Telemark area of Norway invented the Telemark and Christie turns as a means of controlling speeds on downhill descents. Both alpine and cross-country skiing owe their existence to these early inventors. Skiing grew very popular in the 1900s, and the need for different types of equipment and better control on steeper slopes led to the birth of alpine skiing. Alpine skiing disciplines of downhill and slalom debuted at the 1936 Olympic Winter Games in Innsbruck, Austria. Skiing also became a popular recreational sport in the 1930s when ski lifts were invented, and the ski industry began booming in the 1950s. Giant slalom was introduced at the 1952 Winter Olympics in Oslo, Norway, and the Super G debuted at the 1988 Olympics.

Over the years, faster and safer ski equipment has been developed, and skiers have combined this new equipment with improved training and ski techniques to improve the enjoyment of the sport. More than 14 million skiers enjoy alpine skiing and more than 3 million telemark skiing.

The younger cousin of skiing (or, rather, surfing and skateboarding!), snowboarding was invented in 1965 when a surfer built a surfboard for the snow by putting two skis together. One year later production of this prototype became known as the "snurfer," to describe the effect of surfing on snow. Equipment ideas continued to develop; by the early 1980s the design had been refined, and a handful of snowboards were on the market. The sport really took off in the mid-1980s when snowboarding developed a "bad boy" image. Despite being a widely popular sport today among both males and females of all ages, it still retains a bit of its rebellious image and individualistic flavor. In 2000, snowboarding was the fastest-growing sport in the United States, with a growth of over 50 percent. Today snowboarding boasts more than 7.7 million participants.

The sport of snowboarding continues to carve out its own unique path in the competitive arena, debuting at the 1988 Nagano Olympics for the half-pipe or freestyle and giant slalom or alpine competition. Snowboarders practicing the freestyle discipline have their own specific training programs, with alpine snowboarding having its own specific technique and equipment. At the 2006 Winter Olympics in Turin, Italy, snowboarders will compete in the parallel giant slalom, half-pipe, and snowboardcross events for men and women.

At the recreational level, both skiing and snowboarding are highly popular, with participation heavy through the winter months. Skiers and snowboarders can have a wide variety of sporting interests off-season, but they can also train or condition for their sport year-round. Some off-season sports can include mountain biking and endurance sports; for the snowboarding crowd, skateboarding and surfing may be popular sports. Elite skiers and snowboarders of course focus on and do sport-specific training year-round.

While skiing and snowboarding use very different techniques, both are considered to be mainly power sports that require high levels of both anaerobic and aerobic power and conditioning, muscular strength and endurance, flexibility, and skill. Alpine skiers and snowboarders can exercise or train for many hours; however, the activity is intermittent with runs varying in length, with a fair amount of extended time spent returning to the top of the mountain. For the serious freestyle or half-pipe snowboarder, aerobic conditioning is very important. Typically on many training days, they "hike the pike" to return to the top of their training run and may complete as many as 15 runs. In contrast, many recreational skiers and alpine snowboarders enjoy concentrated exercise times on vacations and weekends, during which they spend as much time as possible out on the slopes via chairlift. Optimal conditioning and proper nutritional strategies are essential to maintain energy levels, coordination, and skill through the end of the day to keep enjoyment levels high and injury levels low.

Competitions in these disciplines do require speed and skill, rather than a focus on endurance, as competitors race against the clock, and half-pipe snowboard competitors need a unique set of gymnastics skills. Competitors require expert equipment, sport-specific technique, and the right physiological and psychological profiles. Physiological testing indicates that the profile of most successful world-class skiers includes a number of interrelated factors, though skiers do seem to possess a unique blend of muscle fiber type, agility, coordination, and balance.

Physiological data based on elite alpine skiers indicate that they have a more muscular physique, which provides greater leverage and power when skiing. Heavier body masses are considered an advantage in speed events and sections with low technical difficulty. There has been a trend toward higher body mass in elite skiers with enhanced power training of the upper body. Because racing events in alpine skiing last between 45 seconds and 2.5 minutes, the energy supply during competition is both aerobic and anaerobic. Anaerobic energy provides a substantial part of immediate energy demands during both training and competition. However, elite alpine skiers do require a high aerobic capacity for several reasons: to meet the energy demands of training and competition, to provide a fast and adequate recovery for the intervals between runs and races, and to endure the long stress of a 4- to 5-month race season that includes plenty of traveling. The end of the season also includes the world championship.

Elite skiers undergo a substantial amount of endurance training, often completing 6 to 7 hours of endurance training weekly in the summer months. Aerobic power has been found to be fairly predictive of success in racing. Muscular strength in the lower limbs is also required for current carving techniques and equipment, and strength training is highly sport-specific. Physiological data have also stressed the importance of anaerobic power. Researchers have found skiers to have a high level of abdominal muscular endurance.

NUTRITIONAL DEMANDS OF TRAINING

Whatever the level of training, alpine skiers and snowboarders can benefit by starting a day of training with plenty of wholesome carbohydrate, high-quality protein, and hydrating fluids. Maintaining hydration levels is important on the slopes and at altitude. While breakfast is the most important meal of the day, high-carbohydrate snacks and a quality carbohydrate-containing lunch are also essential to maintain muscle glycogen stores and blood glucose levels. Proper nutrition strategies fuel your muscles for run after repeated run, and steady blood glucose levels maintain your concentration so that you can focus on maintaining your skill and performing safely.

ENERGY REQUIREMENTS

A full day of either skiing or snowboarding can increase daily caloric requirements far beyond basic energy expenditure. For example, a 140-pound (64-kilogram) female alpine skier can burn 7.1 calories per minute skiing at a recreational level. A day of skiing could easily burn over 800 to 1,200 calories. Basic energy expenditure is estimated at 1,700 calories daily, resulting in daily energy needs of 2,500 to 2,900 calories. A male skier weighing 180 pounds (82 kilograms) burns 11.9 calories per minute, with a full day of skiing resulting in over 1,500 to 2,000 calories burned. Total energy needs for the day could reach over 3,700 calories. Of course, how much fuel is required for the day depends on the time it takes to complete a run and the number of runs completed in a full day of skiing. Skiers should not fall too far short on energy needs in order to prevent fatigue at the end of a long day on the slopes. Energy requirements can vary greatly on days when skiers focus on work in the gym or other winter activities. But it is good to be prepared for a full day on the slopes.

Less research is available on the calorie-burning effects of snowboarding. But like skiers, these athletes complete run after repeated run during a full day on the slopes. Currently it is reasonable to assume that alpine snowboarders' level of calorie burning during a day on the slopes is similar to that of alpine skiers, and they can burn several hundred to over 1,000 calories beyond their basic energy requirements during a full day of snow surfing.

Muscle glycogen content of elite skiers has been assessed before and after a day or a few days of skiing on the slopes. Glycogen stores were reduced by 50 percent of starting levels after a day of giant slalom or slalom training, with both Type I and Type II muscle fibers being glycogen depleted. Muscle glycogen utilization can be fairly substantial during a day of leisure or competitive skiing, and starting out for a day on the slopes with suboptimal glycogen stores could have an adverse effect on performance.

BODY COMPOSITION

Body fat levels in alpine skiers are healthy and lower than the general population, but they usually do not reach the very low levels seen in endurance sports such as cross-country skiing. Body fat levels in female alpine skiers average about 21 percent and range from 7 to 14 percent in male alpine skiers. Recent data on elite level skiers found the average female to be at 23 percent body fat (range of 16 to 30 percent) and the average male at 16 percent body fat (range of 9 to 21 percent). Slalom skiers tend to be leaner than skiers in other events, though the ideal body fat for each skier is unique to that skier, with downhill racers having the greatest muscle mass. A muscular physique is considered to be an advantage at the elite level of skiing, and muscular development and strength is certainly an important attribute for the recreational skier.

Body composition for elite female alpine snowboarders is in the 21 to 25 percent body fat range, with males at 9 to 12 percent. Body fat levels in the freestylers tend to be lower, due to the gymnastic-like nature of moving their bodies in the air, with females at 15 to 18 percent and males at 6 to 9 percent.

Skiers and snowboarders should follow a well-formulated training program and match energy and nutrient intake through the various training cycles to arrive at their healthiest and, if appropriate for their goals, most competitive body composition. While body fat contributes no strength or endurance advantage, keeping body fat levels to low healthy norms or below should be adequate for top performance.

If decreased body fat is a goal, efforts to this end should occur before intense training. Many skiers are also likely focused on the muscle-building phase of body composition and should eat appropriately for this phase of training. Any weight loss efforts should be sensible, with a recommended calorie restriction of 200 to 300, and no more than 500, calories daily, particularly if you are in a strength and muscle-building phase of training. Refer to Chapter 5 for healthy, appropriate weight loss guidelines.

» MEAL PLANS FOR COMPETITION

Sport-specific conditioning

■ Morning workout
Breakfast
Protein smoothie:
   Milk, skim, 8 oz. (240 ml)
   Yogurt, 6 oz. (180 ml)
   Protein powder, 1 scoop
   Frozen fruit, 1 c. (240 ml)

**Sport-specific
conditioning workout**
Sports drink, 16 oz. (480 ml)

Recovery breakfast
   Cereal, 1.5 oz. (45 g)
   Soy milk, 8 oz. (240 ml)
   Banana, 1 small

Lunch
   Salad mix, with chicken, 6 oz.
   (180 g)
   Soup, noodle, 1 c. (240 ml)
   Crackers, whole-grain, 8
   Pear, 1 large

Snack
   Yogurt, 6 oz. (180 ml)
   Grapes, 1 c. (240 ml)

Dinner
   Broiled pork chop, 4 oz. (120 g)
   Olive oil, 2 t. (14 ml)
   Sweet potato, 1 large
   Steamed leafy green vegetables, 1 c. (240 ml)
   Salad, 2 c. (480 ml)
   Salad dressing, light, 4 tbsp. (80 ml)

Snack
   Frozen yogurt, 6 oz. (180 ml)
   Fresh fruit, 1 c. (240 ml)

2,400 calories
350 g carbohydrate (58%)
120 g protein (20%)
58 g fat (22%)

**■ Aerobic conditioning and
strength training session
evening workout**
Breakfast
Whole-grain bread, 2 slices
(60 g)
Peanut butter, 4 t. (25 ml)
Jam, 1 tbsp. (20 ml)

Grapefruit, half
Juice, 8 oz. (240 ml)

Snack
Fresh fruit, 1 medium to
large piece

Lunch
Turkey wrap:
   Turkey, 3 oz. (90 g)
   Tortilla, 1 large
   Salsa, veggies, ½ cup
   (120 ml)
   Cheese, low-fat, 1 oz.
   (30 g)
Soup, 1 c. (240 ml)

Preworkout
Bagel, 3 oz. (90 g)
Lean protein, 2 oz. (60 g)
Honey, 1 tbsp. (20 ml)
Yogurt, 6 oz. (180 ml)
Apple, 1 medium

TRAINING DIET COMPOSITION

Because of the likelihood of some glycogen depletion from a day or more of repeated skiing and snowboarding, and possible glycogen depletion from training in the days before hitting the slopes, a diet adequate in carbohydrate should be consumed. Consuming a high-carbohydrate diet the day before a full weekend of skiing or snowboarding is recommended so that the fun and training starts with full muscle glycogen levels. A high-carbohydrate diet should be consumed during a full day on the slopes, especially during successive days of training. Protein requirements are easily met on a well-balanced eating plan, with protein portions and timing important during the strength-training phase that many skiers and snowboarders participate in for their sport. Fat intake should round out energy requirements with healthy fats.

■ **Workout—45 minutes aerobic conditioning, 45 minutes of strength training**
Sports drink, 24 oz. (720 ml) per hour

Post-training
Smoothie:
  Milk, 12 oz. (360 ml)
  Protein powder, 2 scoops
  Frozen fruit, 1 c. (240 ml)

Dinner
Fish, 4 oz.
Olive oil, 4 t. (27 ml)
Kasha, cooked, 1 c. (240 ml)
Vegetable, cooked, 1 c.
Salad, 2 c. (480 ml)
Salad dressing, light, 4 tbsp. (80 ml)

2,700 calories
380 g carbohydrate (56%)
150 g protein (22%)
66 g fat (22%)

■ **Nutrition for a day on the slopes**
Breakfast
Eggs, 2 scrambled
Oatmeal, cooked, 1 c. (240 ml)
Banana, 1 small
Raisins, 1 tbsp. (20 ml)
Yogurt, 6 ounces (180 ml)
Juice, 8 oz. (240 ml)
Water, 16 oz. (480 ml)

Chairlift
Warmed sports drink in insulated bottle

Midmorning snack
Energy bar, 1

Lunch
Hot sandwich:
  Turkey, 2 oz.
  Cheese, 2 oz.
  Bread, whole-grain, 2 slices (60 g)
Chili, vegetarian, 1 c. (240 ml)
Hot chocolate, 8 oz. (240 ml)
Orange, 1 medium

Chairlift
Water or sports drink in insulated bottle

Midafternoon snack
Carbohydrate gel

Dinner
Beef stir-fry:
  Beef, 4 oz. (120 g)
  Mixed vegetables, 1 c. (240 ml)
  Oil, 4 t. (27 ml)
Noodles, cooked, 2 c. (480 ml)

Dessert
Frozen yogurt, 8 oz. (240 ml)
Frozen berries, 1 c. (240 ml)

3,100 calories
430 g carbohydrate (55%)
110 g protein (14%)
105 g fat (31%)

» NUTRITIONAL CONSIDERATIONS AT ALTITUDE

A day on the slopes means a day or several days in a row at altitude. Breathing at high elevations can be challenging, as can exercising, and the higher the elevation, the less dense the air you breathe. This effect results in altitude hypoxia or a reduction of oxygen in your body tissues. Your body can adjust or acclimatize to altitude, though this process can take a few weeks. When you travel quickly to altitude for a weekend or longer stay to ski or snowboard, you may experience symptoms such as rapid heart rate, headache, shortness of breath, fatigue, loss of appetite, decreased urine output, and insomnia. This complex of symptoms is most likely to occur in individuals who reside near sea level and ascend rapidly to high altitude. Symptoms normally develop in 6 to 12 hours, peak at 24 to 48 hours, and subside in 3 to 7 days as your body acclimatizes to altitude.

As you adjust to altitude, your blood volume will return to normal after an initial blood volume drop designed to concentrate the red blood cells that carry oxygen in your blood. You do develop more red blood cells if you stay for longer periods at altitude, and your muscles will begin to extract more oxygen from your blood. Altitude clearly causes metabolic adaptations that affect your nutritional needs. Even relatively moderate elevations of 5,000 feet (1,520 meters) can affect how you should eat and drink.

The air at altitude is extremely dry, and every breath you take results in fluid loss. You also have increased "insensible" fluid losses through your skin. Normally these insensible losses are 0.5 quarts (about 0.5 liter) daily but can increase to 2 quarts (about 2 liters) daily. But your fluid needs don't stop there. Urinary losses are 1 to 2 quarts (about 1 to 2 liters) daily. You will also lose fluid through sweat losses when exercising on the slopes. Replacing your fluid losses at altitude must be a very conscious effort.

When exercising at altitude, you have to consider your calorie and carbohydrate intake, as your basal metabolic rate can increase by as

PERIODIZING YOUR NUTRITIONAL INTAKE

Physical conditioning for skiing and snowboarding is important because most recreational skiers and snowboarders do not spend enough days on the slopes to ski or surf themselves into shape, whereas elite racers can ski and snowboard almost year-round and do sport-specific training. Good aerobic fitness offers many advantages to skiers and snowboarders. When training on the slopes, your muscles are supplied a greater amount of oxygen with less effort. This can help prevent fatigue at the end of the day on the slopes and hopefully prevent injury. Many skiers and snowboarders participate in some general aerobic conditioning and activity in the off-season, and they may even be involved in specific sports training in the warmer months. Leading up to ski and snowboard season, there is a specific process for getting into shape.

much as 40 percent the first few days at altitude, which may be your entire time above sea level. After a few days, your metabolic rate will drop but then remain at 15 percent above normal. Overall, your energy needs at altitude can increase by 200 to 300 calories daily. While this may seem like a welcome increase in energy requirements, your appetite can also decrease at altitude, and it may be possible to undereat by several hundred calories daily. Undereating and losing weight at altitude also does not result in body fat loss but will likely result in loss of valuable protein stores instead.

It is best that the extra calories you consume at altitude come from carbohydrate. A diet adequate in carbohydrate not only reduces the effect of altitude sickness but supports your training efforts and supplies muscle glycogen. Carbohydrate foods are also more easily digested and tolerated than high-fat foods consumed at altitude. Low blood glucose levels can also creep up on you at altitude, so consume snacks as needed when on the slopes. Sports drinks clearly provide both needed carbohydrates and fluids.

Iron is undoubtedly a mineral that deserves your attention at altitude. Athletes training at altitude should have their iron status monitored regularly. Having adequate iron stores ensures that you meet the demands of producing more red blood cells at altitude. Besides emphasizing good sources of iron as listed in Table 1.14, iron supplementation may boost and maintain iron stores. Be careful, though, not to supplement iron to excess, and do so under a physician's supervision, because too much iron can increase oxidation and free radical production in the body.

Focusing on foods high in vitamin C (Table 1.10) and vitamin E (Table 1.11) can also be beneficial as exercising at high altitudes places "oxidative stress" on your body. Exercise at altitude may also raise your vitamin E requirements. Recommendations for vitamin E supplementation are currently at 100 to 200 IU daily.

Off-season

During the off-season, skiers and snowboarders can focus on strength-training and aerobic conditioning activities. The warmer-weather months are likely filled with running, cycling, swimming, gym workouts, and hiking, and any sport in which you enjoy participating such as tennis, racquetball, or squash. It is important that you build and maintain a good aerobic base for both fitness and health. Activities specific to skiing are also recommended, such as walking and running up and down hills and uneven terrain to develop calf and quad muscles, or cycling to develop gluteal muscles. If you are dedicated to another sport other than skiing or snowboarding in the warmer months, chances are that your aerobic base is well developed and that you need to end this training several weeks before the ski and snowboard season. Strength training needs to be coordinated with any of the other sports training that you are involved in, but this time of year is an appropriate time to build strength endurance for skiing. Half-pipe snowboarders can spend time on the trampoline to practice spinning and twisting movement.

Nutrition during this cycle should focus on matching carbohydrate intake with the volume and intensity of your aerobic conditioning as described in Chapter 3. Refer to Table 3.6 for specific carbohydrate amounts based on training time and intensity. It should be fairly easy to match up your requirements with your off-season workout plan.

Protein requirements during this training cycle are easily reached with quality protein foods and good planning. Aim for the higher end of the protein range for longer training days. Fat will round out your energy needs, and you should consume 0.4 to 0.5 gram per pound of body weight (0.8 to 1.0 gram per kilogram). Once your carbohydrate and protein requirements are met, additional calories can be obtained from healthy fats.

For aerobic training sessions lasting longer than 90 minutes, practice the principles of recovery nutrition. Consume 0.5 to 0.7 gram of carbohydrate for every pound of weight (1 to 1.5 grams per kilogram), and for sessions over 90 minutes, consume 10 to 15 grams of high-quality protein. Many times this carbohydrate can be in liquid form, as you also need to consume 20 to 24 ounces of fluid (600 to 720 milliliters) for every pound (0.5 kilogram) of weight lost during training. The same amount of carbohydrate and protein can be consumed again in 2 hours to continue the recovery process.

For strength-training sessions, make sure that you consume 10 to 15 grams of high-quality protein with 25 grams of carbohydrate in the hour before and hour after training. (Nutritional guidelines for muscle building are described in Chapter 5.) When you combine serious strength training with a decent volume of aerobic training, your energy needs can be quite high. Most important, on days when you combine aerobic training with weight training, time your meals and snacks properly for energy and recovery.

While elite skiers and snowboarders find snow training the best way to train year-round for top performance in their sport, this may not be possible for many dedicated recreational and even competitive skiers. If you are very focused on other sports during the skiing and snowboarding off-season, other nutrition references include my prior books, *Sports Nutrition for Endurance Athletes* and *Performance Nutrition for Team Sports*.

Preseason

Once skiers and snowboarders have recovered from summer and fall activities, preseason training can start 4 to 8 weeks before the first ski trip. This preparatory phase includes maintaining your current level of conditioning and focusing on exercises targeted toward the specific movements of skiing and snowboarding. Getting as sport-specific as possible is the key to training at this time, while trying to copy the muscular movements and speeds that you will experience when skiing and snowboarding. Jumping and plyometric exercises are popular among skiers. Snowboarders also develop upper-body movement and more body control forward and back to prepare for surfing on the slopes once ski season begins.

With higher-intensity training, your nutritional focus should be on adequate carbohydrate intake. Training is likely to be focused and not steady state or endurance based, so calorie needs may require adjusting. Maintaining adequate hydration is essential during these workouts, and sports drinks can supply both the fluid and carbohydrate required for repeated movements of high-intensity training.

In-season

During the ski and snowboard season, your focus is to maintain your fitness, flexibility, and strength and to develop any weak areas. Chances are your nutritional needs are varied depending on whether you are spending a full day out on the slopes or working out in the gym during the week while dreaming of powder and blue sky. A 60- to 75-minute workout requires less calorie intake than a full day of skiing or snowboarding. Match up your nutritional needs with training volume and intensity, as described in Chapter 3. While alpine skiers and snowboarders can follow the nutrition recovery guidelines described in Table 3.4, nutritional recovery strategies can differ during a day on the slopes. As previously described, carbohydrate intake is based on volume and intensity of training. However, when you spend a full day on the slopes, recovery strategies also take place between runs, as well as at the midday and evening meal. Snacks can also be incorporated into your nutritional plan on the mountain. Practice the nutritional guidelines outlined here for a full day on the slopes, and maintain hydration, muscle glycogen, and blood glucose levels with a high-carbohydrate breakfast and lunch, and steady carbohydrate snacks during the day. After a long day on the slopes, focus on recovery.

Postseason

During the postseason, you likely are switching gears and prioritizing new sport and fitness goals for the warmer months. Some skiers and snowboarders stay active in their sport for summer camps; others are switching over to late spring and summer sports. Nutritional needs can vary widely depending on your athletic goals, but often in the postseason there is a period of downtime and decreased calorie requirements, along with a concurrent decrease in carbohydrate and protein needs.

CARBOHYDRATE AND FLUID INTAKE BEFORE AND DURING A DAY ON THE SLOPES

A day on the slopes can be hard work, and your nutrition strategies should focus on re-hydrating and refueling throughout the day. Injuries and accidents occur more frequently in the afternoon, perhaps the result of fatigue related to dehydration, muscle glycogen depletion, and low blood glucose levels.

Skiers and snowboarders planning for a full day on the slopes should consume a breakfast filled with wholesome carbohydrate and low-fat sources of protein to top off muscle glycogen stores and provide the liver with plenty of carbohydrate for sustained blood glucose levels during exercise. Consuming carbohydrate before training can help maintain liver glycogen stores and blood glucose levels during the early part of training, and perhaps off-set any difficulty that may be encountered with consuming carbohydrate during training due to cold weather and logistics. Start all days on the slopes adequately hydrated. Consume fluids in the 2 hours before getting to the top of the mountain, with time for a bladder break before hitting the chairlift.

Follow the pre-exercise eating and fluid guidelines described in Chapter 4. Determine how closely you can eat before training on the slopes and what your portion tolerances are. More recreational speeds should allow for decent-sized portions and eating close to the start of exercise, while high-intensity runs should allow for a bit more digestion time. Push carbohydrate portions to your maximum tolerance so that the fuel from your preexercise meal can sustain you for a morning on the slopes. You can also prehydrate before training with water or a sports drink for additional and easily digested carbohydrates. Gels and energy bars are both a quick, well-tolerated snack before training and can also provide a well-tolerated carbohydrate boost when riding the chairlift during a more strenuous day on the slopes.

Your fluid losses when training in the cold and at altitude can be significant and warrant fluid replacement. A sports drink that also provides carbohydrate is the recommended choice. Sports drinks may also minimize urine production when compared to water consumed during training, a helpful tip when training out in the cold. Carry squeeze bottles with a warmer temperature mix. Bottles can be placed at the bottom or top of the mountain to ensure regular fluid and carbohydrate consumption as you lose fluids and carbohydrates with each successive run, or carried in special belts to meet your hydration needs.

While hydration should always be a focus when on the slopes, carbohydrate replacement and snacks can also sustain energy levels. Gels can also pack a carbohydrate punch and are easy to slurp down. Carry gel products close to your body to keep them from freezing. Energy bars, granola bars, bananas, and other carbohydrate treats that pack well in the cold can be carried close to your body for a carbohydrate and blood glucose pickup.

Lunch is also an important meal in the middle of a busy day on the slopes. Warm foods providing plenty of carbohydrate are your best bets, while rounding out the meal with small to moderate portions of lean protein and low-fat choices. Lunch is also a good opportunity to rehydrate for a full afternoon on the slopes. Some warm high-carbohydrate options include soups, breads, chilis, pasta and rice dishes, toasted sandwiches, and baked potatoes. Some cold choices include sandwiches, fruit salad, yogurt with fruit, frozen yogurt, smoothies, and muffins. Alcohol has no place in the lunchtime break, and skiing or snowboarding in the afternoon after consuming alcohol places you and others on the mountain at great risk for serious injury and accidents. Alcohol adversely affects your hydration levels, fine motor skills, and judgment.

Table 8.1 summarizes nutrition guidelines for your various training sessions and training cycles.

COMPETITION NUTRITION

Whatever the type of ski race or snowboard event in which you are competing, it is important that you are well fueled, well hydrated, and physiologically and psychologically comfortable at the start gate. For any event, consider a properly timed high-carbohydrate, low-fat meal. Refer to Table 4.4 for optimal meal timing portions. Practice with food choices and portions before higher-intensity training sessions similar to racing and competition

TABLE 8.1 » NUTRITION FOR TRAINING CYCLES

Training Cycle	Nutrition Strategies
Off-season Focus on strength training and aerobic conditioning and cross-training. Often includes training for running, cycling, hiking, team sports in warmer months. Skateboarders can include mountain biking, surfing, and skateboarding. Build or maintain good aerobic base. Aerobic activities specific to skiing and snowboarding.	Match carbohydrate intake with training volume and intensity (see Table 3.6). Aim for 2-3 g carbohydrate per pound (5-7 g/kg) for low-intensity training several hours and moderate intensity 1 hour. Increase to 3-4.5 g carbohydrate per pound (7-10 g/kg) as volume and intensity increases. For training sessions greater than 75-90 minutes, consume 30-60 g carbohydrate per hour. Protein requirements are 0.45-0.75 g/lb. (1.0-1.6 g/kg). Practice the weight training nutrition guidelines outlined in Chapter 5, and time both protein and carbohydrate intake before and after strength training. Hydrate before, during, and after training.

CONTINUED

TABLE 8.1 continued

Training Cycle	Nutrition Strategies
Preseason Starts 4-8 weeks before the first ski or snowboard trip. Includes maintaining current level of conditioning and focusing on exercises that target the specific movements of skiing and snowboarding to copy muscular movements and speeds. Explosive movements and maximum strength weight lifting. Freestyle snowboarders focus on gymnastic movements.	Practice nutrition guidelines for resistance training as outlined in Chapter 5. Start high-intensity sport-specific training well fueled and well hydrated. Consume a sports drink during sessions to provide fuel for repeated high-intensity efforts. Aim for 0.65-0.9 g/lb. (1.4-2.0 g/kg) of protein. Pay attention to recovery nutrition for high-intensity sessions lasting longer than 75-90 minutes.
In-season The focus is to maintain fitness, flexibility, and strength and develop any weak areas. Often includes weekend days on the slopes and gym and other training workouts during the week.	Start the days on the slopes with a warm high-carbohydrate breakfast and plenty of fluids. Consume a steady supply of an easily consumed carbohydrate source when heading back up the mountain in the form of sports drinks, gels, and energy bars. Pay attention to fluid needs at altitude. Adjust calorie needs for in-season training session in the gym. Practice winter hydration strategies when training outdoors and not on the slopes.
Postseason Often includes a switch-over to late spring and summer sports. Some skiers and snowboarders stay active within their sport with summer camps.	Decrease carbohydrate intake to 2.5-3 g/lb. (5.5-7 g/kg) when training increases. Adjust calorie intake to decreased training level. Protein needs are 0.5-0.6 g/lb. (1.2-1.4 g/kg). Focus on a high-quality diet and experiment with new foods. Adjust nutritional intake to increase carbohydrates and calories when preparing for training in a spring/summer sport.

efforts. Have your pre-race meal well thought out the day of competition. This allows you to top off both muscle and liver glycogen stores and raise blood glucose levels before the race. Skiers and snowboarders should also reduce the fiber content of their meal before competition in anticipation of the pre-race nerves. Choices should be low-fat, easy to digest, with no spicy surprises.

Precompetition
Skiing

Before a day of competition that can include several runs, make sure to consume adequate carbohydrate to fully replenish muscle carbohydrate stores. Whatever the training regimen the day before racing, make sure that you match intake with adequate carbohydrate and calories. Refer to Table 3.6 for carbohydrate guidelines matched to training. Consuming carbohydrate amounts slightly above your requirements ensures that glycogen stores are fully replenished.

Time your pre-race meal to allow plenty of digestion time, ideally with 3 hours before a comfortable time interval, though this may not be practical for your start time. If this time interval is feasible, aim for 1.0 to 1.5 grams of carbohydrate per pound (2 to 3 grams per kilogram). In the hours leading up to the start time, you can maintain blood glucose and fluid levels by sipping a sports drink. Gels can also be consumed to maintain adequate blood glucose levels, which are imperative for adequate concentration, focus, quick decision making, and skill level.

You may need to consume a steady supply of easily digested carbohydrates throughout the day to maintain energy levels through multiple runs. High-carbohydrate energy drinks, sports, gels, and high-carbohydrate energy bars make good choices.

Snowboarding

Snowboarders should also consider their first run time and consume a precompetition meal ample in carbohydrates with plenty of time for digestion. Glycogen loading the day before a competition can ensure that muscle fuel stores are full for competition. Competitive snowboarders often need to complete many qualifying runs in a short period of time to qualify for the final group of competitors. Nutritionally this requires a well-tolerated intake of carbohydrate between runs to maintain blood glucose levels and mental concentration and focus. The snowboarder should then plan carefully to time intake of sports drinks, gels, and energy bars as needed, for regular consumption on competition day.

Competition

On all-important race days, nutrition continues to play a starring role for skiers and snowboarders. For some meal plans for competition, see page 232.

FOOD AND DRINK AFTER A DAY ON THE SLOPES

For many enthusiastic recreational skiers, after-ski intake is an important part of the day and ski culture. Much of the time this includes eating rich meals and consuming alcohol. Alcohol consumption could affect your ability to ski safely the next day, and even overeating

» MEAL PLANS NUTRITION FOR COMPETITION

Competition day

■ Elimination rounds
Breakfast (2–3 hours before warming up)
Hot cereal, 1 c. (240 ml)
Soy milk, 8 oz. (240 ml)
Egg whites, 3
Juice, 8 oz. (240 ml)

Warm-up
Carbohydrate gel
Warmed sports drink

Before run
Carbohydrate gel, 1 packet

Between runs
Energy bars
Warmed sports drinks
Gel packets

Recovery drink
Recovery nutrition
supplement, 16 ounces
(480 ml) (carbohydrate
and protein)

Dinner
Lean beef, 5 oz. (150 g)
Couscous, cooked, 2 c. (480 ml)

Steamed vegetable, 1 c.
Salad, 2 c. (480 ml)
Salad dressing, light, 4 tbsp.
(27 ml)
Hot chocolate, 8 oz. (240 ml)

3,200 calories
520 g carbohydrate (65%)
90 g protein (11%)
85 g fat (24%)

could result in a food hangover that could make you feel groggy and impair your judgment. Alcohol consumption could also cause you to take more risks when skiing, make poor quick decisions, and leave you fatigued.

It is best to think of the evening after skiing and snowboarding as a time of recovery, a time during which you should rehydrate and refuel right after your day on the slopes. A quick refueling high-carbohydrate snack should do the job, and rehydrate with plenty of water. A high-carbohydrate dinner should follow, and any alcohol should be consumed in moderation. You will have a great time on the slopes the next day if you refuel and rehydrate properly and get plenty of sleep.

» NUTRITIONAL REQUIREMENTS FOR INJURY RECOVERY

While snowboarding was originally considered a dangerous and uncontrolled sport, it is now clear that the snowboard injury rates are no different than those of skiing. However, the injuries common to each sport do differ. Injuries are more likely to occur in the afternoon when fatigue sets in and skill is adversely affected.

You may at some point in your skiing or snowboarding career suffer from strains, abrasions, bruising, and fractures. Most likely the speed at which your injury heals is of concern to you. While you may have a rehabilitation program mapped out, the calories and nutrients that you require for this program may differ from your usual eating. What is clear, however, is that protein, fat, carbohydrates, and vitamins and minerals are essential for timely and complete healing of injuries. Weight management issues may also present themselves at the time of an injury due to a marked decrease in energy expenditure.

Nutritional considerations can vary among specific situations and athletes. But often during rehabilitation an athlete fears putting on body fat. Injury often results in significant changes in energy expenditure as a result of a decrease from your usual training program in regard to the types of training and, for a period of time, even the volume and intensity. When you are accustomed to consuming a specific amount of food for your training program, it may be difficult to know how and when to cut back on your caloric intake to achieve the proper caloric balance. Muscle mass may also decrease when you are injured depending on the type of rehabilitation program that you are prescribed. Depending on the type and extent of the injury, caloric expenditure may decrease by several thousand calories per week. An athlete who decreases training volume by 4 hours a week could experience a weekly 1-pound weight gain if usual eating habits are followed.

When recovering from an injury, it is best not to undereat protein and calories. Protein is necessary for the growth and repair of body tissue, supports healthy immune function, and is required for the synthesis of enzymes and hormones. Undereating calories can also lead to increased incidence of infection and slower wound healing.

Regardless of the type of injury, it is important to maintain energy balance. Injured athletes can keep a food record and determine their normal caloric intake. They then can trim anywhere

from 200 to 500 calories or more daily to prevent weight gain if needed. Sometimes intake of carbohydrate and protein amounts need to be decreased slightly to prevent a gain in body fat. Excess dietary fat that was easily burned off in training should also be shaved down. But avoid drastic dietary restrictions so that you don't miss out on needed nutrients. Often some personalized guidance from a sports dietitian can be helpful when you are injured.

In many instances, however, a good resistance and rehabilitation program provides a big calorie advantage. Building muscle takes work and energy, allowing you to consume more calories and somewhat offset the decreased caloric expenditure from normal training for your sport. If these weight-training sessions are intense, consuming carbohydrate during training can facilitate recovery and muscle repair.

After an initial period of healing, athletes often engage in rehabilitation programs that are just as demanding as their usual training, though the program may differ in scope and timing. Your usual meal plan may need to be adjusted to support energy levels at specific training times and encourage tissue repair and muscle-building efforts.

When you are injured, increasing your intake of certain nutrients and perhaps even supplementation may support the healing process. One of the principal functions of vitamin C is collagen synthesis, a core component of scar tissue. Collagen is also required for the formation and maintenance of connective tissue such as cartilage, tendon, and bone. Vitamin C also plays a role in red blood cell synthesis. Load up on some good vitamin C sources as listed in Chapter 2. Fruits and vegetables are abundant in vitamin C and are also lower-calorie foods. Increasing your intake of fruits and vegetables will also provide

CONTINUED

NUTRITIONAL REQUIREMENTS FOR INJURY RECOVERY (CONTINUED)

antioxidants and bioflavonoids that can protect your muscles against damage during exercise and support the healing process.

Other important vitamins include vitamin A, which supports collagen formation and the immune system. B vitamin requirements can increase if there has been trauma and stress associated with the injury.

Minerals also play important roles in injury recovery, including iron and zinc. Zinc is an important component of many enzymes involved in energy metabolism and is required for protein synthesis and wound healing. Zinc from animal protein is best absorbed. Iron, of course, is needed for oxygen transport and the formation of hemoglobin and myoglobin so that the athlete can maintain a high level of rehabilitation training. Good sources are also listed in Chapter 2.

Your protein and calorie requirements can change at specific phases of the rehabilitation process. However, a nutrient-dense diet is a plus at any time after an injury. A good multivitamin mineral supplement high in antioxidants and bioflavonoids can also be useful in supporting healthy food choices.

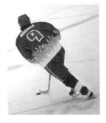

9 Nutrition for Hockey

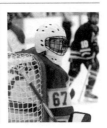

Ice hockey is enjoyed by players of all levels across North America and is extremely popular, with more than 2 million participants in both the United States and Canada. Participation can begin at an early age for boys and girls, at the club, amateur, high school, and collegiate levels. The National Hockey League, formed in Canada in 1920, now consists of thirty professional teams in both the United States and Canada.

Hockey is a unique team sport played on ice. This winter sport is played almost year-round at some level, and the professional hockey season is one of the most physically demanding in regard to training and competitive schedule. Training for ice hockey takes place both on and off the ice.

DEMANDS OF THE GAME

Ice hockey is a demanding sport both aerobically and anaerobically. During a game, hockey is characterized by repeated high-intensity efforts interspersed with periods of moderate activity and rest during play stoppage. While most of the effort during a game is powered by the anaerobic system, using creatine phosphate and muscle glycogen as a fuel, the aerobic system is also crucial for hockey players. The aerobic system fuels a small part of the energy required for intense hockey play and most of the energy at moderate activity levels. Most important, in ice hockey, a well-trained aerobic system is crucial for recovery between plays and during time on the bench. Top players who have more ice time have even less time on the bench, making the aerobic system even more important for recovery.

During a game, hockey players move on the ice at speeds that may reach 30 to 40 miles per hour (48 to 64 kilometers per hour), and their goal shots may send the puck flying at up to 100 miles per hour (160 kilometers per hour). Hockey players must possess muscular strength, muscular endurance, and general aerobic fitness. Hockey of course requires a high level of skating skill, superior strength endurance, and the ability to move explosively, shoot, pass, stop and start, pivot, turn quickly, take one-on-ones, and maneuver while fending off an opponent's body checks. Hockey can also be a very exciting game to watch because of its fast pace and frequent change in action.

During a game, hockey is unique in that player substitutions can be made during play. Except for the goalie, players are usually on the ice for 45 to 90 seconds per shift, with top players perhaps playing a total of 30 cumulative minutes. Players may have 4 to 5 minutes of recovery between shifts, and games last for three 20-minute periods. These high-speed efforts receive fuel from the phosphocreatine and anaerobic glycolysis system, making muscle glycogen an important fuel source.

Hockey training is also very intense and demanding, working both the high-intensity anaerobic systems and the aerobic system. Between bouts of all-out efforts, a well-trained aerobic system improves the player's recovery between hard training efforts and between games. Players may build aerobic fitness through bike riding, stair climbing, and a strength-training program. Hockey-specific conditioning is a very important part of training, and other components of a training program consist of drills, plyometrics, and on-ice skills. A well-conditioned player is able to skate longer without feeling the fatigue that can negatively impact skating technique.

ENERGY REQUIREMENTS

Hockey players have high-energy needs during the season, and they should adjust their caloric intake accordingly for their off-season, preseason, in-season, and postseason training. Hockey players are large and more muscular than in past decades and may have high-calorie needs due to their high body weight. A 180-pound (82-kilogram) hockey player may burn 12 calories per minute during an intense practice, or 600 calories in 50 minutes. These calories would be required in addition to basic daily calorie requirements of 2,300 calories. The player may also participate in other training sessions that require additional calories anywhere from another 500 to 1,000 calories daily. Depending on their playing level and the time of season, male hockey players may require more than 4,000 calories daily.

Female hockey players also need a high amount of calories per pound or kilogram of body weight based on their training program and level of play. For example, a 140-pound (64-kilogram) female hockey player training on and off ice for 90 minutes could require 2,700 to 3,000 calories daily for training and recovery.

BODY COMPOSITION

Body composition and body weight goals need to be individualized to the player, his or her training and competition schedule, and level of play. Often, high-level hockey players have trouble maintaining weight during the season due to the high energy demands of training and competing. They can play several games per week and experience frequent travel, which takes a toll on their body and can result in unwanted weight loss that diminishes their power and performance.

Young hockey players and experienced players often desire to gain muscle mass and should follow the nutritional requirements outlined for weight training in Chapter 5, when following a hockey-specific strength-training program. These hockey players will have higher daily protein and calorie needs, and they need to time meals and snacks appropriately around their weight training and other training sessions. Supplements targeted for muscle building are generally not advised for younger athletes who can focus on whole food choices. Some protein powder supplements can be conveniently used to obtain protein before and after strength training.

Appropriate body composition is also advised for hockey players, as moving excess body fat during play requires more effort and energy. Hockey players should reach body composition goals gradually, as rapid weight loss can decrease power and compromise fuel stores. Players should avoid excess body fat gain in the off-season and begin body fat loss efforts preseason, reaching goals before the competition season. During the season, efforts should focus on maintaining muscle mass.

DIET COMPOSITION

Carbohydrate is the preferred fuel for hockey practice and competition, and players should focus on maintaining adequate carbohydrate in their diet. Carbohydrate depletion can become a significant factor in the quality of workouts and during competition, particularly in the third period of the game when fuel stores run low. Muscles nutritionally fatigue, and players lose speed and strength, which affects their skating technique. As occurs in many team sport competitions, the winning team often consists of the players with the most fuel reserves and energy to score.

Proper nutrition allows hockey players to train harder and longer. Well-conditioned players train their muscles to store more carbohydrate, which increases the player's endurance. One study measured muscle glycogen in elite hockey players in Sweden. Researchers determined that a high-carbohydrate diet, with about 60 percent carbohydrate calories, resulted in a higher level of muscle glycogen before competition than a diet that was lower in carbohydrate (40 percent carbohydrate) and that may typically be followed by hockey players. The higher muscle glycogen levels also translated into improved performance. Players consuming the high-carbohydrate diet had greater skating speed, skated more shifts and longer shifts, and skated a greater distance. The differences between the players on the high-carbohydrate diet and those on the mixed diet were most evident during the third period of the game. Researchers noted that the low pregame muscle glycogen stores could be due not only to insufficient diet but also to inadequate recovery between games.

» EATING WELL ON CAMPUS

Many college food services offer a wide selection of foods for students living in dorms or group home settings such as sororities and fraternities. Campus food courts also provide selections in a variety of locations near classrooms, and of course there is the always-present vending machine. Your challenge is to find items that support your athletic training, recovery, and good health.

Eating on campus presents several challenges to the collegiate athlete. One is the "all-you-can-eat" setting, with unlimited returns to the table and a wide variety of hot and cold food choices that may or may not be prepared with moderate to high amounts of fat. You need to become a savvy consumer at the dorm food service, campus food court, and group home eating, just as you would at any restaurant and fast-food establishment.

While dorm mealtimes are fairly extensive, it is important that you review your class and practice schedule and have a plan of when and where you will eat for each day of the week. Late nights of studying also may result in evening snacking when hunger hits and require that you keep a stash of healthy choices in your room. Remember, you are not on a 9-to-5 schedule and need to be flexible with meal and snack times, while giving yourself the consistent mealtime structure required for a healthy diet.

Although it may be tempting to sleep in, make sure that you always start your day with breakfast. Dorm-style breakfast meals offer a wide variety of choices for ample wholesome carbohydrates and protein. Consider the standard cold and hot cereals, and gravitate toward whole-grain, lower-sugar choices. Skim milk and yogurt add more carbohydrates and high-quality protein to the mix. Make sure to include fruit and whole-grain breads as desired. Peanut butter adds some protein, as do eggs—any style. If you do sleep late, try to catch the tail end of breakfast time. You can also keep some simple breakfast items in your room, such as cereal, milk, fruit, and yogurt, so that skipping breakfast is not necessary.

Breakfast choices often go beyond the simple items frequently consumed at home. Food

Training between games also depletes muscle glycogen stores, and players should pay close attention to their carbohydrate intake when their schedule is filled with practice sessions and competition. One study found that muscle glycogen stores were depleted by 60 percent in varsity players in a single game. Combined with inadequate carbohydrate intake, intense training can result in low muscle glycogen stores that could compromise performance.

Hockey players also have elevated protein requirements as team sport and strength athletes. The required amount of 0.6 to 0.8 gram per pound (1.4 to 1.7 grams per kilogram) daily is easily met in a well-planned diet. Glycogen depletion during practice or a game can also result in protein oxidation during exercise, contributing to a net loss in protein over time. However, a well-planned diet, with appropriate carbohydrate intake, should

fare that was once limited to weekend brunches such as omelets, waffles, pancakes, sausage, and bacon are now available every day. These items can be part of your breakfast choices, with portions kept to reasonable levels.

Most athletes get hungry every 3 to 4 hours and maybe even sooner after practice. While you should make sure that you sit down to lunch and dinner regularly, it is also important to plan some snacks into your sports diet. Quick items like yogurt and fruit can be purchased on campus, as can granola bars and even a sandwich. Carry snacks with you as needed, and stake out various campus locations close to classrooms for healthy choices.

Try not to arrive for your lunch and dinner meals famished. Look over the hot menu for that meal and the cold items that are available. Some food services and group homes often post menus ahead of time. Decide on what looks good and best fits your nutritional needs. Keep an eye out for whole grains, fruits, and vegetables. Try not to arrive to meals overly hungry, as this can make appropriate portioning challenging.

Some of the standard items offered at the food service can include a salad bar, often offering a wide variety of choices, a sandwich bar that may be available at both lunch and dinner, soups, baked potato bars, several hot entrées, and often a decent variety of desserts.

The salad bar can certainly supplement a healthy meal, but choose wisely and adequately if it is your main course. Plenty of fresh vegetables such as carrots, mushrooms, cucumbers, and peppers are great, as are leafy greens such as lettuce and spinach. If the salad is to be a main focus of the meal, be sure to include proteins such as cottage cheese, eggs, tuna, cheese, chickpeas, kidney beans, tofu, and turkey. Prepared salads such as pasta salad, potato salad, and marinated vegetable salads also add carbohydrates but contribute some fat as well, so portion-control these items. Watch out for items loaded with mayonnaise if you are trying not to overdo your fat intake.

Sandwiches remain the main feature of most luncheon meals. Protein choices include turkey, tuna, peanut butter, and ham. Gravitate toward

CONTINUED

whole-grain bread, but also vary your choices with pita bread and sandwich wraps. Round out your sandwich with a bowl of soup, fruits, vegetables, and yogurt or a glass of milk. Higher-calorie items would include large bagel or submarine sandwiches, French fries, and milkshakes. Baked potato bars, like sandwich bars, can provide a nice balance of protein and carbohydrate. Spuds can be topped with vegetables, cheese, yogurt, chili, turkey, and sauces.

Hot entrées are available at both lunch and dinner and can run the gamut from healthy stir-fries to fried entrées, though a wider variety of healthy entrées seem to be offered at more dorm food services in recent years. Ask questions about how the foods are prepared, and request sauces on the side and specific portions.

Veggie and turkey burgers make good low-fat choices, as do pasta plates with red sauces, grilled or broiled fish, and other grilled meats. Regularly offered sides often include steamed rice, baked potatoes, skim milk and yogurt, fresh fruit, and soups.

Desserts are often in abundant supply at the dorm food service. A self-serve frozen yogurt machine and side toppings make a popular choice. Ice cream, cakes, and pies may also be available on a regular basis but are probably highest in calories. More reasonable options include fruit bars, yogurt bars, and Popsicles, as well as sorbet and baked or fresh fruit. Set limits on desserts to once daily or several times weekly depending on your energy needs.

prevent this from happening. Healthy fats should provide the remainder of calories to meet energy needs in the diet.

IMPORTANT NUTRITION STRATEGIES FOR HOCKEY
Hydration, Fluid Replacement, and Carbohydrate Intake

Despite playing on the ice in relatively cooler temperatures than do other team sports participants, hockey players can incur high sweat losses during practice and a game. During their high-intensity training, an increase in body temperature is seen, and the result is a high sweat rate. The amount of equipment and pads that hockey players wear also increases their risk for dehydration. Goalies are even more susceptible to dehydration because of the heavier weight of their equipment. Dehydration compromises performance long before fuel depletion, so hockey players should monitor their sweat losses during various types of practice sessions and training intensities. Significant weight loss during a training session indicates that players are not drinking adequately and not keeping up with their sweat losses.

Hockey players need to drink fluids on a schedule before, during, and after practice to maintain adequate hydration levels. Strategies can be individualized to sweat rates during on-ice practices, weight-training sessions, general conditioning training, aerobic training, and off-ice anaerobic training. Various types of training sessions offer different opportunities to drink during training. Players should appreciate that these opportunities to drink should be taken full advantage of in an effort to maximize performance and recovery.

Training and games place a high demand on muscle glycogen for fuel, and the fluids consumed should contain carbohydrate. Sports drinks, providing a good balance of fluid and carbohydrate, should be the beverage of choice during intense training sessions. Sports drinks also help players maintain adequate blood glucose levels, which is important for concentration and maximizing the rapid reaction times during play. Players should be aware that maintaining optimal hydration allows fluids to empty more quickly from the stomach and can prevent delayed stomach emptying and the feeling of fluid sloshing in the stomach during intense efforts.

During games and intense practices, hockey players can also consume high-carbohydrate gels. These supplements offer a concentrated source of carbohydrate that quickly raises blood glucose levels and provides fuel between periods. One gel packet should be consumed with at least 8 ounces (240 milliliters) of water.

In addition to drinking during practice and games, hockey players should make an effort to rehydrate after games, especially if they have lost more than 1 percent of their body weight, or about 2 pounds for a 180-pound player (1 kilogram for an 82-kilogram player). Rehydration choices should include a drink that contains some sodium. Players should drink 20 ounces (600 milliliters) for every pound (0.5 kilogram) of weight lost. Concentrated carbohydrate drinks provide carbohydrate for glycogen replenishment, fluid for rehydration, and sodium to enhance the rehydration process.

Some hydration and carbohydrate replacement strategies specific to the hockey player include the following:

- Check morning weight several times weekly to determine whether daily hydration is adequate.
- Drink 14 to 20 ounces (400 to 600 milliliters) of fluid in the 2 hours before practice or a game. Stop drinking 30 to 60 minutes before a game to empty your bladder.
- Start drinking early. This strategy is particularly important if breaks in practice occur at greater time intervals.
- Take small sips of fluid during practice or the game when you are on the bench, about 4 to 6 ounces (120 to 180 milliliters) whenever possible.
- Practice drinking during training sessions that simulate competition conditions.
- Monitor your weight before and after exercise to assess how effectively you replace fluids.

- Fluid should be nearby and easily accessible. Players should have their own individual squeeze bottle to drink from during practice.
- Consume 8 ounces (240 milliliters) or more of a sports drink between periods during games, or consume one carbohydrate gel and 8 ounces (240 milliliters) of water.

» MEAL PLANS FOR TRAINING

Training diet

■ Morning conditioning afternoon hockey practice

Breakfast (6:30 a.m.)
Breakfast, cereal, 2 c. or 3 oz. (90 g)
Milk, skim, 12 oz. (360 ml)
Orange juice, 8 oz. (240 ml)
Banana, 1 small
Toast, 2 slices (60 g)
Margarine, 2 t. (15 ml)
Jam, 2 tbsp. (40 ml)

Conditioning (7:30 a.m.)
Water to maintain hydration

Snack (8:30 a.m.)
Yogurt, 6 oz. (180 ml)
Peach, 1 medium

Lunch (12:00 p.m.)
Turkey sub:
    Turkey, 6 oz. (180 g)
    Bread, 2 slices (60 g)
    Mayo, 2 t. (15 ml)
Juice, 12 oz. (360 ml)
Yogurt, 6 oz. (180 ml)

Snack (3:00 p.m.)
Granola bar, 1
Apple, 1 medium

During practice
24 oz. sports drink (720 ml)

Dinner (7:00 p.m.)
Lean beef, 4 oz. (120 g)
Baked potato, 1 large or 10 oz. (300 g)
Mixed vegetables, 1 c. (240 ml)
Garden salad, 2 c. (480 ml)
Dressing, light, 4 tbsp. (60 ml)

Snack
Milk, 8 oz. (240 ml)
Crackers, whole-grain, 8 small

3,500 calories
500 g carbohydrate (57%)
135 g protein (15%)
109 g fat (28%)

■ Hockey training diet hard evening practice

Breakfast (7:30 a.m.)
Grits, cooked, 1 c. (240 ml)
Raisins, 2 tbsp. (40 ml)
Yogurt, nonfat, plain, 6 oz. (180 ml)
Cashews, 2 t. (12 ml)

Lunch (11:30 a.m.)
Tuna, 4 oz. (120 g)
Pita bread, 1 round or 2 oz. (60 g)
Celery, pepper, carrots, 2 c. (480 ml)
Apple juice, 12 oz. (360 ml)

Pretraining snack (3:00 p.m.)
Bagel, 4 oz. (120 g)
Nut butter, 2 tbsp. (40 ml)
Apple, 1 large

During practice
40 oz. (1,200 ml) sports drink

Recovery shake (6:30 p.m.)
Milk, 12 oz. (360 ml)
Yogurt, 6 oz. (180 ml)
Frozen berries, 1 c. (240 ml)

Dinner (8:00 p.m.)
Pork tenderloin, 4 oz. (120 g)
Rice, cooked, 1½ c. (360 ml)
Corn, ½ c. (120 ml)
Mushrooms, ¼ c. (60 ml)
Bread, 2 slices (60 g)
Olive oil, 4 t. (30 ml)
Sherbet, 1 c. (240 ml)
Raspberries, 1 c. (240 ml)

3,300 calories
520 g carbohydrate (63%)
110 g protein (13%)
88 g fat (24%)

- Rehydrate with at least 40 ounces (1,200 milliliters) of a carbohydrate drink after practice or competition.

The sample meal plan on page 242 provides some training diet menus that provide guidelines for meals, snacks, and fluid intake around training.

Fluid Intake in Young Players

Young hockey players also need to keep up with their fluid losses during practice. Players can become dehydrated during practice sessions lasting under 1 hour. Sports drinks are still the preferred choices during these practice sessions and games, as research indicates that a sports drink can enhance intermittent, high-intensity exercise lasting only 60 minutes. Flavored drinks also improve hydration efforts among young athletes.

Nutritional Strategies Around Competition

Precompetition

Hockey players can time their eating before practice and particularly competition to maximize their fuel stores, especially body carbohydrate stores, and minimize any unwanted gastrointestinal side effects. A high-carbohydrate pregame meal can top off muscle glycogen and fill liver glycogen stores. Meal timing is essential, and most players should be comfortable consuming 150 to 200 grams of carbohydrates about 2 to 3 hours beforehand. Small amounts of easily digested protein such as skim milk, soy milk, and poultry can be consumed. Other protein choices that are often well tolerated before competition include peanut butter and low-fat cheeses in small amounts. Fats such as oils and spreads should be kept to reasonable amounts for easy digestion.

Meal timing should reflect personal tolerances and game timing. Players may want to have a larger midday meal the day of an evening game and a light, easily digested meal or large snack 2 to 3 hours beforehand. While meal and snack timing should reflect game time and personal tolerances, players should appreciate that their carbohydrate intake for the day should be adequate to ensure recovery from the last practice session and fill glycogen stores prior to the game. Experiment with various sports nutrition products such as liquid meal replacements, gels, and a high-carbohydrate drink in the 2 to 3 hours prior to the game. Products should be tested in practice and never on game day.

Postgame Recovery

Because hockey players may play several games in a week, participate in weekend tournaments, or have a busy schedule of both practices and games, postgame recovery should be optimized to replenish muscle glycogen stores prior to the next training session or game.

Within 30 minutes of a game, the athlete should consume 0.5 gram of carbohydrate per pound body weight (1 gram per kilogram). This recovery snack can also include 15 to 20 grams of protein. These carbohydrate and protein amounts can be repeated with a meal or snack in 2 hours to continue the muscle glycogen replenishment process. The meal plan below provides some sample menus for various game start times, including fluids to be consumed during competition, as well as recovery meals and snacks.

» MEAL PLANS FOR GAME DAY

Competition diet

■ **Evening game at 7:00 p.m.**
Breakfast (8:30 a.m.)
Oatmeal, cooked, 1 c. (240 ml)
Egg, 1
Toast, 1 slice (30 g)
Margarine, 2 t. (15 ml)
Juice, 8 oz. (240 ml)

Lunch (1:00)
Baked chicken, 6 oz. (180 g)
Rice, cooked, 2 c. (480 ml)
Vegetables, cooked, 1 c. (240 ml)
Milk, 12 oz. (360 ml)
Frozen yogurt, 12 oz. (360 ml)
Fruit, 1 c. (240 ml)

Pregame snack (4:00 p.m.)
Sandwich:
  Bread, 2 slices (60 g)
  Honey, 2 tbsp. (40 ml)
  Peanut butter, 4 t. (30 ml)
  Water, 16 oz. (480 ml)

Game
4-6 oz. (120-180 ml) sports drink every shift
16 oz. (480 ml) sports drink between periods

Postgame
High-carbohydrate recovery drink, 16 oz. (480 ml)

Dinner (10:00 p.m.)
Pasta, cooked, 3 c. (720 ml)
Meat sauce, 1 ½ c. (360 ml)
Salad, 2 cups (480 ml)
Dressing, light, 4 tbsp. (80 ml)
Bread, 2 slices (60 g)

4,100 calories
600 g carbohydrate (60%)
130 g protein (13%)
120 g fat (27%)

■ **Hockey game with 3:00 p.m. start time**
Breakfast (8:00 a.m.)
Cereal, 1.5 oz. (45 g)
Milk, skim, 8 oz. (240 ml)
Strawberries, 1 c. (240 ml)
Juice, 12 oz. (360 ml)
Eggs, scrambled, 2
Toast, 2 slices (60 g)
Peanut butter, 4 t. (27 ml)

Lunch (12 noon)
Roast turkey, 4 oz. (120 g)
Bread, 2 slices (60 g)
Mayo, light, 2 tbsp. (40 ml)
Pretzel, 1.5 oz. (45 g)
Orange, 1 medium
Juice, 12 oz. (360 ml)

Pregame
Gel, 1 packet
Sports drink, 24 oz. (360 ml)

During game
4-6 oz. (120 to 180 ml) on the bench
8 oz. (240 ml) between periods

Postgame
Carbohydrate recovery drink, 12 oz. (360 ml)

Dinner (7:00 p.m.)
Chicken and bean burrito, 1 large

3,200 calories
530 g carbohydrate (66%)
120 g protein (15%)
67 g fat (19%)

» EATING WELL ON THE ROAD

Hockey players and other athletes competing for their sport in high school and in college, as well as winter sport athletes traveling for competition, may frequently be required to make healthy food choices on the road. It is important to consider how traveling affects your precompetition nutrition program and plan accordingly. Special meals can be ordered on airlines with advanced notice. When traveling by road or plane, try to bring your own bottled water for consumption in order to maintain hydration. Make healthy choices at airports whenever possible. Aim for turkey sandwiches or wraps for lower-fat choices and plenty of carbohydrates. Choose low-fat frozen yogurt, fruit juice, soft pretzels, low-fat milk, baked potatoes, and smoothies. Plan ahead and pack some of your favorite non-perishable items such as energy bars, granola bars, cereals, packets of instant breakfast mix, dried fruit, whole-grain crackers, powdered sports drinks, meal replacements, instant soups, fruit juice, and any items that travel safely.

You can also investigate the food options at your destination before you leave. Call ahead to your accommodation and find out about food establishments in the area. Internet searches can also provide valuable travel information.

Outlined here are some healthier suggestions for various meal and snack choices when eating on the road.

Meal	Food Choices
Breakfast	Choose dry and cooked cereals, juices, fresh fruit, waffles, French toast, and pancakes. Keep margarine and butter to a minimum. Order low-fat or skim milk and low-fat yogurt. Bagels and muffins with small amounts of peanut butter and jam are good choices as well. Order omelets made with egg whites and go easy on the cheese, while asking for vegetable fillings.
Lunch	Try to frequent restaurants that have low-fat sandwiches made from poultry or lean meats. Lower-fat tuna salads may be available. Go easy on the cheese, and ask for extra vegetable toppings whenever possible. Choose salads covered with lean protein, baked potatoes, and chili. Choose the regular-sized hamburger or cheeseburger, and split a small French fry serving with a teammate.
Dinner	Choose lean meats, fish, or poultry that is broiled, grilled, baked, or blackened. Ask that potatoes, rice, pasta, or noodles be prepared with less fat. Consume breads and rolls, and go easy on the margarine or butter. Have fruit for dessert whenever possible. Order salad with dressing on the side.
Snacks	Try fresh fruit, dried fruit, granola bars, and energy bars. Buy milk chugs and low-fat yogurt whenever possible. Snack on low-fat crackers, instant soups, and pretzels. Drink water and other fluids.

PERIODIZING YOUR NUTRITION PLAN

As a hockey player, your training program likely changes throughout the year depending on your level of competition and your participation in school, club, or recreational hockey programs, as well as training in another sport. You have a lot to accomplish in your yearly training program including aerobic conditioning, anaerobic conditioning, developing strength and power, building muscular endurance, while developing quickness, agility, speed, and flexibility on the ice.

Generally hockey players use the off-season to build a base for both aerobic fitness and strength. In the preseason, training shifts to more high-intensity training, speed, and intervals, and hockey-specific training. During the season, the hockey player focuses on preparing for competition and maintaining fitness and developing any weaker areas. Depending on whether you are a high school, collegiate, masters, or professional athlete, you may compete several times a week, in weekend tournaments, or only once weekly, all of which affects your training program and recovery time. Postseason is a rest period and varies in length for hockey players.

These cycles in your training program all require adjustments in your diet composition, and meal timing as described in Table 9.1. During the off-season with a focus on aerobic condition, your energy needs can decrease. In the preseason, your energy intake increases and nutrient requirements build, and your focus is on recovery from higher-intensity training and nutritional practices conducive to muscle building. During the competitive season, eat to maintain muscle mass and recovery from training and competition. (Specific nutritional recovery strategies and amounts for various types of training sessions are described in more detail in Table 3.4.)

At all times during the training cycle, replace fluid and carbohydrate during and after training. Dehydration can occur during different training levels of exercise; it is just the degree of dehydration that distinguishes various types of workouts. Chapter 4 outlines strategies for fluid and fuel consumption during training and competition.

CREATINE AND HOCKEY PLAYERS

Creatine is often a popular ergogenic aid with hockey players who want to build muscle and improve strength. One study of elite ice hockey players looked at the performance effects of creatine loading for 5 days, followed by a 10-week maintenance dose. Over this study period, an improvement was seen in on-ice sprint performance. Further studies specific to ice hockey training and performance are needed.

One of the side effects of creatine loading is an immediate weight gain, most likely fluid gain. Hockey players may not like training with this additional weight. Concerns with

TABLE 9.1 » PERIODIZING YOUR HOCKEY NUTRITION PLAN

Training Cycle	Nutrition Strategies
Off-season	Consume moderate carbohydrate, high protein, low fat. Follow nutrition guidelines for strength training. Ensure adequate carbohydrate intake for light aerobic conditioning. Replace fluid losses during training.
Preseason	Consume moderate to high carbohydrate, moderate protein, low fat. Continue nutrition strategies specific to strength training sessions. Replace carbohydrate and fluids with a sports drink during interval and high-intensity training. Practice immediate recovery nutrition after high-intensity training lasting longer than 60-90 minutes. Monitor weight to assess hydration status and fluid replacement strategies
In-season	Consume high carbohydrate, moderate to high protein, adequate fat for energy. Practice fluid and carbohydrate replacement during practice and competition. Eat an optimal precompetition meal. Practice recovery nutrition after training and competition. Ensure daily hydration.
Postseason	Consume moderate carbohydrate, moderate protein, low fat. Ensure basic hydration. Replace sweat losses. Maintain healthy body weight.

creatine use in young athletes and possible harmful side effects persist. There is also concern that use of such supplements in young athletes may encourage use of more harmful supplements and illegal supplements. Young hockey players should follow the proper nutritional guidelines for muscle building and strength as outlined in Chapter 5.

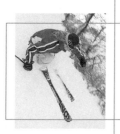

Appendix A: Glycemic Index of Foods

High-Glycemic Foods (GI > 70)

Food	Serving Size	Grams Carbohydrate (CHO) per Serving	Glycemic Load per Portion	Index for 50 g
Glucose	(test portion)	50	–	100
Potato, instant, mashed	5 oz. (150 g)	22.8	22.1	97
Baguette	1 oz. (30 g)	15.9	15.1	95
Potato, baked	6.5 oz. (200 g)	29	27.3	94
Rice, instant	5 oz. (200 g)	42	36.5	87
Cornflakes	1 oz. (30 g)	25	21.5	86
Pretzels	2 oz. (60 g)	39	32.2	83
Rice Krispies	1 oz. (30 g)	29	24	82
Waffles	2 oz. (60 g)	24.7	19.2	76
Doughnut	1.6 oz. (47 g)	19	14.3	76
Total cereal	1 oz. (30 g)	25	19	76

GLYCEMIC INDEX OF FOODS continued

Food	Serving Size	Grams Carbohydrate (CHO) per Serving	Glycemic Load per Portion	Index for 50 g
Waffle	2 oz. (60 g)	25	19.3	76
Soda crackers	0.8 oz. (25 g)	17.8	13.1	74
Cheerios	1 oz. (30 g)	25	18.5	74
Watermelon	8 oz. (240 g)	12	8.6	72
Bagel, white	2.25 oz. (70 g)	35.5	25.5	72
Millet	5 oz. (150 g)	34.8	24.7	71
Bread, white	2 oz. (60 g)	26.8	18.8	70
Pancakes, from mix	2.7 oz. (80 g)	32.5	21.8	67
Moderate-Glycemic Foods (GI 55–70)				
Croissant	1.9 oz. (57 g)	14.7	22	67
Shredded Wheat	1 oz. (30 g)	21.7	14.6	67
Cream of Wheat	1 oz. (30 g)	20	13.2	66
Pineapple	4 oz. (120 g)	9.6	6.3	66
Oat kernel bread	2 oz. (60 g)	25.6	16.6	65
Raisins	2 oz. (60 g)	42.7	27.3	64
Rye crispbread	1 oz. (30 g)	16	10.1	63
Muffin	1.9 oz. (57 g)	27.7	17.2	62
Corn, sweet	2.6 oz. (80 g)	16	9.5	62
Ice cream	1.6 oz. (50 g)	9.9	6.1	62
Couscous	5 oz. (150 g)	14.3	8.7	61
Bran muffin	1.9 oz. (57 g)	20.9	12.5	60
Spaghetti, white, durum wheat	6 oz. (180 g)	44.3	25.6	58
Pita bread	1 oz. (30 g)	16	9.2	57
Orange juice	9 oz. (264 g)	21	12	57
Muesli	2 oz. (60 g)	32	17.9	56
Oat bran, raw	2 oz. (60 g)	30	16.5	55
Popcorn	2 oz. (60 g)	19	10.5	55
Pumpernickel bread	1 oz. (30 g)	13.4	7.4	55
Low-Glycemic Foods (GI <55)				
Pound cake	1.75 oz. (53 g)	25	13.4	54
Buckwheat	5 oz. (150 g)	28.8	14.6	51
Bread, whole-grain	2 oz. (30 g)	23	12	51

CONTINUED

GLYCEMIC INDEX OF FOODS continued

Food	Serving Size	Grams Carbohydrate (CHO) per Serving	Glycemic Load per Portion	Index for 50 g
Banana, ripe	4 oz. (120 g)	23.9	12.1	50
All-Bran	2 oz. (60 g)	36.8	18.4	50
Rice, brown	5 oz. (150 g)	47.7	23.9	49
Porridge oatmeal	8 oz. (250 g)	20.3	9.9	48
Sweet potato	5 oz. (150 g)	26	12.5	48
Bulgur	5 oz. (150 g)	26	11.9	46
Lactose	(test portion)	50	-	43
Chickpeas	5 oz. (150 g)	21	8.6	42
Grapefruit juice	8 oz. (260 g)	15.7	7.5	41
Pear, Bartlett	4 oz. (120 g)	11.3	4.6	40
Apple juice	8 oz. (243 g)	26	10.4	40
Apple	4 oz. (120 g)	14.6	5.9	33
Apricots, dried	2 oz. (60 g)	25	8	32
Fettucine	4 oz. (120 g)	30	9.6	32
Yogurt, fruited	6.5 oz. (200 g)	33	10.9	32
Milk, skim	8 oz. (259 g)	13	4.1	32
Spaghetti, whole-meal	4 oz. (120 g)	30	9.6	28
Peach	8 oz. (240 g)	15	4.2	28
Lentils	5 oz. (150 g)	14.9	4.1	28
Kidney beans	5 oz. (150 g)	24	5.5	23
Fructose	(test portion)	50	-	20

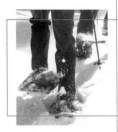

Appendix B: Facts about Vitamins and Minerals

» FACTS ABOUT VITAMINS AND MINERALS

Vitamins	DRIs	Major Sources	Major Functions
WATER-SOLUBLE			
Thiamin (vitamin B1)	**Males** 14-70 yrs: 1.2 mg **Females** 14-70 yrs: 1.1 mg	Wheat germ, whole-grain breads and cereal, organ meats, lean meats, legumes	Energy production from carbohydrate, essential for healthy nervous system
Riboflavin (vitamin B2)	**Males** 14-70 yrs: 1.3 mg **Females** 14-18 yrs: 1.0 mg 18-70 yrs: 1.1 mg	Milk and dairy products, green leafy vegetables, lean meats, beans	Energy production from carbohydrates and fats, healthy skin
Niacin (nicotinamide, nicotinic acid)	**Males** 14-70 yrs: 16 mg **Females** 14-70 yrs: 14 mg	Lean meats, fish, poultry, whole grains, peanuts	Energy production from carbohydrate, synthesis of fat, blocks release of FFA

CONTINUED

FACTS ABOUT VITAMINS AND MINERALS continued

Vitamins	DRIs	Major Sources	Major Functions
Vitamin B6 (pyridoxine)	**Males** 14-50 yrs: 1.3 mg 51->70 yrs: 1.7 mg **Females** 14-18 yrs: 1.2 mg 19-50 yrs: 1.3 mg 50->70 yrs: 1.5 mg	Liver, lean meats, fish, poultry, legumes, bran cereal	Role in protein metabolism, necessary for formation of hemoglobin and red blood cells, synthesis of essential fatty acids, required for glycogen breakdown
Vitamin B12 (cobalamin)	**Males** 14->70 yrs: 2.4 mcg **Females** 14->70 yrs: 2.4 mcg	Lean meats, poultry, dairy products, eggs	Formation of red blood cells, metabolism of nervous tissue, involved in folate metabolism, formation of DNA
Folic acid (folate)	**Males** 14->70 yrs: 400 mcg **Females** 14->70 yrs: 400 mcg	Green leafy vegetables, legumes	Role in red blood cell and DNA formation
Biotin	**Males** 14-18 yrs: 25 mcg 19->70 yrs: 30 mcg **Females** 14-18 yrs: 25 mcg 19->70 yrs: 30 mcg	Meats, legumes, milk, egg yolk, whole grains	Role in metabolism of carbohydrate, protein, fat
Pantothenic acid	**Males** 14->70 yrs: 5 mg **Females** 14->70 yrs: 5 mg	Liver, lean meats, eggs, salmon, all animal and plant foods	Role in metabolism of carbohydrate, protein, fat
Vitamin C	**Males** 14-18 yrs: 75 mg 19->70 yrs: 90 mg **Females** 14-18 yrs: 65 mg 19->70 yrs: 75 mg	Citrus fruits, green leafy vegetables, broccoli, peppers, strawberries, potatoes	Essential for connective tissue development, role in iron absorption, antioxidant, role in wound healing
FAT-SOLUBLE RDAs			
Vitamin A (retinol, provitamin carotenoids)	**Males** 14->70 yrs: 900 mcg **Females** 14->70 yrs: 700 mcg	Liver, milk, cheese, fortified margarine, carotenoids in plant foods (orange, red, deep green in color)	Maintains healthy tissue in skin and mucous membranes, essential for night vision; plays role in bone development

CONTINUED

FACTS ABOUT VITAMINS AND MINERALS continued

Vitamins	DRIs	Major Sources	Major Functions
Vitamin D (cholecalciferol)	**Males** 14-50 yrs: 5 mcg 50-70 yrs: 10 mcg >70 yrs: 15 mcg **Females** 14-50 yrs: 5 mcg 51-70 yrs: 10 mcg >70 yrs: 15 mcg	Vitamin D-fortified milk and margarine, fish oil, action of sunlight on skin	Increases intestinal absorption of calcium; promotes bone and tooth formation; plays a role in preventing colon cancer and autoimmune diseases, such as type 1 diabetes and rheumatoid arthritis
Vitamin E (tocopherol)	**Males** 14->70 yrs: 15 mg **Females** 14->70 yrs: 15 mg	Vegetable oils, margarine, green leafy vegetables, wheat germ, whole-grain products	Formation of red blood cells, antioxidant
Vitamin K (phylloquinone)	**Males** 14-18 yrs: 75 mcg 19->70 yrs: 120 mcg **Females** 14-18 yrs: 75 mcg 19->70 yrs: 90 mcg	Liver, soybean oil, spinach, cauliflower, green leafy vegetables	Essential for normal blood clotting

Minerals	DRIs	Major Sources	Major Functions
MAJOR MINERALS			
Calcium	**Males** 14-18 yrs: 1,300 mg 19-50 yrs: 1,000 mg 50->70 yrs: 1,200 mg **Females** 14-18 yrs: 1,300 mg 19-50 yrs: 1,000 mg 51->70 yrs: 1,200 mg	Milk, cheese, yogurt, ice cream, dried peas and beans, dark green leafy vegetables	Bone formation, enzyme activation, nerve impulse transmission, muscle contraction
Phosphorus	**Males** 14-18 yrs: 1,250 mg 19->70 yrs: 700 mg **Females** 14-18 yrs: 1,250 mg 19->70 yrs: 700 mg	Protein foods: meat, poultry, fish, eggs, milk, cheese, dried peas and beans, whole grains	Bone formation, cell membrane structure, B vitamin activation, component of ATP-CP, and other important organic compounds

CONTINUED

FACTS ABOUT VITAMINS AND MINERALS continued

Minerals	DRIs	Major Sources	Major Functions
Magnesium	**Males** 14-18 yrs: 410 mg 19->70 yrs: 420 mg **Females** 14-18 yrs: 360 mg 19-30 yrs: 310 mg 31->70 yrs: 320 mg	Milk, yogurt, dried beans, nuts, whole grains, tofu, green vegetables, chocolate	Role in protein synthesis, glucose metabolism, muscle contraction
TRACE MINERALS			
Iron	**Males** 14-18 yrs: 11 mg 19->70 yrs: 8 mg **Females** 14-18 yrs: 15 mg 19-50 mg.: 18 mg 50->70 yrs: 8 mg	Organ meats, lean meats, poultry, shellfish, dried peas and beans, whole-grain products, green leafy vegetables	Hemoglobin formation, oxygen transport
Zinc	**Males** 14->70 yrs: 11 mg **Females** 14-18 yrs: 9 mg 19->70 yrs: 8 mg	Organ meats, meat, fish, poultry, shellfish, nuts, whole-grain products	Part of enzymes involved in energy metabolism, immune function
Copper	**Males** 14-18 yrs: 890 mcg 19->70 yrs: 900 mcg **Females** 14-18 yrs: 890 mcg 19->70 yrs: 900 mcg	Organ meats, meat, fish, poultry, shellfish, nuts, bran cereal	Role in use of iron and hemoglobin by body, involved in connective tissue formation and oxidation
Fluoride	**Adequate intake** **Males** 14-18 yrs: 3 mg 19->70 yrs: 4 mg **Females** 14->70 yrs: 3 mg	Milk, egg yolks, drinking water, seafood	Helps form teeth and bones
Selenium	**Males** 14->70 yrs: 55 mcg **Females** 14->70 yrs: 55 mcg	Meat, fish, poultry, organ meats, seafood, whole grains and nuts from selenium-rich soil	Part of antioxidant enzyme

CONTINUED

FACTS ABOUT VITAMINS AND MINERALS continued

Minerals	DRIs	Major Sources	Major Functions
Chromium	**Adequate intake** **Males** 14-50 yrs: 35 mcg 50->70 yrs: 30 mcg **Females** 14-18 yrs: 24 mcg 19-50 yrs: 25 mcg 50->70 yrs: 20 mcg	Organ meats, meats, oysters, cheese, whole-grain products, beer	Enhances insulin function as glucose tolerance factor
Iodine	**Males** 14->70 yrs: 150 mcg **Females** 14->70 yrs: 150 mcg	Iodized table salt, seafood, water	Part of thyroxine, which plays a role in reactions involving cellular energy
Manganese	**Adequate Intake** * **Males** 14-18 yrs: 2.2 mg 19->70 yrs: 2.3 mg **Females** 14-18 yrs: 1.6 mg 19->70 yrs: 1.8 mg	Beet greens, whole grains, nuts, legumes	Part of essential enzyme systems
Molybdenum	**Males** 14-18 yrs: 43 mcg 19->70 yrs: 45 mcg **Females** 14-18 yrs: 43 mcg 19->70 yrs: 45 mcg	Legumes, cereal grains, dark green leafy vegetables	Part of essential enzymes involved in carbohydrate and fat metabolism

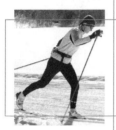

Appendix C: Comparison of Sports Nutrition Products

COMMERCIAL SPORTS DRINKS (8-OZ. OR 240-ML SERVING)

Product	Type of Carbohydrate	Carbohydrate Concentration (%)	Calories	Carbohydrate (g)	Sodium (mg)
Accelrade	Sucrose, fructose, maltodextrin (also contains small amounts branched chain amino acids)	7.75	93	17	127
All Sport	Fructose, sucrose	7	70	19	55
Body Fuel	Maltodextrin, fructose	7	70	17	70
Cytomax	Fructose, maltodextrin, polylactate, glucose	8	83	19	70
Endura	Glucose polymers, fructose	6	60	15	92

CONTINUED

COMMERCIAL SPORTS DRINKS (8-OZ. OR 240-ML SERVING) continued

Product	Type of Carbohydrate	Carbohydrate Concentration (%)	Calories	Carbohydrate (g)	Sodium (mg)
Exceed	Glucose polymer, fructose	7	70	17	50
Gatorade	Sucrose, glucose	6	50	14	110
Gatorade Endurance Drink	Sucrose, glucose	6	60	15	200
Gookinaid	Glucose, fructose	5	43	10	69
GU20	Maltodextrin, fructose	5.5	52	13	120
Hydra Fuel	Glucose polymer, fructose, glucose	7	66	16	25
Met-Rx ORS	Rice syrup solids, glucose	8	70	19	125
Perform	Glucose, fructose, maltodextrins	7	60	16	110
Performance	Maltodextrin, fructose	10	100	25	115
PR Solution	Maltodextrin, fructose	12.5	120	30	50
Power Ade	Fructose, sucrose	6	55	14	50
PowerBar Endurance Sports Drink	Maltodextrin, dextrose, fructose	7	70	17	160
Red Bull	Sucrose, glucose	12	112	28	215
Revenge	Maltodextrin, amylopectin starch	9	90	23	100
Warp Aide	Fructose, maltodextrin	8	70	19	80
Coca-Cola	High-fructose corn syrup, sucrose	12	108	29	9
Orange juice	Fructose, sucrose	11-15	112	26	2.7
Water		0	0	0	0

RECOVERY DRINKS

Product	Serving Size	Calories	Carbohydrate (g)	Protein (g)	Fat (g)
Boost	8-oz. (240-ml) can	240	33	15	6
EndoroxR4 (vanilla)	2 scoops (74 g) for 12 oz. (360 ml)	260	50	13	1
Ensure	8-oz. (240-ml) can	250	40	9	6
Gatorade Energy Drink	12 oz. (360 ml)	310	78	0	0
Gatorade Nutrition Shake	11-oz. (325-ml) can	360	55	20	8
Metabolol Endurance Formula	1 packet (52 g)	200	24	14	5
Metabolol II	1 packet (66 g)	260	40	18	3
Met-Rx (vanilla)	1 packet (72 g)	250	20	37	2.5
Endura Optimizer	2 scoops (78 g)	280	58	12	1
Physique	½ cup (57 g)	210	38	14	0.5
UltraFuel	16 oz. or 2 scoops (480 ml)	400	100	0	0

CARBOHYDRATE GELS

Product	Serving Size	Calories	Carbohydrate (g)	Sodium (mg)
Accel Gel	1.4 oz (41-g) packet	90	20 (plus 5 g protein)	95
Carb BOOM	1.4 oz (41-g) packet	110	27	50
Clif Shot	1.1 oz (32-g) packet	100	37	50
Gu	1.1 oz (32-g) packet	100	30	20
Power Gel	1.1 oz (41-g) packet	110	33	50

GLYCEMIC INDEX OF SELECTED SPORTS NUTRITION PRODUCTS AND CARBOHYDRATE SOURCE

Product	Glycemic Index
DRINK	
Gatorade	89
XLR8	68
Powerade	65
Cytomax	62
Allsport	53
CARBOHYDRATE SOURCE	
Fructose	22–24
Galactose	22–24
Honey	55
Sucrose	65
Glucose	100
Maltodextrin	105

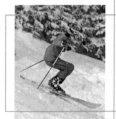

Appendix D: Sample Menus

Sample menus of varying calorie and carbohydrate levels are provided here. You can adjust portions and make substitutions as desired to raise or lower calorie and carbohydrate intake. The vegetarian menus can be used by animal protein eaters to obtain additional meal ideas. Vegetarians can utilize the animal protein-containing menus by making plant protein substitutions. Use the food lists provided in Chapter 6 to make substitutions for ingredients that are not available.

SAMPLE MENUS

**2,200 calories,
290 g carbohydrate
(51%)
143 g protein (25%)
60 g fat (24%)**

Cooked grain cereal,
1 c. (240 ml)
Banana, 1 small
Cottage cheese,
½ c. (120 ml) or egg, 1
Nuts, 1 tbsp. (15 ml)

Recovery smoothie:
   12 oz. dairy milk (360 ml)
   Frozen fruit, 1 c. (240 ml)

Low-fat tuna salad,
3 oz. (100 g)
Bread, 2 slices (60 g)
Lentil salad or pasta salad,
½ c. (120 ml)

Salmon, 6 oz. (180 g)
Buckwheat or rice, cooked,
1 c. (240 ml)
Asparagus, 1 c. (240 ml)
Salad, 2 c. (480 ml)
Olive oil, 2 t. (20 ml)
Salad dressing, 2 tbsp. (30 ml)

Sorbet or frozen yogurt,
½ c. (120 ml)
Peach, 1 medium

**2,500 calories
415 g carbohydrate
(64%)
110 g protein (17%)
53 g fat (53%)**

Oatmeal, 1 c. cooked (240 ml)
Apple, 1 medium
Juice, 8 oz. (240 ml)

Yogurt, 6 oz. (180 ml)
Strawberries, 1 c. (240 ml)

Chicken, 3 oz. (100 g)
Whole-grain bread,
2 slices (60 g)
Pretzels, ¾ oz. (22 g)
Pear, 1 large

Bagel, 3 oz. (90 g)
Peanut butter, 1 t. (8 ml)

Beef strips, 3 oz. (100 g)
Noodles, 2 c. cooked (480 ml)
Bread, 1 slice (30 g)
Olive oil, 2 t. (15 ml)
Mixed vegetables, 1 c. (240 ml)

**2,600 calories
335 g carbohydrate
(50%)
139 g protein (21%)
83 g fat (28%)**

Muesli, ¾ c. (180 ml)
Apple, 1 medium
Raisins, 2 tbsp. (30 ml)
Soy or dairy milk, 1 c. (240 ml)
Almonds, 2 t. (15 ml)

Granola bar, 1 medium
Peach, 1 medium

Chicken tacos:
   Chicken, 3 oz. (100 g)
   Kidney or pinto beans,
   ½ c. (120 ml)
   Rice, 1 c. (240 ml)
   Tortillas, corn, 2 small
   Oil, 2 t. (30 ml)

Papaya, 1 whole
Crackers, 2 oz. (60 g)
Cream cheese, 2 tbsp. (40 ml)

Risotto:
   Beef, 4 oz. (120 g)
   Broccoli, 1 c. (240 ml)
   Rice, 1 ½ c. cooked (360 ml)
Bread, 2 slices (60 g)
Oil, 2 t. (15 ml)

CONTINUED

SAMPLE MENUS continued

3,200 calories
480 g carbohydrate (59%)
147 g protein (18%)
90 g fat (24%)

Waffles, 4 squares
Syrup, ½ c. (120 ml)
Berries, 1 c. (240 ml)
Hard-boiled egg, 1
Soy or dairy milk,
12 oz. (360 ml)

Roast turkey, 3 oz. (100 g)
Avocado or hummus, 2 tbsp.
(30 ml)
Toasted pita, 1 round
Plums, 3 medium
Soy or dairy milk, 8 oz.
(240 ml)
Nonfat yogurt, 6 oz. (180 g)

Pasta, 3 c. cooked
Marinara sauce, 1 ½ c.
(360 ml)
Lean beef, 3 oz. (100 g)
Bread, 2 slices (60 g)
Salad, 2 c. (480 ml)
Olive oil, 3 t. (20 ml)
Salad dressing, 2 tbsp.
(30 ml)

3,200 calories
488 g carbohydrate (59%)
146 g protein (18%)
87 g fat (24%)

Raisin bran, 1 ½ c.
Milk, 8 oz. (240 ml)
Grapefruit, 1 whole
Bagel, 3 oz. (100 g)
Low-fat cheese, 2 oz. (60 g)

Recovery smoothie:
 Milk, skim, 16 oz. (480 ml)
 Granola, ½ c. (120 ml)
 Banana, 1 large

Peanut butter, 1 tbsp. (15 ml)
Jam, 2 tbsp. (30 ml)
Bread, 2 slices (60 g)

Orange, 1 medium
Yogurt with fruit, 8 oz.
(240 ml)

Grilled chicken, 6 oz. (180 g)
Sweet potatoes, 10 oz. (300 g)
Peas, 1 c. cooked (240 ml)
Bread, 2 slices (60 g)
Olive oil, 5 t. (50 ml)
Fruit salad, 1 c. (240 ml)

Sorbet, 1 c. (240 ml)
Strawberries, 1 c. (240 ml)

4,300 calories
610 g carbohydrate (56%)
168 g protein (15%)
137 g fat (28%)

Bran flakes, 1 c. (240 ml)
Milk, 1 c. (240 ml)
English muffin, 2
Melted low-fat cheese, 2 oz.
(60 g)
Smoothie:
 Soy milk, 12 oz., (360 ml)
 Banana, 1
 Wheat germ, 1 tbsp. (15 ml)

Sports drink, 40 oz. (1200 ml)

Beef and Bean burritos:
 Beef, 8 oz. (240 g)
 Rice, ½ c. cooked (120 ml)
 Beans, 1 c. (240 ml)
 Tortillas, 2 large
 Salsa, 1 c. (240 ml)
 Canola oil, 4 t. (30 ml)

Gingersnaps, 6
Juice, 8 oz. (240 ml)

Tofu stir-fry:
 Tofu, 4 oz. (120 g)
 Brown rice, cooked,
 1 ½ c. (360 ml)
 Sweet peppers, broccoli,
 1 c. cooked (240 ml)
 Sesame seed oil, 1 tbsp.
 (15 ml)

Granola bar, 1
Ice cream, 1 c. (240 ml)
Chocolate syrup, 2 tbsp.
(30 ml)
Nuts, 2 t. (15 ml)

CONTINUED

SAMPLE MENUS continued

2,200 calories
340 g carbohydrate
(60%)
99 g protein (18%)
56 g fat (22%)

Orange juice, 1 c. (240 ml)
French toast, 2 slices
Syrup, ½ c. (120 ml)
Strawberries, 1 c. (240 ml)

Low-fat cheese, 2 oz. (60 g)
Bread, 2 slices (60 g)
Tomato, 1 whole
Yogurt with fruit, 1 c. (240 ml)
Pear, 1 whole

Crackers, 8 small
Hummus, ½ c. (120 ml)
Milk, skim, 8 oz. (240 ml)

Rice, cooked, 1 ½ c. (360 ml)
Shrimp, 6 oz. cooked (180 g)
Red pepper, 1 whole
Broccoli, 1 c. cooked (240 ml)
Sesame seed oil, 1 tbsp. (15 ml)

Frozen yogurt, 1 c. (240 ml)
Fruit slices, ½ c. (120 ml)

2,400 calories
346 g carbohydrate
(58%)
99 g protein (17%)
68 g fat (26%)

English muffin, 1 whole
Cream cheese, 2 tbsp. (30 ml)
Jam, 2 tbsp. (30 ml)
Grapefruit juice, 12 oz. (360 ml)
Egg, 1 whole

Pinto beans, ½ c. (120 ml)
Rice, cooked, 1 c. (240 ml)
Tortilla, 1 whole
Salsa, 4 tbsp. (60 ml)
Cheese, 1 oz. (30 g)
Avocado, ¼ whole

Granola bar, 1
Peaches, 2
Almonds, 1 tbsp. (15 ml)

Pasta, cooked, 2 c. (480 ml)
Lean beef, 3 oz. (100 g)
Marinara sauce, 1 c. (240 ml)
Green salad, 2 c. (480 ml)
Salad dressing, 2 tbsp. (30 ml)

Frozen yogurt, 1 c. (240 ml)
Blueberries, ½ c. (120 ml)

2,700 calories
380 g carbohydrate
(55%)
130 g protein (19%)
86 g fat (27%)

Oatmeal, cooked, 1 ½ c. .
(360 ml)
Skim milk, 8 oz. (240 ml)
Wheat germ, 4 tbsp. (60 ml)
Bread, 2 slices (60 g)
Jam, 2 tbsp. (30 ml)
Orange juice, 8 oz. (240 ml)

Chicken, 4 oz. (120 g)
Bread, whole grain, 2 slices
(60 g)
Mayonnaise, light, 2 tbsp.
(30 ml)
Rice and bean salad, ½ c.
(120 ml)
Grapes, 1 c. (240 ml)

Energy bar, 1
Banana, 1
Yogurt with fruit, 8 oz.
(240 ml)

Tofu, 6 oz. (180 g)
Asian noodles, cooked, 2 c.
(480 ml)
Vegetables, 2 c. (480 ml)
Sesame seed oil, 2 tbsp.
(30 ml)

CONTINUED

SAMPLE MENUS continued

3,000 calories
430 g carbohydrate
(58%)
176 g protein (23%)
63 g fat (19%)

Bagel, 4 oz. (120 g)
Peanut butter, 2 tbsp. (30 ml)
Citrus juice, 12 oz. (360 ml)
Banana, 1 whole
Yogurt, plain, 1 c. (240 ml)

Tuna, 4 oz. (120 g)
Mayonnaise, 1 tbsp. (15 ml)
Pita bread, 1 large (60 g)
Pretzels, 1½ oz. (45 g)
Raw vegetable salad, 1 c.
(240 ml)
Soy or dairy milk, 12 oz.
(360 ml)
Peach slices, 1 c. (240 ml)
Granola, low-fat, ¼ c. (60 ml)

Halibut, 8 oz. (240 g)
Buckwheat, cooked, 1½ c.
(360 ml)
Asparagus, 1 c. (240 ml)
Canola oil, 2 t. (15 ml)

Sorbet, 1 c. (240 ml)
Fig cookies, 3 small

3,700 calories
630 g carbohydrate
(68%)
130 g protein (14%)
75 g fat (18%)

Grits, cooked, 1 c. (240 ml)
Raisins, 2 tbsp. (30 ml)
Yogurt, nonfat, plain, 1 c.
(240 ml)
Dried cherries, 10
Cashews, 1 tbsp. (15 ml)

Hummus, ½ c.
Pita bread, 2 rounds
Celery, pepper, carrots, 2 c.
(480 ml)
Apple juice, 12 oz. (360 ml)

Bagel, 2 oz. (60 g)
Nut butter, 2 tbsp. (30 ml)
Apple, 1 large

Pork tenderloin, 8 oz. (240 g)
Rice, cooked, 1½ c. (360 ml)
Corn, ½ c. (120 ml)
Mushrooms, ¼ c. (60 ml)
Bread, 2 slices (60 g)
Olive oil, 4 t. (15 ml)

Sherbet, 1 c. (240 ml)
Raspberries, 1 c. (240 ml)

4,500 calories
775 g carbohydrate
(67%)
140 g protein (12%)
105 g fat (21%)

Pancakes, 4 small
Maple syrup, ¾ c. (180 ml)
Banana, 1 large
Raisins, 2 tbsp. (30 ml)
Nuts, 1 tbsp. (20 ml)
Soy milk, 12 oz. (360 ml)

Sports drink, 40 oz. (1200 ml)

Burrito:
    Chicken, 5 oz. (150 g)
    Rice, cooked, 2 c. (480 ml)
    Pinto beans, 1 c. (240 ml)
    Avocado, ¼ whole
    Salsa, ½ c. (120 ml)

Linguine, cooked, 3 c. (720 g)
Mixed vegetables, 1 c. (240 ml)
Bread, 2 slices (60 g)
Olive oil, 2 tbsp. (30 ml)
Salad, 2 c. (480 ml)
Salad dressing, 2 tbsp. (30 ml)

Frozen yogurt, 2 c. (480 ml)
Cookies, 2
Strawberries, 1 c. (240 ml)

SAMPLE VEGETARIAN MENUS

2,200 calories,
348 g carbohydrate
(62%)
95 g protein (17%)
53 g fat (21%)

Farina, cooked, 1 c. (240 ml)
Skim milk, 8 oz. (240 ml)
Nuts, 1 tbsp. (15 ml)
Apple, 1
Orange juice, 12 oz. (360 ml)

Soy burger, 1 patty
Bun, 1 whole
Cheese, low-fat, 1 oz. (30 g)
Lentil or bean salad, ½ c.
(120 ml)
Vegetables, raw, 1 c. (240 ml)
Avocado, ¼ whole

Kidney beans, 1 c. (240 ml)
Rice, cooked, 1 c. (240 ml)
Tortilla, 1 large
Green salad, 1 c. (240 ml)
Salad dressing, 2 tbsp. (30 ml)

Granola bar, 1 whole
Peach, 1 whole
Yogurt with fruit, 8 oz. (240 ml)

2,400 calories
390 g carbohydrate
(63%)
105 g protein (17%)
56 g fat (20%)

Muesli, ¾ c. (180 ml)
Soy or dairy yogurt, 8 oz.
(240 ml)
Blueberries, 1 c. (240 ml)

Garbanzo beans, ⅓ c. (80 ml)
Salad greens/vegetables, 3 c.
Pita, 1 large (60 g)
Cheese, low-fat, 2 oz. (60 g)
Grapefruit juice, 8 oz. (240 ml)

Energy bar, 1 medium
Apple, 1

Tempeh, ¾ c. (180 ml)
Rice, 1½ c. cooked (360 ml)
Broccoli, cooked, 1 c. (240 ml)
Sesame seed oil, 1 tbsp. (15 ml)

Orange, 1 medium
Almond, 2 t. (15 ml)

3,000 calories
475 g carbohydrate
(67%)
102 g protein (14%)
60 g fat (19%)

Waffles, 2 small
Maple syrup, 4 oz. (120 ml)
Raspberries, 1 c. (240 ml)
Skim milk, 1 c. (240 ml)

Hummus, ½ c. (120 ml)
Rice, cooked, ½ c. (120 ml)
Lentil salad, ½ c. (120 ml)
Pita bread, 1 large (60 g)
Carrots and celery, 2 c.
(480 ml)

Bagel, 4 oz. (120 g)
Cheese, low-fat, 2 oz. (60 g)
Apple, 1

Tofu, 4 oz. (120 g)
Soba noodles, cooked, 2 c.
(480 ml)
Greens, cooked, 1 c.
Sesame seed oil, 1 tbsp. (15 ml)

Pear, 1 large

CONTINUED

SAMPLE VEGETARIAN MENUS continued

2,900 calories
470 g carbohydrate
(62%)
113 g protein (15%)
78 g fat (23%)

Pancakes, 4 small
Syrup, 6 tbsp. (90 g)
Raisins, 2 tbsp. (30 ml)
Apple juice, 8 oz. (240 ml)
Eggs, 2 whole

Soy or dairy yogurt with fruit,
8 oz. (240 ml)
Almonds, 2 tbsp. ((30 ml)

Bean soup, 1 ½ c.
Rye crackers, 4
Vegetable salad, 1 c. (240 ml)
Soy milk, 12 oz. (360 ml)

Potato, 1 large
Kidney beans, 1 c. (240 ml)
Cheese, low-fat, 1 oz. (30 g)
Green salad, 2 c. (480 ml)
Salad dressing, 3 tbsp. (45 g)

Frozen yogurt, 1 c. (240 ml)
Banana, 1 large

3,600 calories
635 g carbohydrate
(68%)
134 g protein (14%)
73 g fat (18%)

Bran flakes, 1 ½ c. (360 ml)
Wheat germ, 2 tbsp. (30 ml)
Soy or dairy milk, 8 oz.
(240 ml)
Peach, 1 medium

Recovery drink:
Juice, 12 oz. (360 ml)
Yogurt, 1 c. (240 ml)
Banana, 1 whole

Nut butter, 2 tbsp. (30 ml)
Bread, 2 slices (60 g)
Bean soup, 1 c. (240 ml)
Raw vegetables, 1 c.

Tofu, 8 oz. (240 g)
Peas, 1 c. (240 ml)
Noodles, 2 c. (480 ml)
Rolls, 2 (60 g)
Vegetable oil, 2 tbsp. (30 ml)
Green salad, 2 c. (480 ml)
Salad dressing, 2 tbsp. (30 ml)

Sports drink, 40 oz. (1,200 ml)

3,300 calories
550 g carbohydrate
(65%)
120 g protein (14%)
77 g fat (21%)

Oatmeal, cooked, 1 ½ c.
(360 ml)
Skim milk, 1 c. (240 ml)
Wheat germ, 2 tbsp. (30 ml)
Orange juice, 12 oz. (360 ml)
Yogurt, 1 c. (240 ml)
Apple, 1 large

Sports drink, 40 oz. (1,200 ml)

Thin-crust pizza, easy cheese,
3 slices
Green salad, 2 c.(480 ml)
Salad dressing, 2 tbsp. (40 ml)
Soy milk, 8 oz. (240 ml)

Pretzels, 2 oz. (60 g)
Hummus, ½ c. (120 ml)
Raw vegetables, 1 c. (240 ml)

Spaghetti, cooked, 3 c.
(720 ml)
Marinara sauce, 2 c. (480 ml)
Parmesan cheese, 3 tbsp.
(45 ml)
Italian bread, 2 slices (60 g)
Olive oil, 1 tbsp. (20 ml)

Sorbet, 1 ½ c. (360 ml)
Fig bars, 2

Selected Bibliography

Åkermark, C, et al. 1996. Diet and muscle glycogen concentration in relation to physical performance in Swedish elite ice hockey players. *International Journal of Sport Nutrition* 6(3): 272–284.

Armstrong, LE. 2002. Caffeine, body fluid-electrolyte balance, and exercise performance. *International Journal of Nutrition and Exercise Metabolism* 12(2): 189–206.

Balsom, PD, et al. 1999. Carbohydrate intake and multiple sprint sports: With special reference to football (soccer). *International Journal of Sports Medicine* 20(1): 48–52.

Bangsbo, JL, et al. 1992. The effect of carbohydrate diet on intermittent exercise performance. *International Journal of Sports Medicine* 13: 152–157.

Beals, K. 2004. *Disordered Eating Among Athletes.* Champaign, IL: Human Kinetics.

Bladin, C, et al. 2004. Snowboarding injuries. *Sports Medicine* 34(2): 133–139.

Børsheim, E, et al. 2004. Effect of amino acid, protein, and carbohydrate mixture on net muscle protein balance after resistance exercise. *International Journal of Sport Nutrition and Exercise Metabolism* 14(3): 255–271.

Bosco, C, et al. 1997. Effect of oral creatine supplementation on jumping and running performance. *International Journal of Sports Medicine* 18(5): 369–372.

Broad, EM, et al. 1996. Body weight changes and voluntary fluid intakes during training and competition sessions in team sports. *International Journal of Sport Nutrition* 6(3): 307–320.

Burke, L, Deakin, V. 2000. *Clinical Sports Nutrition.* Sydney: McGraw-Hill.

Burke, LM, et al. 1993. Muscle glycogen storage after prolonged exercise: Effect of the glycemic index of carbohydrate feedings. *Journal of Applied Physiology* 75: 1019–1023.

Burke, LM, et al. 1996. Muscle glycogen storage after prolonged exercise: Effect of frequency of carbohydrate feedings. *American Journal of Clinical Nutrition* 64: 115–119.

Burke, LM, et al. 2004. Carbohydrate and fat for training and recovery. *Journal of Sports Sciences* 22(8): 15–30.

Burns, RD, et al. 2004. Intercollegiate student athlete use of nutritional supplements and the role of the athletic trainers and dietitian in nutrition counseling. *Journal of the American Dietetic Association* 104(2): 246–249.

Catlin, D, et al. 2000. Trace contamination of over-the-counter androstenedione and positive urine test results for a nandrolone metabolite. *Journal of the American Medical Association* 284: 2618–2621.

Connolly, DA. 2002. The energy expenditure of snowshoeing in packed versus unpacked snow at low-level walking speeds. *Journal of Strength and Conditioning Research* 16(4): 606–610.

Connolly, DA, et al. 2002. Changes in selected fitness parameters following six weeks of snowshoe training. *Journal of Sports Medicine and Physical Fitness* 42(1): 14-18.

Coyle, E. 2004. Fluid and fuel intake during exercise. *Journal of Sports Sciences* 22(8): 39–55.

Crowe, MJ, et al. 2003. The effects of B-hyrdoxy-B-methylbutarate (HMB) and HMB/creatine supplementation on indices of health in highly trained athletes. *International Journal of Nutrition and Exercise Metabolism* 13(2): 184–197.

Dalleck, LC, et al. 2003. Energy cost and physiological responses of males snowshoeing with rotating and fixed toe-cord designs in powdered snow conditions. *Ergonomics* 46(9): 875–881.

Davis, JM, et al. 1997. Carbohydrate drinks delay fatigue during intermittent, high-intensity cycling in active men and women. *International Journal of Sports Nutrition* 7(4): 261–273.

Dubnov, G, Constantini, NW. 2004. Prevalence of iron depletion and anemia in top-level basketball players. *International Journal of Nutrition and Exercise Metabolism* 14(1): 30–37.

Febbraio, MA, et al. 1996. Carbohydrate feedings before prolonged exercise: Effect of glycemic index on muscle glycogenolysis and exercise performance. *Journal of Applied Physiology* 81: 1115–1120.

Gleeson, M, et al. 2004. Exercise, nutrition, and immune function. *Journal of Sports Sciences* 22(8): 115–125.

Haff, GG, et al. 2000. Carbohydrate supplementation attenuates muscle glycogen loss during acute bouts of resistance exercise. *International Journal of Sport Nutrition and Exercise Metabolism* 10(3): 326–339.

Hagel, BE, et al. 2004. Injuries among skiers and snowboarders in Quebec. *Epidemiology* 15(3): 279–286.

Heyward, VH, Stolarczyk, LM. 1996. *Applied Body Composition Assessment.* Champaign, IL: Human Kinetics.

Hogg, P. 2003. Preparation for skiing and snowboarding. *Australian Family Physician* 32(7): 495–498.

Ivy, JL, et al. 1988. Muscle glycogen storage after different amounts of carbohydrate ingestion. *Journal of Applied Physiology* 64(5): 2018–2023.

Ivy, JL, et al. 1988. Muscle glycogen synthesis after exercise: Effect of time of carbohydrate ingestion. *Journal of Applied Physiology* 64(4): 1480–1485.

Izquierdo, M, et al. 2002. Effects of creatine, supplementation on muscle power, endurance, and sprint performance. *Medicine and Science in Sports and Exercise* 34(2): 332–343.

James, AP, et al. 2001. Muscle glycogen supercompensation: Absence of gender-related difference. *European Journal of Applied Physiology* 85(6): 533–538.

Jones, AM, et al. 1999. Oral creatine supplementation improves multiple sprint performance in elite ice-hockey players. *Journal of Sports Medicine and Physical Fitness* 39(3): 189–196.

Kenefick, RW, et al. 2004. Hypohydration effects on thermoregulation during moderate exercise in the cold. *European Journal of Applied Physiology* 92(4–5): 565–570.

Kirwan, JP, et al. 1988. Carbohydrate balance in competitive runners during successive days of intense training. *Journal of Applied Physiology* 65(6): 2601–2606.

Knapik, JJ, et al. 2002. Energy cost during locomotion across snow: A comparison of four types of snowshoes with snowshoe design consideration. *Work* 18(2): 171–177.

Kovacs, EMR, et al. 2002. Effect of high and low fluid intake on post-exercise rehydration. *International Journal of Sport Nutrition and Exercise Metabolism* 12: 14–23.

Kreider, RB, et al. 1998. Effects of creatine supplementation on body composition, strength, and sprint performance. *Medicine and Science in Sport and Exercise* 30(1): 73–82.

Larsson, P, et al. 2002. Physiological predictors of performance in cross-country skiing from treadmill tests in male and female subjects. *Scandinavian Journal of Medicine and Science in Sports* 12(4): 347–353.

Lemon, P, et al. 1992. Protein requirements and muscle mass/strength changes during intensive training in novice bodybuilders. *Journal of Applied Physiology* 73: 767–775.

Miller, SL, et al. 2003. Independent and combined effects of amino acids and glucose after resistance exercise. *Medicine and Science in Sports and Exercise* 35(3): 449–455.

Millet, GP, et al. 2003. Energy cost of different skating techniques in cross-country skiing. *Journal of Sports Science* 21(1): 3–11.

Minehan, M, et al. 2002. Effect of flavor and awareness of kilojoule content of drinks on preference and fluid balance in team sports. *International Journal of Sport Nutrition and Exercise Metabolism* 12(1): 81–92.

Mognoni, P, et al. 2001. Heart rate profiles and energy cost of locomotion during cross-country skiing races. *European Journal of Applied Physiology* 85(5): 62–67.

Murray, R. 1995. Fluid needs in hot and cold environments. *International Journal of Sport Nutrition* 5: S62–73.

Neumayer, G, et al. 2003. Physical and physiological factors associated with success in professional skiing. *International Journal of Sports Medicine* 24(8): 571–575.

Nicholas, CW, et al. 1995. Influence of ingesting a carbohydrate–electrolyte solution on endurance capacity during intermittent, high-intensity shuttle running. *Journal of Sports Science* 13(4): 283–290.

Nicholas, C, et al. 1997. Carbohydrate intake and recovery of intermittent running capacity. *International Journal of Sport Nutrition* 7(4): 251–260.

Parkin, J, et al. 1997. Muscle glycogen storage following prolonged exercise: Effect of timing of ingestion of high glycemic index food. *Medicine and Science in Sport and Exercise* 29: 220–224.

Pettersson, U, et al. 2000. Bone mass in female cross-country skiers: Relationship between muscle strength and different BMD sites. *Calcified Tissue International* 67(3): 199–206.

Rosenbloom, CA, ed. 2000. *Sports Nutrition: A Guide for the Professional Working with Active People.* Chicago: American Dietetic Association.

Roy, B, Tarnopolsky, M, et al. 1998. Influence of differing macronutrient intakes on muscle glycogen resynthesis after resistance exercise. *Journal of Applied Physiology* 84(3): 890–896.

Roy, R, et al. 1997. Effect of glucose supplement timing on protein metabolism after resistance training. *Journal of Applied Physiology* 82(6): 1882–1888.

Schneider, PL, et al. 2001. Physiological responses to recreational snowshoeing. *Journal of Applied Physiology Online* 4(3): 45–52.

Sherman, WM, et al. 1989. Effects of 4 h preexercise carbohydrate feedings on cycling performance. *Medicine and Science in Sports and Exercise* 21(5): 598–604.

Sherman, WM, et al. 1991. Carbohydrate feedings 1 h before exercise improves cycling performance. *American Journal of Clinical Nutrition* 54: 866–870.

Shirreffs, S, et al. 1996. Post-exercise rehydration in man: Effect of volume consumed and drink sodium content. *Medicine and Science in Sports and Exercise* 28(10): 1260–1271.

Shirreffs, SM, et al. 2004. Fluid and electrolyte needs for preparation and recovery from training and competition. *Journal of Sports Sciences* 22(8): 57–63.

Siefert, JG, et al. 1998. The physiological effects of beverage ingestion during cross-country ski training in elite collegiate skiers. *Canadian Journal of Applied Physiology* 23(1): 66–73.

Simard, C, et al. 1988. Effects of carbohydrate intake before and during an ice hockey game on blood and muscle energy substrates. *Research Quarterly for Exercise and Sport* 59: 144–147.

Slater, G, et al. 2001. B-hyrdoxy-B-methylbutarate (HMB) supplementation does not affect changes in strength or body composition during resistance training in trained men. *International Journal of Nutrition and Exercise Metabolism* 11(3): 384–396.

Smith Rockwell, M, et al. 2001. Nutrition knowledge, opinions, and practices of coaches and athletic trainers at Division I University. *International Journal of Nutrition and Exercise Metabolism* 11(2): 174–185.

Stuempfle, KJ, et al. 2002. Hyponatremia in a cold weather ultraendurance race. *Alaska Medicine* 44(3): 51–55.

Stuempfle, KJ, et al. 2003. Change in serum sodium concentration during a cold weather ultra-distance race. *Clinical Journal of Sport Medicine* 13(3): 171–175.

Tarnopolsky, MA, MacLennan, DP. 2000. Creatine monohydrate supplementation enhances high intensity exercise performance in males and females. *International Journal of Sport Nutrition and Exercise Metabolism* 10(4): 452–463.

Tarnopolsky, MA, et al. 1997. Postexercise protein–carbohydrate and carbohydrate supplements increase muscle glycogen in men and women. *Journal of Applied Physiology* 83(6): 1877.

Tarnopolsky, MA, et al. 2001. Gender differences in carbohydrate loading are related to energy intake. *Journal of Applied Physiology* 91: 225–230.

Tipton, KD, Wolfe, RR. 2004. Protein and amino acids for athletes. *Journal of Sports Science* 22(1): 65–79.

Welde, B, et al. 2003. Energy cost of free technique and classical cross-country skiing at racing speeds. *Medicine and Science in Sports and Exercise* 35(5): 818–825.

Welsh, RS, et al. 2002. Carbohydrates and physical/mental performance during intermittent exercise. *Medicine and Science in Sports and Exercise* 34(4): 723–731.

White, AT, Johnson, SC. 1991. Physiological comparison of international, national, and regional alpine skiers. *International Journal of Sports Medicine* 12(8): 374–378.

Yaspelkis, B, et al. 1993. Carbohydrate supplementation spares muscle glycogen during variable-intensity exercise. *Journal of Applied Physiology* 75: 1477–1485.

Index

About the Author

Monique Ryan, MS, RD, LDN, is a nationally recognized nutritionist with over twenty years of experience. She is founder of Personal Nutrition Designs, a nutrition consulting company based in the Chicago area. Started in 1992, Personal Nutrition Designs provides nutrition programs for diverse groups of people with an emphasis on long-term follow-up and support programming.

Monique was a member of the Performance Enhancement Team for USA Triathlon, USA Cycling (Women's Road Team), and Synchro Swimming USA up to the 2004 Athens Olympic Games. She has worked with the Timex Multisport Team, and was the nutritionist for the Saturn Cycling Team from 1994 to 2000. Monique has also consulted with professional baseball and basketball players and other team and winter sport athletes competing at the high school, collegiate, and recreational levels. Monique also lectures extensively on sports nutrition to coaches, trainers, and amateur athletes who train at all levels. She has presented across the U.S., Canada, Brazil, and Australia. She currently consults with the Chicago Fire soccer champions.

Monique is a prolific nutrition writer and is also the author of *Performance Nutrition for Team Sports* and *Sports Nutrition for Endurance Athletes*. She is the author of over 150 published articles. Monique has a Bachelor of Science degree in Nutrition and Dietetics and a Master of Science Degree in Nutrition. She completed her clinical training at Northwestern Memorial Hospital Medical Center in Chicago and is a registered dietitian (RD) licensed in the state of Illinois (LDN). Monique is a member of the American College of Sports Medicine (ACSM) and is an ACSM Health Fitness Instructor. Monique has competed in the sports of road cycling and mountain biking, and currently participates in a variety of endurance and winter sports.